Rainer Sundmacher

# Color Atlas of Herpetic Eye Diseases

## A Practical Guide to Clinical Management

Rainer Sundmacher

# Color Atlas of Herpetic Eye Diseases

## A Practical Guide to Clinical Management

With 211 Figures and 6 Tables

Springer

**Rainer Sundmacher, MD**
Professor Emeritus
University Eye Hospital
Moorenstraße 5
40225 Düsseldorf
Germany

ISBN 978-3-540-69462-5 e-ISBN 978-3-540-69463-2
DOI 10.1007/978-3-540-69463-2

Library of Congress Control Number: 2008940421



Cover design: Frido Steinen-Broo, eStudio Calamar, Spain
Illustrations: Albert R. Gattung & Regine Gattung-Petith, Edingen-Neckarhausen, Germany
Production & Typesetting: le-tex publishing services oHG, Leipzig, Germany

Printed on acid-free paper

9 8 7 6 5 4 3 2 1

Springer.com

# Foreword

This book is more than an atlas and a text. It has what clinicians want most: experience.

Actual case examples are analyzed by a specialist who has arguably treated more patients with ocular herpes than any other ophthalmologist. Not merely an inventory of viral keratitis, this sourcebook explains the ins and outs of infection and inflammation due to herpes simplex virus, varicella-zoster virus and other herpes viruses.

Herpetic eye disease needs a descriptive vocabulary, and the author provides a sensible classification. His distinctive terminology updates outmoded jargon, creating a new norm. Professor Sundmacher communicates with clarity, continuity and style.

The book's strength is in its details. Therapeutic decision-making is based on clinical research, often the author's own pioneering trials. For medical and surgical dilemmas, practice-based advice springs from a pragmatic explanation of virology, immunology and wound healing.

The proficiency and scope of this authoritative resource leads me to rephrase a century-old maxim: 'To know herpes is to know ophthalmology.'

Kirk R. Wilhelmus, MD PhD
Houston, Texas USA

# Foreword

It is a pleasure to write a foreword for this beautiful atlas of ocular disease caused by herpes viruses. I first met Professor Rainer Sundmacher in Freiburg many years ago when he set up an inspirational meeting on these viruses. Since that time in the early 1980s, he has worked tirelessly on the management of viral disease of the external eye. Virus research has exploded in recent years, and in particular great strides have been made in the development of antiviral therapy. It is therefore an appropriate time to produce an atlas of these diseases, which can cause serious visual loss. The book also provides detailed advice on treatment and therapy.

It is the external disease caused by herpes simplex and varicella zoster virus that is most frequently seen by ophthalmologists. This book highlights many of the difficult problems that are encountered in the diagnosis and management of these viruses. The detailed and vivid photographs illustrate the main features of these viruses, and the analysis of each photograph provides unique insights in a clinical setting. Such insights will be useful to those involved in the management of viral diseases of the eye. There are uplifting accounts of clinical treatments that can lead to successful outcomes, although at the same time caution is urged, since these treatments can cause damage to the eye if not carefully monitored by clinicians. This volume will enable those who are not experts in corneal and external disease to recognize conditions that may be foreign or new to them, and thus can be recommended to benefit A&E departments, where there is no ophthalmological immediate supervision. On the other hand, the atlas will be valuable to both trainees and consultants because of the considerable expertise and experience that the authors have gathered in their clinical careers.

David Easty, MD FRCS FRCOphth.
Professor Emeritus of Ophthalmology
University of Bristol, UK

# Acknowledgements

Firstly, I owe thanks to Professor Reiner Thomssen, virologist in Göttingen, who inspired my interest in this field, and who was really disappointed when I had to leave him to start a clinical career in ophthalmology under the supervision of Professor Günter Mackensen in Freiburg. I remember Günter Mackensen with warmest respect for trusting my abilities and responsibility as a young resident and for his lasting interest in all my herpes and keratoplasty projects. These could not have been performed without numerous co-workers, all of whom deserve thanks. Their names are documented in the publications of our group. Especially important help came from the virologist Dieter Neumann-Haefelin and Annegret Mattes, who were responsible for the virological part of my Freiburg studies, while the medical photographer H. Preuninger supplied an impressive basis of thousands of slides from my herpes patients. I look back with warmest memories on the long series of experimental and clinical interferon studies. They would not have been possible without the trustful and generous help of Professor Kari Cantell, from Helsinki, the only person worldwide who was able to supply highly purified leukocyte interferon for clinical studies.

In regards to my research done in Düsseldorf, I would like to especially thank Thomas Reinhard, who made the most valuable contributions in the fields of keratoplasty, secondary glaucoma, and systemic immunotherapy after keratoplasty, to which Alexander Reis added important experimental work. The clinical slide collection was further augmented by Helen Baseler, Gerlinde Westphal, and Kerstin Bisgiel.

My research work on herpes would have been impossible without the input from the many publications worldwide and from personal contacts and discussions with international herpes researchers. As I cannot even roughly name the most important publications of my colleagues, I would like to thank – *pars pro toto* – some of the attendees of the First International Symposium on Herpetic Eye Diseases, held in Freiburg in 1980. I have learned a great deal from all of them and owe them a lot: J. R. Baringer, O. P. van Bijsterveld, K. Cantell, E. De Clercq, J. Colin, L. M. T. Collum, D. J. Coster, D. L. Easty, M. G. Falcon, C. S. Foster, B. R. Jones, H. E. Kaufman, R. J. Marsh, P. C. Maudgal, J. McGill, T. C. Merigan, G. O. H. Naumann, A. B. Nesburn, J. O. Oh, W. H. Prusoff, H. Shiota, G. Smolin, H. M. J. Völker-Dieben, G. O. Waring III, and K. R. Wilhelmus.

This atlas would not have been finished without the constant pressure of my colleagues attending the herpes, cornea, and keratoplasty courses, which I have been teaching over the last decades. Whether they are really to be thanked for this pressure, must be left to the judgement of the reader.

I am grateful to Hartmut Hengel for the introductory virological chapter, to Johannes Stammen for help with the chapter on anterior segment CMV disease, to Thomas Reinhard for his work on presumed EBV disease, and to Lutz Hansen for the well-illustrated chapter on posterior segment diseases caused by herpes viruses.

I thank my family, whose continuous love and support for my professional work made this possible.

Finally, it is a pleasure to thank Springer and staff, especially Marion Philipp and Martina Himberger and Nadja Kroke for their excellent editing work.

Freiburg
September 2008

Rainer Sundmacher
Professor Emeritus of Opthalmology
University of Düsseldorf, Germany

# Contents

# List of Contributors

**Rainer Sundmacher, MD**
Professor Emeritus
University Eye Hospital
Moorenstraße 5
40225 Düsseldorf
Germany

**Lutz L. Hansen, MD**
Professor
Head of Retinology Section
University Eye Hospital
Kilianstraße 5
79106 Freiburg
Germany

**Hartmut Hengel, MD**
Professor
Head of Department of Virology
University Clinics
40225 Düsseldorf
Germany

**Thomas Reinhard, MD**
Professor, Medical Director
University Eye Hospital
Kilianstraße 5
79106 Freiburg
Germany

**Johannes Stammen, MD**
University Eye Hospital
40225 Düsseldorf
Germany

# Introduction

When I started ophthalmologic residency in 1970, the knowledge of herpetic eye diseases was very limited. Its pathophysiology was mostly only suspected. Medical antiviral therapy had just started (idoxuridine eye drops), and prophylaxis against the frequent viral recurrences was not available. Steroids appeared to be the only remedy against the downhill course of the disease in many individuals, though this remedy was a rather double-edged one. In quite a number of cases, eyes were blinded from herpetic corneal scars and secondary glaucoma. Attempts to restore vision by keratoplasty were equally frustrating because various risks of such a surgical procedure were at most borderline understood, and if they would have been, no drugs except for steroids would have been available to successfully deal with the numerous complications.

Nowadays, after decades of medical and surgical progress, the outcomes are much more positive. Effective topical and systemic antiviral drugs, ever improving systemic immunosuppressive agents, and clinical herpes specialists who are experts in their field allow prevention of blindness in herpes patients.

While this ideal description may hold true at present for some of the "developed" areas of the world, it is certainly not the case for the major part of the world population which does not have access to qualified ophthalmologists and advanced medical and surgical care.

However, the population in the "developed" countries cannot be sure to maintain its current high standard in herpes care. Ironically, it is just the high level of herpes control achieved in the last decades that now exerts a negative feedback: topical and systemic antiviral agents combined with steroids seem to be so effective and readily available that disastrous downhill courses have become rare, and, if they do occur, specialists are available to offer helpful advice. The pharmaceutical industry is highly content with the status achieved, seeing no need to invest into further development of anti-herpetic agents. Consequently, research money for herpes projects has become rather scarce. Young scientists prefer to start out on different, currently better funded research grounds, and the still practicing older herpes specialists are mostly left alone with no successors to devote themselves to further development of this area.

While this situation has certainly not yet been noted by the majority of practicing ophthalmologists, university clinicians clearly suggest that we have a shortage not only of herpes specialists but of anterior segment specialists in general: seven out of ten ophthalmological chairs in Germany have lately been given to retinal surgeons. Anterior segment specialists may become increasingly rare. It will presumably take years before we can expect a turnaround of clinical herpes research and the emergence of a new research and teaching generation.

Meanwhile, the only thing we can do is to document our current understanding of treatment and prophylaxis of herpetic ocular diseases in such a way that it would serve the general ophthalmologist seeking help for patients' actual problems and the potential science candidate looking out for interesting unsolved topics to work on. Both items are addressed in this atlas. The practitioner may use it like a cook book. To find help, continuous reading from the beginning to the end is not necessary, although it is, of course, recommended for a better understanding of the topic. Depending on one's individual level of knowledge in these fields, one may either start directly from the index and follow on to the page offering a solution to the problem, or – if the problem in itself is still undetermined – one may find the solution by quickly referring to the pictures. From there, the picture-associated text with the headings *clinic, diagnosis, differential diagnosis,* and *therapy,* provides detailed information. Reference is frequently made to pictures, which are relevant for differential diagnosis.

For those interested in the evidence for the statements or recommendations provided or problems and phenomena that are currently unsolved, I have included my judgement either *expressis verbis* or by the chosen wording, e. g., *study-proven, is, can be, may be, probably, speculative, general experience, personal experience, etc.* Primarily for these readers, some *selected references* are included at the end of each chapter. Using these as a starting point for individual literature search, it should be easy to obtain quick access to the complete scientific background of most but not all herpes problems. Some topics, such as neonatal herpes and vaccination, have been omitted. They would have been out of the scope of an atlas.

Being one of the clinical herpes specialists who performed quite a number of double-blind controlled therapy studies, I may say that evidence-based medicine is, of course, of utmost importance, but only in areas where adequate studies are practically feasible. In the herpes field, this has *sufficiently* been the case with dendritic keratitis only. Unfortunately, dendritic keratitis is the least significant clinical problem we face in ocular herpes. A much larger number of other herpetic eye diseases have still to be managed by practical experience and "personal conviction" only. This "unscientific" situation becomes even more critical as many details of our view of herpes pathophysiology must still be classified as "speculative belief", irrespective of how probable they may be. This makes this atlas partly a personal creed based on four decades of practical and scientific work and on experiences from the follow-up of thousands of herpes patients.

## Conference Proceedings and Books on Herpetic Ocular Disease


Blodi FC (1984) Herpes simplex infections of the eye. Contemporary issues in ophthalmology, vol. 1, Churchill Livingstone, NY, pp 171

Easty DL (1985) Virus disease of the eye, Lloyd-Luke, London, pp 350

Easty D, Hill T, Shimeld C (1991) Proceedings of the International Conference on Herpetic Eye Diseases, 25th-27th July 1990, Oxford, England. Suppl to Curr Eye Res vol 10, 211 pp

Maudgal PC, Missotten L (1985) Herpetic eye diseases, Proceedings of the international symposium at Leuven 1984, Doc Ophthalmol Proc Ser vol 44, W Junk Publ, Dordrecht, pp 447

Oh, JO, Dawson CR (1987) International conference on herpetic eye diseases, Curr Eye Res 6, no 1, spec. issue, pp 286

Oh JO, O´Connor GR (1976) Symposium on herpesvirus infections. Surv Ophthalmol 21, no 2, pp 137

Pouliquen Y, Colin J et al (1983) L´herpes oculaire. Bull Soc d´Ophtal Fr, num. spec., pp 335

Sundmacher R (1981) Herpetic eye diseases. Internationales Symposium der Deutschen Ophthalmologischen Gesellschaft 1980, Bergmann, München, pp 522

# Common Characteristics and Distinct Features of Human Pathogenic Herpesviruses

*Hartmut Hengel*

Chapter

1

## 1.1 Hallmarks of Herpesvirus Infections

The members of the family of the *herpesviridae* are phylogenetically very old viruses that co-evolved over millions of years with their hosts. Depending on the type of the target cell that is entered by the virion, herpesviruses can take two different paths of infection. Virus progeny is generated only in productively infected cells. This type of infection is associated with host cell lysis. In contrast, other cells repress lytic viral gene expression and preserve the herpesviral genome for a very long time, a state that is called latency. However, herpesvirus latency can be reversed to a productive infection mode, i.e., the herpesviral genome replicates and produces an infectious virus. These basic principles of herpesvirus biology imply that: 1) herpesvirus *disease* manifestations must be distinguished form herpesvirus *infection*, 2) diseases can occur already during primary replication, but also a long time after primary infection as a result of virus reactivation, and 3) recurrent disease manifestations can occur due to the lifelong infection.

This chapter very briefly introduces the nature of herpesviruses and their life-style. It concentrates on those family members of the human herpesviruses (HHV) that cause severe herpetic eye diseases.

## 1.2 Virus Taxonomy and Herpesviral Subfamilies

The membership in the family is based on the common architecture of the virion (comprising an icosahedral capsid surrounding the core, a largely unstructured tegument, and an outer lipid bilayer envelope) and a double-stranded DNA genome ranging from 124 to 235 kbp. To date, nine distinct members of the *herpesviridae* have been known to cause infection in humans as their natural hosts (see Table 1.1), which are subdivided into three subfamilies, *alpha*, *beta*, and *gamma*. Based on these criteria, remarkably divergent viruses have been included in the herpesvirus family. While the alpha *herpesviridae* are

Table 1.1 Human pathogenic herpesviruses

| Designation | Synonym | Abbreviation | Genome size (Kbp) | Subfamily | Site of latency |
|---|---|---|---|---|---|
| Human HV1 | Herpes simplex virus 1 | HSV-1 | 152 | $\alpha$ | Sensory neurons in ganglia (e.g. ganglion trigeminale Gasseri) |
| Human HV2 | Herpes simplex virus 2 | HSV-2 | 155 | $\alpha$ | Sensory neurons in ganglia (e.g. sacral and vagal ganglia) |
| Human HV3 | Varicella zoster virus | VZV | 125 | $\alpha$ | Dorsal root ganglia neurons, trigeminal ganglia neurons, ganglia of the autonomic nervous system |
| Human HV4 | Epstein-Barr virus | EBV | 172 | $\gamma 1$ | Memory B lymphocyte |
| Human HV5 | Cytomegalovirus | CMV | 235 | $\beta$ | CD34+ hematopoietic stem cell |
| Human HV6A | HHV-6 variant A | HHV-6A | 170 | $\beta$ | CD34+ hematopoietic stem cell, monocytes? |
| Human HV6B | HHV-6 variant B | HHV-6B | 168 | $\beta$ | CD34+ hematopoietic stem cell, monocytes? |
| Human HV7 | | HHV-7 | 145 | $\beta$ | CD4+ T lymphocytes ? |
| Human HV8 | Kaposi's sarcoma associated HV | HHV-8 | 210 | $\gamma 2$ | B lymphocyte |

usually neuroinvasive, the beta subfamily members display a broader cell tropism that includes myelomonocytic cells, while the gamma herpesviruses are typically lymphotropic.

## 1.3 General Themes of Human Herpesvirus Infections

Besides the virion structure and the length of the dsDNA genomes, human herpesviruses share further biological characteristics, which are important for the understanding of their infection and disease.

**Latency and recurrent infection:** Upon primary infection, herpesviruses invariably establish a lifelong latent state of infection in a specific type of target cell. Latent viral genomes persist as closed circular episomal DNA in the nucleus as long as lytic gene expression is repressed, i. e., no infectious virus can be recovered from latently infected tissue. Latent genomes are transcriptionally active by expressing a limited set of genes, but they become periodically reactivated for transcribing lytic genes and producing infectious progeny which then spreads from cell to cell. Recurrences occur in the presence of both cell-mediated and humoral immune responses (i. e., antibodies). Depending on the particular herpesvirus, conditions of the host and the site of virus shedding reactivation events can occur without clinical symptoms but also lead to disease. The herpesvirus produced during the reactivation episode can be transmitted to a new host which becomes primary or superinfected.

**Gene expression:** During productive (lytic) infection, herpesviral genes are transcribed in a temporal order and assigned to three distinct classes, i. e., *immediate early*, *early,* and *late*. Depending on the particular virus, one herpesviral replication cycle takes between 20 and 100 hours. The transcriptional program of the host cell becomes completely altered or even shut off during productive herpesvirus infection.

**Cell lysis**: In most tissues, virus replication is lytic, i. e., it is accompanied by the destruction of the infected cell.

**Immune control:** The latent state and replication of the herpesviruses are controlled by cellular immunity. Of particular importance are cytotoxic CD8 + T lymphocytes, cytokine-producing CD4 + T lymphocytes, as well as natural killer (NK) cells. Accordingly, immunocompromised patients lacking effective cell-mediated immune defence are prone to frequent and extensive phases of reactivation that often lead to overt disease.

**Immune evasion:** The herpesviruses are equipped with many genes that subvert immunity. Generally, T cell recognition, NK cell recognition, interferon responses, and apoptosis of infected cells are avoided by all herpesviruses. Moreover, the $\beta$- and $\gamma$-viruses have acquired former host genes ("molecular piracy"), which modify the immune response. Among these are cytokines like CMV-encoded and EBV-encoded IL-10 that down-regulate antiviral immune responses and inflammation. Moreover, the $\beta$-herpes subfamily expresses chemokines as well as chemokine receptors that exploit the host immune response: virus-encoded chemokine-receptors mediate chemotaxis and promote the spread of infected cells.

**Enzymes involved in nucleic acid metabolism:** To achieve a high yield of genome replication, the herpesviruses express virus-specific arrays of enzymes that support DNA synthesis, such as thymidine kinases, ribonucleotide reductases, and DNA polymerases. Such enzymes allow for the therapeutic inhibition of viral replication by antiviral drugs.

## 1.4 Distinct Features of Human Herpesviruses

Human pathogenic herpesviruses also differ in many regards, and some of these private features account for the virus-specific pathogenesis and disease pattern. These properties include the attachment of HHV virions to target cell receptors and the host cell tropism of infection. In addition, the site of latency, the pattern of reactivation, and the spread of recurrent infection critically determine the clinical picture of herpesvirus diseases. The alpha-herpesviruses HSV and VZV target neuronal ganglion cells as a site of latency and are competent for trans-neuronal spread during the primary and recurrent phase of infection. Despite sharing neuroinvasiveness as an unique property, the frequency of reactivation events between both viruses differs considerably (see Fig. 1.1). The unequal reactivation events of HSV and VZV have direct consequences for boosting of antiviral immunity. The higher frequency of reactivation events by HSV results in efficient *endogenous* boosting that maintains immune memory. In contrast, efficient boosting of VZV-specific memory responses relies to a larger extent on exposure with *exogenous* VZV (i. e., household contacts of children undergoing varicella). Waning of VZV-immunity over a life-time leads to increased risk of herpes zoster.

### Detailed analysis of Fig. 1.1

In some children, primary HSV-1 infection presents itself as herpetic gingivostomatitis, but does not cause clinical symptoms in the majority of infected individuals (semicircle with checker board pattern). Primary replication is followed by intermitted phases of latent and reactivated HSV infection. Reactivation events are frequent and can occur without clinical manifestations (white semicircles) or cause disease, e. g., herpetic keratitis (blue semicircles). Primary VZV replication results in chickenpox in almost all patients (blue semicircles), followed by usually only one episode of recurrent VZV infection. In most cases, recurrent VZV replication involves the skin (e. g., as zoster ophthalmicus), but can also present as disease without skin manifestation (zoster sine herpete). *x*-axis: time; *y*-axis: amount of infectious virus progeny produced.

Finally, there is still preliminary but growing evidence supporting the notion that genetic variabilities within most or even all of the members of the HHV substantially contribute to the development and manifestation of specific herpesviral diseases.

Some of the virus-specific features of those HHV which are implicated in herpetic eye diseases are described below, i. e., HSV-1/2, VZV, CMV, and EBV.

**Cell tropism and virus spreading**

**HSV-1/2:** Virion attachment and virus entry are mediated by a number of viral glycoproteins, specifically the cell surface

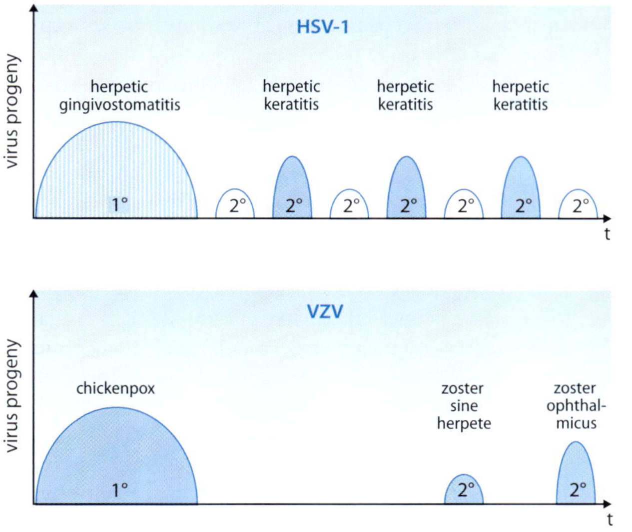


Fig. 1.1 Typical pattern of latent and productive infection of Herpes simplex virus 1 (HSV-1, *top panel*) and varicella zoster virus (VZV, *lower panel*) in the immunocompetent host

molecules nectin-1, the herpes virus entry mediator (HVEM, a member of the tumor necrosis factor receptor family), and 3-O-sulfated heparan sulfates. HSV shows a strong tropism to neuronal cells, but also lymphocytes, endothelial cells, fibroblasts, and epithelial cells of the skin and mucosa. Following local spread in the tissue at the primary site of infection, HSV enters sensory neurons by fusion at the axonal termini. The nucleocapsid of the virus is carried by retrograde axonal transport along microtubules to the nucleus in the cell body of the neuron.

**VZV:** Insulin degrading enzyme (IDE) was identified as a cellular receptor of cell-free as well as cell-associated VZV binding to the glycoprotein, gE, of the virion. VZV has a similar tropism to HSV, which includes neurons, lymphocytes, fibroblasts, and epithelial cells of the skin and mucosa. Unlike other herpesvirus infections, primary infection with VZV, varicella, is contracted by inhalation of infectious aerosol. Based on its particular tropism for T lymphocytes, the virus has established a cell-associated viremia. Thus, VZV can access neurons either hematogenously or by centripetal neural transport after entry at axonal termini in mucocutaneous lesions.

**CMV:** CMV usually enters the body via mucosal sites. Virion entry involves $\beta 1$ integrin expression on target cells. Upon local replication in epithelial cells, fibroblasts, and smooth muscle cells, the virus spreads to endothelial cells. Detached endothelial cells establish cell-associated viremia to visceral organs and the bone marrow. There, infection of stroma cells and cells of the myelomonocytic lineage occurs, including megacaryocytes and CD34+CD38-hematopoietic progenitor cells, where CMV establishes a latent state of infection. Remarkably, CMV displays a pronounced tropism to retinal pigment epithelial cells in vitro.

**EBV:** The virus binds via its outer envelope glycoprotein gp350/220 to CD21, which is also the receptor for the C3d component of complement. Major histocompatibility class II molecules represent a further entry receptor used by the virus. EBV entry to B lymphocytes is thought to differ from entry to polarized epithelial cells. The EBV integral membrane protein, BMRF2, which binds to $5\beta 1$ integrin, is implicated in this process. Oral and lingual epithelium is likely to be the primary target of orally transmitted virus. In parallel, EBV colonization of the B lymphocyte pool takes place, where latent EBV genomes are found in the CD27+B cell memory subset at a low frequency of approx. $10^{-5}$ infected cells. Colonization of the B cell pool is necessary and sufficient for EBV persistence. EBV genome carrying B cells have the capacity to seed throughout the lymphoid system and to migrate back to oropharyngeal sites. Primary (i.e., infectious mononucleosis) and latent EBV infection is under strict control of antiviral T cells recognizing latent and lytic antigens, respectively.

**Latency and reactivation patterns**

**HSV-1/2:** In a fraction of infected neurons of a ganglion which harbor 10 to 30 copies of latent HSV genomes per cell, productive infection becomes periodically reactivated. Nucleocapsids are carried by anterograde axonal transport along microtubules to axon terminals where the egress of enveloped infectious particles takes place, allowing for trans-synaptic and further intercellular spread (e.g., to cells of the conjunctiva and cornea). Virus gene expression and replication in neurons is controlled by T cells and interferon-$\gamma$. The latent virus is frequently reactivated after local stimuli, such as injury to tissues innervated by neurons harboring latent HSV, by corneal scarification, or by systemic factors (e.g., exposure to UV light, physical or emotional stress, hormonal imbalance, and hyperthermia).

**VZV:** Latent VZV genomes are readily detected in trigeminal ganglia and dorsal root ganglia. In some cases, latent VZV is also found in geniculate ganglia, olfactory bulbs, and ganglia of the autonomic nervous system. In trigeminal ganglia, VZV and HSV genomes can be detected in the same neuron. Reactivation and shedding of VZV from neurons along cutaneous nerve pathways typically presents itself as herpes zoster, although reactivation can also lack a vesicular rash and cause neuritis (zoster sine herpete, e.g., Bell's palsy).

**CMV:** Latent CMV genomes can be reactivated from CD34+ hematopoietic stem cells, identifying this cell type as the principal site of latency. The viral load produced during primary CMV replication correlates with the copy number of latent genomes present in organs and the relative risk of recurrent disease. Moreover, CMV latency and reactivation is controlled by T lymphocytes, NK cells, and IFN$\gamma$, but also endocrine factors, as reflected by the increasing probability to shed virus during pregnancy and lactation. Depending on the extent of reactivated infection, the virus can be found in almost all organs including white blood cells. The reactivated virus is disseminated via infected myelomonocytic and endothelial cells to peripheral sites where the virus spreads locally from cell to cell. Shedding of cell free virus occurs from the salivary glands into saliva and mammary glands and into breast milk. Further sites of extensive virus shedding are the genital and urethral tracts.

**EBV:** EBV is spread by the oral route. Shedding of EBV detectable in saliva as a result of reactivation and replication at oropharyngeal sites occurs frequently in immunocompetent carriers. In immunologically compromised patients, EBV induces various tumors and oral hairy leukoplakia, a replicative lesion of the immunocompromised host on the lateral borders of the tongue.

**Epidemiology**

Human herpesviruses are ubiquitous agents distributed worldwide but restricted to humans as their natural host. Seroepidemiological studies have determined the prevalence of virus-specific IgG in many countries, indicating the frequency of infection within a defined population. Geographic location, socioeconomic status, and age are the primary factors that influence the acquisition of infection. HSV-1, VZV, and EBV are found in 80–99% of the adult population in all countries, while the seroprevalence of CMV infection ranges from 50% (Western Europe) to 99% (African and Asian countries). HSV-2 is found less frequently than HSV-1, in 20% to 70% of adults depending on socioeconomic status, race, and geographic location.

## References


Cohen JI, Straus SE, Arvin AM (2007) Varicella-Zoster-Virus. In: Knipe, D.M., Holey, P.M. (eds.): Fields Virology, 5th ed. Lippincott Williams & Wilkins, Philadelphia, pp 2773–2818

Ekstrand MI, Enquist LW, Pomeranz LE (2008) The alpha-herpesviruses: molecular pathfinders in nervous systems circuits. Trends Mol Med 14: 134–140

Hengel H, Brune W, Koszinowski UH (1998) Immune evasion by cytomegalovirus – survival strategies of a highly adapted opportunist. Trends Microbiol 6: 190–197

Mocarski ES (2002) Immunomodulation by cytomegaloviruses: manipulative strategies beyond evasion. Trends Microbiol 10: 332–339

Mocarski ES, Shenk T, Pass, RF (2007) Cytomegalovirus. In: Knipe, D.M., Holey, P.M. (eds.): Fields Virology, 5th ed. Lippincott Williams & Wilkins, Philadelphia, pp 2701–2772

Polic B, Hengel H, Krmpotic A, Trgovcich J, Pavic I, Lucin P, Jonjic S, Koszinowski, UH (1998) Hierarchical and redundant lymphocyte subset control precludes cytomegalovirus replication during latent infection. J Exp Med 188: 1047–1054

Rickinson AB, Kieff E (2007) Epstein-Barr Virus. In: Knipe, D.M., Holey, P.M. (eds.): Fields Virology, 5th ed. Lippincott Williams & Wilkins, Philadelphia, pp 2655–2700

Roizman B, Knipe DM, Whitley RJ (2007) Herpes simplex viruses. In: Knipe, D.M., Holey, P.M. (eds.): Fields Virology, 5th ed. Lippincott Williams & Wilkins, Philadelphia, pp 2501–2602

Thomas SL, Wheeler JG, Hall AJ (2002) Contacts with varicella or with children and protection against herpes zoster in adults: a case-control study. The Lancet 360: 678–682

# Herpes Simplex Virus (HSV) Diseases of the Anterior Segment and the Adnexa

*Rainer Sundmacher*

Chapter **2**

## Core Messages

- In **viral** herpetic diseases, replicating HSV can be isolated from the affected structures and antiviral treatment is always the basis of therapy.
- In **metaherpetic** diseases, i. e., in non-viral healing disorders after preceding viral disease, antiviral therapy increases the healing problems and is, therefore, mostly contraindicated.

The vast majority of ocular HSV diseases affect the anterior segment of the eye and its adnexes. Diseases of the posterior segment are relatively rare (see Chap. 6).

The topographical classification of HSV anterior segment diseases used here was first presented at the International Symposium on Herpetic Eye Diseases in Freiburg, 1980, and has since proven to be very practical and helpful for diagnosis and therapy (Fig. 2.1). In topographical order, on the left-hand side it lists the HSV diseases in which replicating HSV can regularly be isolated from the affected structures, and for which antiviral treatment forms the basis of therapy. On the right-hand side, the topographically corresponding metaherpetic diseases are depicted, i. e., the non-viral healing disorders after preceding viral herpetic disease. Although minimal virus replication or persistence may still be demonstrable in some of these conditions, e. g., by PCR techniques, the term metaherpetic signifies that virus replication pathophysiologically and therapeutically no longer plays a significant role. Antiviral therapy increases metaherpetic healing problems and is, therefore, mostly contraindicated. The numbers in Fig. 2.1 correspond to the subsequent sections in which each clinical picture is described in detail.

The *viral* HSV diseases addressed on the left-hand side are the following:

2.3 HSV blepharitis and HSV intermarginal blepharitis
2.4 HSV conjunctivitis
2.5 Epithelial HSV keratitis (punctate, dendritic, geographic)
2.6 Interstitial HSV keratitis and ulcerating HSV keratitis
2.7 HSV endotheliitis and disciform keratitis
2.8 HSV trabeculitis and glaucoma
2.9 HSV iritis
2.10 HSV scleritis

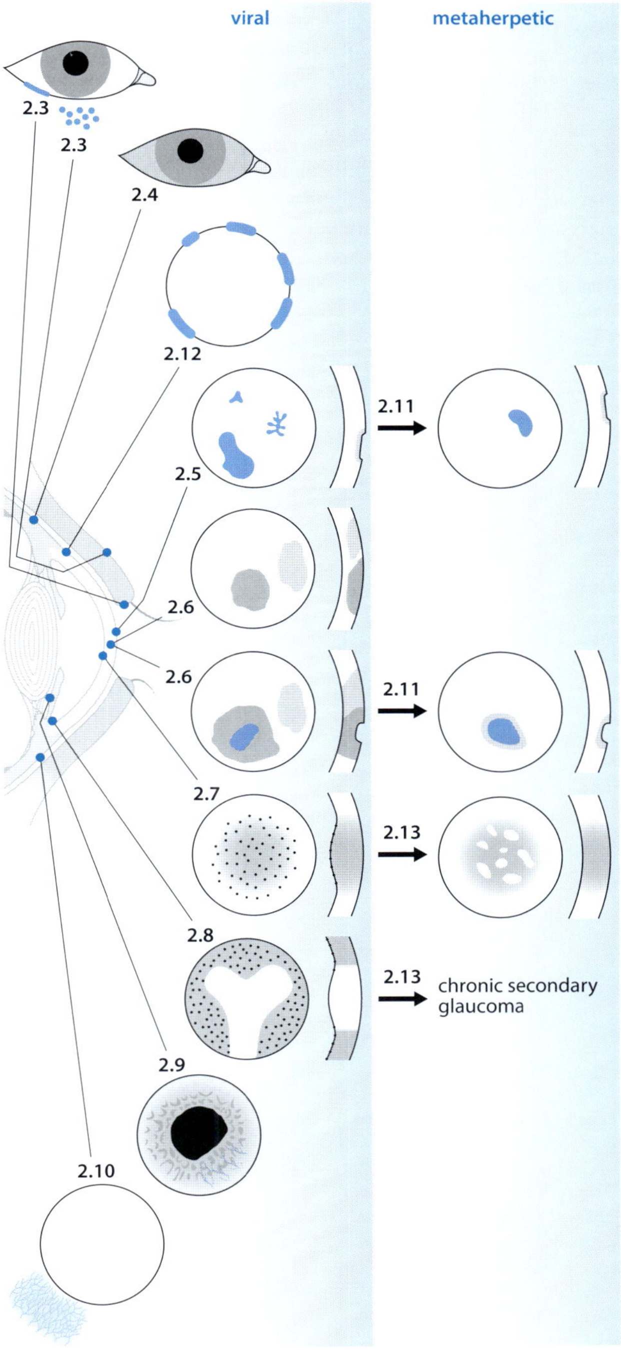


Fig. 2.1 Topographical classification of HSV viral and metaherpetic diseases of the anterior segment of the eye (see text)

HSV limbitis is the only clinical disease that by itself is pathognomonic for primary infection; it is therefore described in the special section on primary infection (Sect. 2.12) together with the other variants of this clinical specialty.

Viral HSV diseases of the lacrimal duct system have not been included in this atlas due to the lack of diagnostic visual criteria. Some references are listed in the section on blepharitis (Sect. 2.3). The topic of neonatal herpes has also been omitted, as it is more adequately addressed in textbooks on obstetrics and pediatrics.

Under the heading "metaherpetic" on the right-hand side of Fig. 2.1, the following diseases are addressed:

2.11 Superficial (epithelial) and deep metaherpetic ulcers
2.13 Metaherpetic scars and bullous keratopathy as well as metaherpetic chronic glaucoma

Often, more than one cellular layer or circumscribed area is affected. All diseased sites should be completely identified and analysed as to their viral or metaherpetic contribution to actual disease before a pathophysiologically based therapy plan is established.

## References

Holland EJ, Schwartz GS (1999) Classification of herpes simplex virus keratitis. Cornea 18: 144–154

Liesegang TJ (1999) Classification of herpes simplex virus keratitis and anterior uveitis. Cornea 18: 127–143

Sundmacher R (1981) A clinico-virologic classification of herpetic anterior segment diseases with special reference to intraocular herpes. In: R Sundmacher (ed) Herpetic Eye Diseases. Bergmann, Munich, pp 203–208

Sundmacher R (1987) Clinical aspects of herpetic eye diseases. Current Eye Res 6: 183–188

Sundmacher R, Neumann-Haefelin D (1976) Keratitis metaherpetica. Klinische und virologische Befunde. Klin Monatsbl Augenheilk 169: 728–737

# Pathophysiology

Section

2.1

## Core Messages

- Primary ocular HSV infection is followed by HSV latency in V1 of the trigeminal ganglion. From there, endogenous neuronal viral recurrences may lead to HSV disease in the area of primary infection.
- As primary HSV infection is mostly subclinical and passes unrecognized, pathophysiologically, most first observed attacks of HSV eye disease are first endogenous recurrences already.
- The most evident trigger for HSV recurrences is stress.

The most important pathophysiologic characteristic of herpes simplex viruses is their ability to get access to peripheral sensory neurons and hide away in a latent status in the nuclei of the associated neural ganglion cells, from where they may cause endogenous neuronal viral recurrences leading to various forms of peripheral herpetic disease (Fig. 2.2).

Some knowledge of the pathophysiological background helps a better understanding of many clinical observations and is the best basis for therapy and prophylaxis. Clinically, the most important are the following:

*Primary HSV infection typically affects the orofacial area and passes mostly subclinically.*

HSV is mostly transmitted by contact – digitally, by caressing, or by sexual contact. Primary infection used to start in early childhood in the orofacial area by close contact with persons suffering from infectious HSV blisters (Fig. 2.103). The improving hygienic living conditions in "developed countries" have continuously shifted the average age of primary infection from early childhood to older age groups. This is accompanied by an increasing frequency of sexually transmitted primary HSV infections, not only in the genital area but also in the orofacial area, thus increasing the percentage of HSV-2 rather than of HSV-1 viruses involved. This can create a therapeutic problem, because HSV-2 may be more pathogenetic than most HSV-1 strains, and the susceptibility towards antiviral agents may also be worse. The vast majority of primary infections pass subclinically or as such a mild disease that herpes etiology is not suspected. The likely explanations for this phenomenon are complex and not well understood; individually different natural resistance of the primarily infected host cells against HSV infections, different pathogenicity of different HSV strains, different infectious doses, an excellent regeneration power of the primary infected superficial epithelial cells, and, last but not least, the individually different kinetics and efficiencies of the

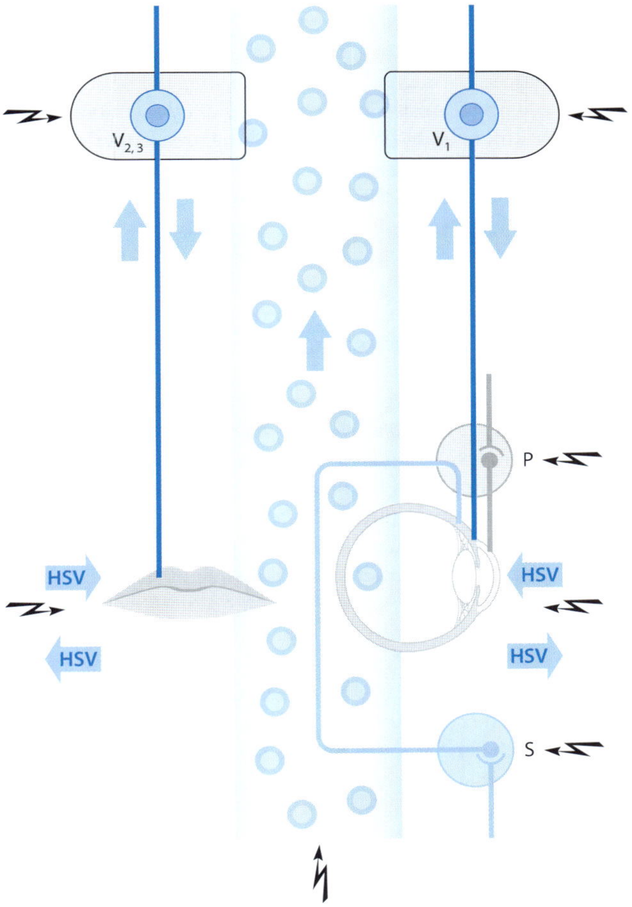


Fig. 2.2 Primary HSV infection, latency, and endogenous neuronal recurrences of HSV diseases in the facial area and the eye (see text)

evolving immune responses of the host may work together to inhibit clinical manifestation of disease after primary infection. In recurrent HSV disease, we are dealing with established immunology, and antiherpetic immunology is far from being only beneficial. Often, cellular immunology is the main reason why recurrent HSV disease is so severe.

*Once cellular immune defence has fully developed after primary infection, relative immunity exists against superinfections of healthy epithelial surfaces.*

When the level of cellular anti-HSV immunity has reached full efficiency after about 2 weeks following the primary infection, simple contamination of intact surfaces with HSV normally does not lead to superinfections. Neither can new primary infection sites be easily created by the already latently present endogenous virus, nor can new contaminating viruses easily break the immune defence. It is only if an infectious virus is forced through the epithelium into the subepithelial tissues, e.g., by a misled injection needle, by a contaminated surgeon's knife, or by vigorous rubbing that superinfection with establishment of a second site of recurrent HSV disease is possible anywhere in the integument – with "old" and "new" virus strains. The same holds true for the situation when virus is spilled into the cul de sac of a healthy eye from neighboring HSV lid blisters. As long as the eye remains non-irritated and its epithelial surface intact and as long as no vigorous rubbing is exerted, there is sufficient surface protection and no superinfection is possible.

*Herpetic ocular disease is a rare event compared with labial herpes. Unilateral ocular herpes normally stays unilateral. Only exceptionally is recurrent HSV eye disease bilateral.*

For ocular herpes to become established, the surface of an eye must be primarily infected *before* this has happened elsewhere in the orofacial area. This sequence of events is quite unusual. Normally, the orofacial area is infected first, and thereafter ocular HSV superinfection becomes difficult, as described above. The fact that primary ocular infection typically starts unilaterally is probably related to unilaterally directed caressing habits. The fact that it normally does not spread to the other eye in the course of primary infection may be explained by the fact that HSV shedding is too sparse in the course of subclinical primary infection. Possibly, an early increasing efficiency of immunity confers sufficient protection to the partner eye against small load HSV contaminations. If primary infection is clinically manifested, then cross contamination and early infection of the partner eye are more likely, and such patients are at a higher risk to develop bilaterally recurrent ocular herpes – an exception from the rule.

*Except for the rare clinical manifestations of primary infection (see Sect. 2.12), all HSV diseases – also the ones first observed – pathophysiologically represent recurrences with fully established cellular immune response.*

*Recurrences manifest themselves characteristically in the area of primary infection.*

HSV has the special ability to gain access to peripheral sensory nerve endings. Once it has invaded the neurons in the course of primary infection, the virus particles travel with the bidirectional endoneuronal plasma flow. Some reach the nuclei of the ganglion cells serving the infected area and there they start endonuclear replication. This may or may not lead to cytolysis of the ganglion cells with subsequent infection of neighboring ganglion and glia cells. This phase of virus replication ends quickly with increasing efficiency of the immune defence, limiting the viral spread to a topographically strictly limited area, e.g., the ophthalmic section of the trigeminal ganglion. Viral spread to other sections of the trigeminal ganglion is not the rule. Thus, labial herpes and ocular herpes do not cause one another on the ganglion level. After virus spread in the ganglion has been halted, HSV "retreats" into its ganglion host cell nucleus and there it "disappears" as naked, not easily detectable, virus DNA attached to the host cell DNA in a status of neuronal latency. For peripheral disease to occur, the virus DNA must find a way to again replicate complete viruses, which are thereafter re-transported within the associated sensory neurons to the site of primary infection and its vicinity, as depicted in Fig. 2.3.

*Not every person harboring HSV in the ganglia will experience recurrent disease. It appears that only about 1/3 of the population is at risk for recurrences and that stress is the trigger and not immunologic insufficiency.*

Only 1/3 of people belonging to professional groups with a nearly 100% infection risk, e.g., dentists and dentistry students, have been reported to suffer from recurrent labial herpes. This indicates, that 2/3 of the population seem to be genetically equipped with a sufficiently strong latency control for herpes virus, whereas in 1/3 of the population this latency control can be overcome by an individual exposure to stress that is too high. In spite of wide-spread belief, immunologic insufficiency could not be confirmed to be the primary cause for HSV recurrences. Therefore, "immune-strengthening" strategies have

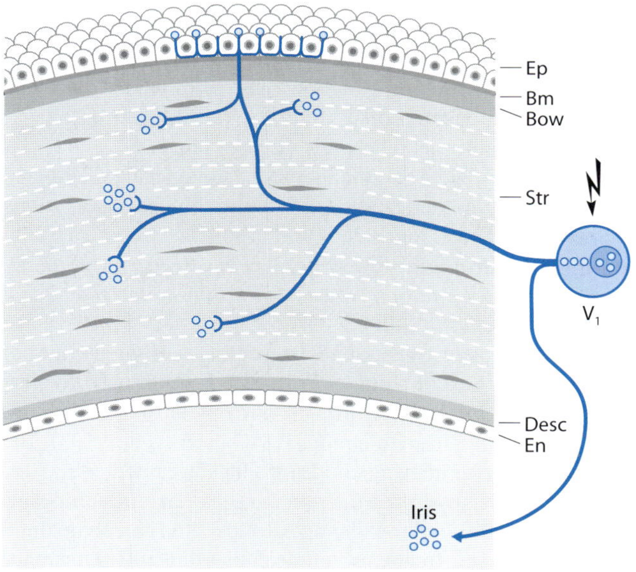


Fig. 2.3 Endogenous HSV recurrences with intra-axonal transport of HSV particles from ganglion cells in V1 back to the area of primary infection. There, clinical disease may or may not develop depending on the accessible target cells and the natural and immunologic defence mechanisms present

no scientific basis in therapy and prophylaxis of herpetic eye disease.

A molecular explanation for a person's relative resistance to herpes disease has not yet been found. Worldwide HLA correlation studies have not resulted in uniform results. It seems that different human races and populations have developed different genetic markers in their evolutionary battle with the herpes viruses, which themselves are not a uniform mass, but are made up of innumerable different strains with different pathogenic potential for different persons. This makes it difficult to disclose general interrelations on a molecular level.

*The sources of pathogenic stress are multiple and mostly not identifiable by the patient himself. However, they probably all end in the same biochemical pathway, which is not yet sufficiently understood.*

Although stress is now accepted as the basic trigger for recurrences, the majority of herpes patients are unable to identify their individual (psychological) stress. As self-analysis is impossible for most patients, it is of little practical help to advise them that their herpes recurrences are stress-triggered, and that they should work on eliminating stress. They may need professional help. Much easier to analyze and to handle are those rarer situations where herpes disease follows severe somatic stress, e. g., the acute onset of high degree fever, or easily conceivable stress situations like severe emotional shock after the death of a beloved person, or exhausting situations like extremely long air travel with severe sleep deficit. It is especially interesting that the time lag between onset of such identifiable causal situations and the first notice of a clinical herpes recurrence by the patient is always in the same range: about 3 days. In this time period, a long sequence of events must have taken place; virus latency control must have been overcome. Virus genes must have coded for production of the complete sequence of virus proteins and virus nucleic acids, and virus particles must have assembled. The virus must then have had time to travel with the axoplasma flow the long way down to the nerve endings, where they have to be set free. In the peripheral tissue, the viruses must have attached to new peripheral host cells, invaded their nucleus, and there must have again started a complete virus replication cycle. The infected peripheral host cells must have undergone cytolysis, or they must at least have expressed sufficient amounts of HSV specific antigens in their cell membranes in order to elicit significant cellular immune reactions. Only with sufficiently strong immune reactions, does inflammation reach the level of clinical notice. It seems that the time required for this complex sequence of events is well in the range of the observed time lag between onset of causal stress and first notice of HSV disease.

*Signals transferred via the sensory nerves and blood-bound signals – humoral as well as cellular ones – probably both play a role in herpes latency control and recurrences. A role for the autonomous nerve system has also been demonstrated experimentally (see the lightning symbols in Fig. 2.2).*

The exact biochemical regulation of latency control and initiation of recurrences, i. e., the biochemical nature of the signals and their precise transmission ways, are not known in detail and are at best suspected. The lightning symbols in Fig. 2.2 indicate at how many sites destabilizing influences on latency control can be envisioned with subsequent endoganglionic recurrent virus production. There are definitely additional cerebral sites from which the observed strong influence of emotion is exerted on latency control and recurrences. While viremia does not seem to play a significant role in virus transport and dissemination of disease in ocular herpes, the blood certainly plays a role in the transport of stress factors and T cells, which become operative in the ganglia. The autonomous nerve system has also been demonstrated to be involved in HSV recurrences in one way or another. Experimentally, epinephrine applied to the cornea causes recurrent HSV shedding in mice. Although epinephrine seems to fit well into our stress hypothesis, the signal transmission ways remain obscure. Even more unclear is the way in which trauma at the site of primary infection may trigger an endogenous recurrence, e. g., dendritic keratitis after a corneal foreign body, or herpetic iritis after cataract surgery. Although rare, such causal sequences have been observed and call for prophylactic measures if surgery in eyes infected with herpes is necessary.

*Corneal sensitivity decreases concomitantly with an increasing number of HSV recurrences. Testing corneal sensitivity is nonetheless only of limited value for differential diagnosis.*

Reduction of corneal sensitivity in the course of diseases that accompany infection and functional incapacitation of corneal sensory nerves comes as no surprise. It is more important to point out why reduced corneal sensitivity is usually diagnostically less helpful than one would expect:

1. Corneal sensitivity is very different in the periphery, the mid-periphery and the centre of the normal cornea. Also, the general level of corneal sensitivity varies considerably inter-individually. The safest way to estimate the level of sensitivity in a diseased eye is to test for comparison the healthy cornea exactly at the corresponding topographic site, and this is not easy to do.
2. Sensitivity reduction is limited to the area supplied by the diseased neurons. This may be only a small part of the cornea and may be missed in testing, especially at the beginning of a series of recurrences.
3. Quantitative esthesiometrics is to be preferred. Without considerable experience, however, its results are barely better than those achieved qualitatively with a simple cotton tip.
4. After a disease attack, sensitivity can be recovered considerably, depending on the amount of permanent damage to the sensory ganglia. After a first dendritic attack, sensitivity may totally return to normal after a while. It seems that adjacent dendrites grow into the denervated area and they substitute function there.
5. All non-herpetic inflammatory diseases, which destroy corneal structures and lead to significant scars, also considerably reduce corneal sensitivity.
6. Sensitivity testing helps in differential diagnosis only in those situations, therefore, when etiologically unclear small infiltrations lie in an otherwise clear corneal stroma. If sensitivity is found to be significantly reduced in comparison to the same exact topographic area of the partner eye, then a herpes diagnosis becomes likely.

*Neurotrophic corneal disorders are another sequela of ganglionic involvement in recurrent ocular herpes. They are the main reason for trophic metaherpetic ulcers.*

The exact pathophysiology of neurotrophic disease has remained disputed in spite of all studies performed. For practical purposes it suffices to accept that sensitivity reduction is closely correlated with neurotrophic disease. Complete surgical cutting of the ophthalmic nerve leads to most severe trophic corneal disease. Similar severe disease is observed after complete loss of sensitivity in severe zoster. Compared with these two diseases, neurotrophic disturbances in HSV ocular disease tend to be mild but still severe enough to cause metaherpetic superficial and deep corneal ulcers (see Sect. 2.11).

While sensory nerve damage is the endogenous reason for metaherpetic neurotrophic disease, inadequate toxic topical therapy may practically be even more important as the ultimate exogenous trigger for clinical manifestation (see Sect. 2.2).

*HSV, like any virus, has a specialized host cell range preferring some cell types more than others.*

HSV attaches to and multiplies in some cells better than in others. This is the case with all viruses, but it is often overlooked when considering pathophysiology in HSV eye disease. Corneal epithelium allows HSV replication more effectively and quicker than keratocytes and endothelial cells do. Also, HSV feels more comfortable in iris cells deriving from the optic cup (i. e., iris muscle cells and iris pigment epithelium) than in iris stroma cells or the vascular endothelium. First infection of keratocytes in clear corneal stroma is a slow and mostly limited event, while recurrent stromal disease tends to become more severe and persistent with increasing inflammatory infiltration. These basic differences in virus-cell interactions are further modified by different virus loads set free at different sites, as well as by different efficiencies of the natural and immunologic defences available at a certain time at different sites. Therefore, Fig. 2.3 illustrates only some *potential sites* of infection. The *probability* of infection and subsequent disease at a certain site are dependent on many determinants, of which some – inflammatory infiltrates – can be therapeutically manipulated.

*There is still no general agreement on the topics of latency and persistence of HSV in the cornea.*

One has to find an explanation for the clinical observation that HSV can "survive" in a clinically "quiet" cornea and after prolonged time cause recurrent corneal disease, even without neuronal connections to the trigeminal ganglion. Some researchers have called this peripheral latency. Others have preferred to call it peripheral persistence. I prefer the latter term.

It is debatable whether or not HSV can hide in keratocytes, endothelial cells, or some other infiltrated cells in the cornea in the same fashion as it does in ganglion cells, i. e., as naked DNA in peripheral cell nuclei, from where it recurs and causes disease. I doubt it and, therefore, I will not speak of corneal latency. In my opinion, it seems more probable that in such cases we are dealing with a very restricted, very slow infection, a *persistent* infection, which results in expression of some HSV antigens on the cell membranes, but does not lead to significant cell death by viral cytolysis alone. Lysis of the host cells is only brought about by reactive cellular anti-HSV immune attacks. Consequently, the best *symptomatic* treatment of such conditions is an adequate suppression of destructive immune activity – and this really helps, even in the long run. *A strictly causal monotherapy*, however, i. e., eradication of the persistent HSV infection by antiviral monotherapy, offers little or no chance of healing. There is a simple general rule: the less viral turnover, the less chances for efficient antiviral therapy. With peripheral HSV persistence, the viral turnover seems to be minimal, and so are the chances for successful antiviral monotherapy.

*Cellular immune reaction has a Janus-faced character in HSV ocular disease. It is absolutely necessary and helpful in superficial epithelial herpes. With all deep herpetic forms, however, the collateral side effects of irreversible destruction of the transparent optical system prevail and call for adequate therapeutic limitation and counteraction.*

As long as HSV infection is limited to the epithelial layer of the cornea in dendritic keratitis, a powerful cellular immune reaction is optimal. The quicker all infected cells are attacked and destroyed, the better. Epithelial infiltration by immune cells is by no means disadvantageous. The cellular debris is washed away with the tear flow. Healthy epithelial neighbor cells glide over quickly, and the lost epithelial layers are replaced by mitosis, restoring an epithelial layer, which is identical to the infected lost one. Therefore, with pure dendritic keratitis, everything that impairs cellular immune reaction, above all steroids, is disadvantageous.

On the other hand, everything that strengthens cellular immune reactions, e. g,. topical interferon (see Sect. 2.2), is helpful.

With deep forms of corneal herpetic disease, the situation is totally different. The immunological battle field attracts more and more inflammatory infiltrates of different cells. These initiate a malicious cycle of cell death and new infiltration, resulting in severe functional destruction of the cornea. Therefore, the problem with deep herpetic disease is: How indispensable is cellular immune reaction for the termination of viral reproduction and what is its overall value as compared to its simultaneous destructive side effect on a clear optical tissue? Both aspects have to be weighed against each other, but optimal functional preservation or restitution of the optic system must have priority over quick eradication of the HSV infection. Deep viral diseases, therefore, call for an intelligently adapted combination therapy of antiviral agents *plus* steroids (see Sect. 2.2).

## References


Babu JS, Thomas J, Kanangat S, Morrison LA, Knipe DM, Rouse BT (1996) Viral replication is required for induction of ocular immunopathology by herpes simplex virus. J Virol 70: 101–107

Bak IJ, Markham CH, Cook ML, Stevens J (1977) Intraaxonal transport of herpes simplex virus in the rat central nervous system. Brain Res 136: 415–429

Banerjee K, Biswas PS, Kamaragurn U, Schoenberger SP, Rouse BT (2004) Protective and pathological roles of virus-specific and bystander CD8 + T cells in herpetic stromal keratitis. J Immunol 173: 7575–7583

Buchman TG, Roizman B, Nahmias AJ (1979) Demonstration of exogenous reinfection with herpes simplex virus type-2 by restriction endonuclease fingerprinting of viral DNA. J Infect Dis 140: 295–304

Carter C, Dyson H, Easty DL (1985) Herpes simplex virus infection of corneal cells in vitro. In: PC Maudgal, L Missotten (eds): Herpetic Eye Diseases. Doc Ophthalmol Progr Ser vol 44, Dr W Junk Publ., Dordrecht, pp 9–14

Carter C, Easty DL (1981) The influence of antiviral immunity in epithelial herpetic keratitis. In: R. Sundmacher (ed): Herpetic Eye Diseases. Bergmann, Munich, pp 111–116

Centifanto-Fitzgerald YM, Yamaguchi T, Kaufman HE, Togon M, Roizman B (1982) Ocular disease pattern induced by herpes simplex virus is genetically determined by a specific region of the viral DNA. J Exp Med 155: 475–489

Cook SD, Brown SM (1986) Herpes simplex virus type 1 persistence and latency in cultured rabbit corneal epithelial cells, keratocytes, and endothelial cells. Br J Ophthalmol 70: 642–650

Cook SD, Hill JH (1991) Herpes simplex virus: molecular biology and the possibility of corneal latency. Surv Ophthalmol 36: 140–148

Dawson CR, Togni B, Thygeson P (1966) Herpes simplex virus particles in the nerves of rabbit corneas after epithelial inoculation. Nature 211: 316–317

Freeman ML, Sheridan BS, Bonneau RH, Hendricks RL (2007) Psychological stress compromises CD8+ T cell control of latent herpes simplex type 1 infections. J Immunol 179: 322–328

Garweg JG, Halberstadt M (2002) Zur Pathogenese der herpetischen Keratitis. Klin Monatsbl Augenheilkd 219: 477–486

Hendricks RL, Janovicz M, Tumpey TM (1992) Critical role of corneal Langerhans cells in CD4- but not in CD8-mediated immunopathology in herpes simplex virus-1-infected mouse corneas. J Immunol 148: 2522–2529

Hendricks RL, Tumpey TM (1991) Concurrent regeneration of T lymphocytes and susceptibility to HSV-1 corneal stromal disease. Curr Eye Res 10 (Suppl): 47–53

Herpetic Eye Disease Study Group (2000) Psychological stress and other potential triggers for recurrences of herpes simplex virus eye infections. Arch Ophthalmol 118: 1617–1625

Holbach LM, Font RL, Wilhelmus KR (1991) Recurrent herpes simplex keratitis with concurrent epithelial and stromal involvement. Immunohistochemical and ultrastructural observations. Arch Ophthalmol 109: 692–695

Kaufmann HE, Azcuy AM, Varnell ED, Sloop GD, Thompson HW, Hill JM (2005) HSV-1 DNA in tears and saliva of normal adults. Invest Ophthalmol Vis Sci 46: 241–247

Kaye SB, Baker K, Bonshek , Maseruka H, Grinfeld E, Tullo A, Easty DL, Hart CA (2000) Human herpesviruses in the cornea. Br J Ophthalmol 84: 563–571

Kaye SB, Lynas C, Patterson A, Risk JM, Mc Carthy K, Hart CA (1991) Evidence for herpes simplex viral latency in the human cornea. Br J Ophthalmol 75: 195–200

Kaye SB, Madan N, Dowd TC, Hart CA, Mc Carthy K, Patterson A (1990) Ocular shedding of herpes simplex virus. Br J Ophthalmol 74: 114–116

Koelle DM, Ghiasi H (2005) Prospects for developing an effective vaccine against herpes simplex virus infection. Curr Eye Res 30: 929–942

Kwon SS, Gangarosa LP, Green K, Hill JM (1982) Kinetics of ocular herpes simplex virus shedding induced by epinephrine iontophoresis. Invest Ophthalmol Vis Sci 22: 818–821

Lang A, Nikolich-Zugich J (2005) Development and migration of protective CD8+ T cells into the nervous system following ocular herpes simplex virus-1 infection. J Immunol 174: 2919–2925

Lenhard V, Haug P, Kirchner H, Hallermann C, Mattes A, Sundmacher R (1981) HLA phenotypes in patients with herpetic keratitis. In: R Sundmacher (ed) Herpetic eye disease. Bergmann, Munich, pp 95–97.

Lewis ME, Leung WC, Jeffrey VM, Warren KG (1984) Detection of multiple strains of latent herpes simplex virus type 1 within individual human hosts. J Virol 52: 300–305

Liesegang TJ (1989) Epidemiology of ocular herpes simplex. Natural history in Rochester, Minn, 1950 through 1982. Arch Ophthalmol 107: 1160–1165

Liesegang TJ (2001) Herpes simplex virus epidemiology and ocular importance. Cornea 20: 1–13

Martin RG, Dawson CR, Jones P, Togni B; Lyons C, Oh JO (1977) Herpesvirus in sensory and autonomic ganglia after eye infection. Arch Ophthalmol 95: 2053–2056

Mintsioulis G, Dawson CR, Oh JO, Briones O (1979) Herpetic eye disease in rabbits after inoculation of autonomic ganglia. Arch Ophthalmol 97: 1515–1517

Missotten L (1994) Immunology and herpetic keratitis. Eye 8: 12–21

Mitchell BM, Bloom DC, Cohrs RJ, Gilden DH, Kennedy PG (2003) Herpes simplex virus-1 and varicella-zoster virus latency in ganglia. J Neurovirol 9: 194–204

Nesburn AB, Dickinson R, Radnotti M, Radnotti MT (1976) Experimental reactivation of ocular herpes simplex in rabbits. Surv Ophthalmol 21: 185

Neumann-Haefelin D, Lenz T, Sundmacher R (1979) Strain characteristics and features of ocular infection of herpes simplex virus type 1 isolates. Med Microbiol Immunol 167: 239–250

Neumann-Haefelin D, Sundmacher R (1981) Herpes viruses – common properties and heterogeneity. In: R Sundmacher (ed) Herpetic eye disease. Bergmann, Munich, pp 3–12

Neumann-Haefelin D, Sundmacher R, Wochnik G, Bablok B (1978) Herpes simplex virus types 1 and 2 in ocular disease. Arch Ophthalmol 96: 64–69

Ohara PT, Chin MS, Vail JH (2000) The spread of herpes simplex virus type 1 from trigeminal neurons to the murine cornea: an immunoelectron microscopy study. J Virology 74: 4776–4786

Openshaw H, McNeill JI, Lin XH, Niland J, Cantin EM (1995) Herpes simplex virus DNA in normal corneas: persistence without viral shedding from ganglia. J Med Virol 46: 75–80

Pavan-Langston D, Rong BL, Dunkel EC (1989) Extraneuronal herpetic latency: animal and human corneal studies. Acta Ophthalmol Suppl 192: 135–141

Pepose JS, Keadle TL, Morrison LA (2006) Ocular herpes simplex: changing epidemiology, emerging disease patterns, and the potential of vaccine prevention and therapy. Am J Ophthalmol 141: 547–557

Posavad CM, Koelle DM, Corey L (1998) Tipping the scales of herpes simplex virus reactivation: the important responses are local. Nat Med 4: 381–382

Price RW, Katz BJ, Notkins AL (1975) Latent infection of the peripheral autonomic nervous system with herpes simplex virus. Nature 257: 686–688

Rager-Zisman B, Quan PC, Rosner M, Moller JR, Bloom BR (1987) Role of NK cells in protection of mice against herpes simplex virus-1 infection. J Immunol 138: 884–888

Remeijer L (2002) Human herpes simplex virus keratitis: The pathogenesis revisited. (Doctoral thesis, Erasmus University Rotterdam)

Remeijer L, Maertzdorf J, Buitenwerf J, Osterhaus ADME, Verjans GMGM (2002) Corneal herpes simplex virus type 1 superinfection in patients with recrudescent herpetic keratitis. Invest Ophthalmol Vis Sci 43: 358–363

Sabagga EMH, Pavan-Langston D, Bean KM, Dunkel EC (1988) Detection of HSV nucleic acid sequences in the cornea during acute and latent ocular disease. Exp Eye Res 47: 545–553

Severin M (1965) Die Hornhautsensibilität bei herpetischer Keratitis. Klin Monatsbl Augenheilkd 146: 683–695

Shimeld C, Hill TJ, Blyth WA, Easty DL (1990) Passive immunization protects the mouse eye from damage after herpes simples virus infection by limiting spread of virus in the nervous system. J Gen Virol 71: 681–687

Souza PM, Holland EJ, Huang AJ (2003) Bilateral herpetic keratoconjunctivitis. Ophthalmology 110: 493–496

Streilein JW, Dana R, Ksander BR (1997) Immunity causing blindness: five different paths to herpes stromal keratitis. Immunol Today 18: 443–449

Sundmacher R (1977) Die Pathophysiologie der Herpes simplex Rezidive. Klin Monatsbl Augenheilk 170: 613–621

Thomas J, Rouse BT (1997) Immunopathogenesis of herpetic ocular disease. Immunol Res 16: 375–386

Warren KG, Brown SM, Wroblewska Z, Gilden D, Koprowski H, Subak-Sharpe JH (1978) Isolation of latent herpes simplex virus from the superior cervical and vagus ganglions of human beings. N Engl J Med 289: 1068–1069

Wilhelmus KR, Falcon MG, Jones BR (1981) Bilateral herpetic keratitis. Br J Ophthalmol 65: 385–387

Wu L, Morahan PS (1992) Macrophages and other non specific defences: role in modulating resistance against herpes simplex virus. In: Rouse BT (ed). Herpes simplex virus: pathogenesis, immunobiology and control. Springer, Heidelberg/NY, pp 89–110

# Basics of Therapy



## Core Messages

Herpetic eye diseases may be divided into four therapeutic groups (see Fig 2.4):

| group | therapy |
|---|---|
| **A** viral superficial (epithelial) | antiviral agents |
| **B** viral deep | antiviral agents *plus* steroids |
| **C** metaherpetic superficial (epithelial) | conservative resurfacing |
| **D** metaherpetic deep | surgical reconstruction |

In Fig. 2.4 herpetic ocular diseases are divided into viral (left-hand side) and non-viral metaherpetic ones (right-hand side). Drawing a second division line between superficial forms of disease, which primarily affect the epithelium (upper part), and deep subepithelial ones (lower part), results in four groups of diseases whose basic therapy can be systemized. This makes basic therapeutic decisions easy.

Table 2.1 extends the therapy scheme with more disease-associated specifications, but still remains basic.

Practical therapy of individual cases requires case-adapted specifications and modifications, which cannot be systemized and are suggested and discussed in different clinical sections.

As basic therapy for groups I–IV, the following measures are efficient:

## 2.2.A Antiviral Agents for Superficial (Epithelial) Viral Disease

Thousands of molecules have presumably been tested in vitro for antiherpetic activity, but only some of these have made their way to animal models, and only a few have been promising enough for controlled studies in humans, of which K. R. Wilhelmus has written an excellent critical review. Study details and the abundant literature on this topic may be found

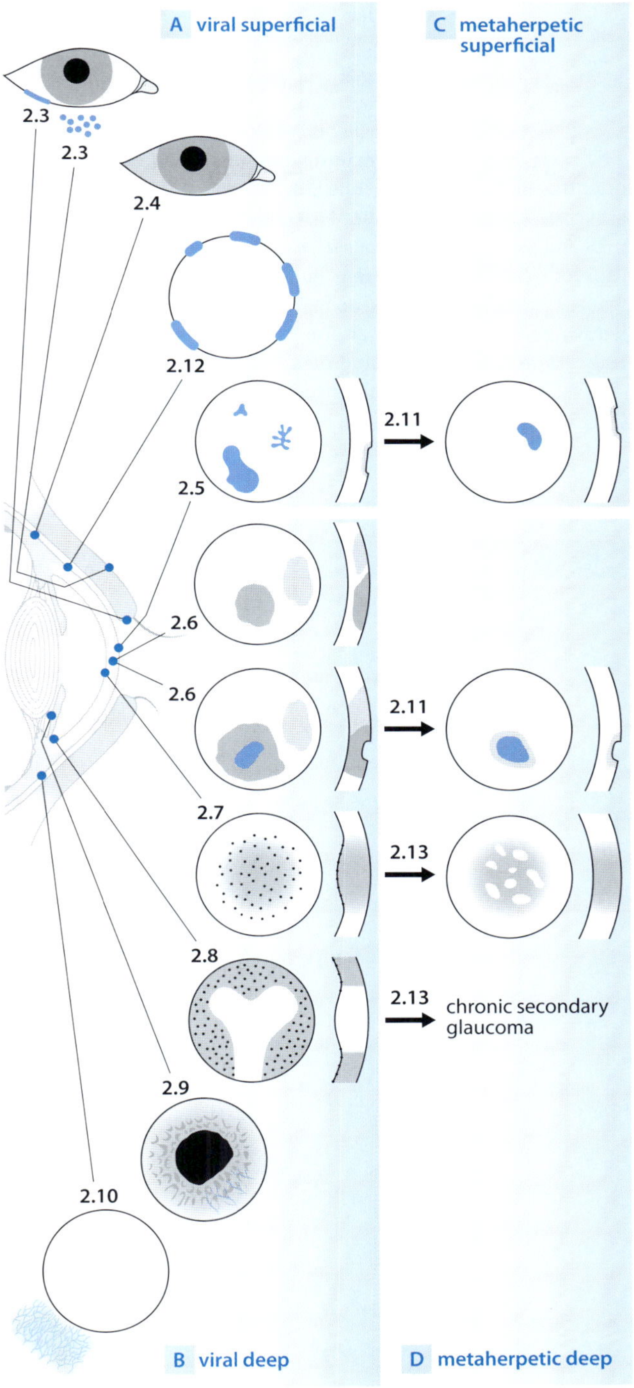


Fig. 2.4 The four therapy groups of herpetic eye disease (see text)

in this work. For the purposes of this atlas, the discussion is focused on four topics:

1. Trifluorothymidine (TFT) and Aciclovir (ACV)
2. Bromovinyldeoxyuridine (BVDU), a potential alternative
3. The lasting value of mechanical debridement
4. The potential value of topical interferon in combination with topical antiviral agents

## 2.2.A.1 Trifluorothymidine (TFT) and Aciclovir (ACV)

TFT eye drops and ACV ointment are by far the most frequently used topical anti-herpetic drugs on the market. They serve most requirements for a successful topical therapy of corneal epithelial herpetic disease, and the further development of different anti-herpetic drugs has therefore come mostly to a standstill. Although both drugs act equally well on dendritic keratitis from the statistical point of view, there are practically important differences (Table 2.2).

TFT and ACV are both active against the broad spectrum of HSV-1 and HSV-2 herpes virus strains, with TFT's binding specificity for its viral target enzyme being lower than ACV's binding specificity. The consequences are twofold:

- In terms of topical toxicity, ACV has advantages over TFT.
- In terms of maximally broad antiviral activity and minimal risk of development of resistant herpes strains, TFT should theoretically have some advantage over ACV.

For practical purposes, other differences may be more important:

- Patients' compliance is much higher with eye drops than with ointment, a plus for TFT in all cases where we are dealing with epithelial herpes only.
- ACV ointment scores in a different field. While TFT molecules cannot penetrate in sufficient amounts into the corneal stroma through an intact corneal epithelium, ACV has this property. ACV ointment is thus superior to TFT eye drops in all cases of dendritic keratitis that are combined with deep corneal herpes requiring simultaneously deep antiviral drug activity.
- Special cases of dendritic keratitis, which cannot reliably be treated with topical drugs (e.g., uncooperative children or mentally retarded adults), may equally efficiently be cured by a *systemic* ACV regime, which is another plus for ACV.

Table 2.1 Basic therapy of the herpetic diseases as depicted in Fig. 2.4

| No | Group/disease | Basic therapy/comments |
|---|---|---|
| **A** | **Viral superficial (epithelial)** | **Antiviral agents** |
| 2.3 | HSV blepharitis | (optional) |
| 2.3 | HSV intermarginal blepharitis | (optional) |
| 2.4 | HSV conjunctivitis | (only occasionally necessary) |
| 2.5 | Epithelial HSV keratitis (punctate, dendritic, geographic) | Topical antiviral drugs |
| 2.12 | HSV limbitis (primary infection) | Systemic antiviral drugs |
| **B** | **Viral deep** | **Antiviral agents *plus adequate* steroids** |
| 2.6 | Interstitial HSV keratitis | Topical antiviral drugs (must penetrate corneal epithelium) plus topical steroids, |
| 2.6 | Ulcerating HSV keratitis | Case-adapted systemic and topical combinations required |
| 2.7 | HSV endotheliitis and disciform keratitis | As with 2.6, eventually systemic antiviral agents in the beginning |
| 2.8 | HSV trabeculitis and glaucoma | Systemic combination therapy plus additional glaucoma therapy required |
| 2.9 | HSV iritis | Systemic antiviral drug plus topical steroids |
| 2.10 | HSV scleritis | Systemic combination therapy |
| **C** | **Metaherpetic superficial (epithelial)** | **Conservative resurfacing** |
| 2.11 | Metaherpetic epithelial ulcer | Artificial tears, therapeutic contact lenses (*no* antiviral drugs, if possible) |
| **D** | **Metaherpetic deep** | **Surgical reconstruction** |
| 2.11 | Metaherpetic deep ulcer | Amnion cover or related surgical measures, keratoplasty |
| 2.13 | Herpetic scars, bullous keratopathy | Keratoplasty |
| 2.13 | Metaherpetic chronic glaucoma | Trabeculectomy (therapy refractive cases only) |

Table 2.2 Some practically important differences of the antiviral substances TFT, ACV, and BVDU for therapy of dendritic keratitis

| | TFT | ACV | (BVDU) |
|---|---|---|---|
| Antiviral activity against | HSV-1 and -2 | HSV-1 and -2 | HSV-1 *only* |
| Topical preparations | Eye drops | Eye ointment | Eye drops* |
| Topical side effects | Reported | Very rare | Not known |
| Penetration into stroma | Insufficient | Sufficient | Sufficient |
| Systemic side effects | Considerable | Very rare | Very rare with short term therapy |
| Systemic therapy | No | Yes | Yes** |

* not yet available for topical therapy as a licensed product
** licensed for systemic VZV therapy in the EU

As a matter of fact, neither drug is equally available worldwide, and a differential choice according to the special requirements of an individual case cannot be made everywhere. While this may not be very important from a statistical point of view, it may matter individually, and the therapeutic recommendations in the atlas section will therefore primarily be guided by an unlimited access to all therapeutic options.

### 2.2.A.2 Bromovinyldeoxyuridine (BVDU), a Potential Alternative

Since the time of its first scientific presentation decades ago, bromovinyldeoxyuridine (BVDU) has been one of the most promising anti-herpetic drugs. My personal experiences date back to a controlled field study in which BVDU eye drops proved to be as efficient as TFT eye drops in the treatment of dendritic keratitis. Although they are equally active on a statistical basis, the failures in both study groups were in different fields, reflecting the different pharmacological and pharmacokinetic characteristics of the drugs. That would have made a licensing of BVDU eye drops attractive for a differentiated therapy. However, pharmaceutical companies then made decisions from the economic point of view, and the project was silently dropped. Admittedly, the use of BVDU involves some risks. Its greatest strength – a rather favorable virus enzyme specificity – is also its potential weak point: BVDU is highly active against HSV-1 strains (about 95% of the strains affecting the eye), but inefficient against HSV-2 strains. That means that every 20th herpes patient would be left untreated if given BVDU, unless reliable and cheap laboratory methods become available to determine quickly, before the start of therapy, which HSV type is involved. Provided that this is the case, BVDU eye drops may become an interesting alternative to TFT and ACV in the topical herpes therapy, with the advantage of less toxicity than TFT and a better patients' compliance than compliance to ACV with equally as deep activity as ACV. For the time being, BVDU remains only a second line drug for all those cases where viral resistance against ACV is suspected, which is not often the case. Also, it must not be forgotten that BVDU itself should be at least as prone for the selection of resistant virus strains as ACV. Nonetheless, the availability of highly active BVDU *eye drops,* which penetrate through intact epithelium into the corneal stroma without damaging epithelial regeneration, would certainly enrich our therapeutic armamentarium.

### 2.2.A.3 The Lasting Value of Mechanical Debridement

Therapy of dendritic keratitis by simple debridement of the dendritic epithelial areas was the therapeutic gold standard for 50 years before iododexoxyuridine (IDU) became available – the first not yet very specific and sometimes toxic antiviral agent (H. E. Kaufman). Some 100 years ago, Grüter was the first to recommend thermocautery with the aid of a rounded hollow metallic handpiece streamed by heated steam. The diseased epithelial areas can thus be exactly demarcated with the epithelium adhering to the heated tip, and undesired thermal effects on corneal stroma and endothelium avoided by only slightly touching the area. The overall results with this purely physical method are stunningly good (Fig. 2.5). About 70% of all dendrites heal within 3 days, 80% within 1 week, and "only" 20% take a longer course with local recurrences, necessitating repeated debridements with prolonged healing thereafter.

It is these 20% of complicated courses – and not primarily the average healing time – that are important when evaluating and comparing the efficiencies of different therapies. Although the average healing time after simple debridement is not necessarily worse than that after antiviral drug therapy, the latter is, without a doubt, much more effective and preferable, because the percentage of serious therapy failures – i. e., corneal destructions and scars – is considerably reduced.

Unfortunately, the certainty with which this judgement is expressed cannot rely on the results of controlled comparative studies, which have never been performed. The reader has to trust my conviction based on extended experiences with debridement. Even today, it will be difficult to meet the excellent *average* healing times after debridement alone. It is important, though, that no unnecessary additional physicochemical damage is involved as is the case with the additional use of iodine or lactic acid.

There is no iatrogenic damage to be feared, if "minimal wiping debridement (mwd)" with a cotton tipped applicator (Barry R. Jones) is used to remove most – but certainly not all – of the virus-loaded epithelial cells.

The question remains as to how to reduce 20% of prolonged healing with debridement to about zero by additional applica-

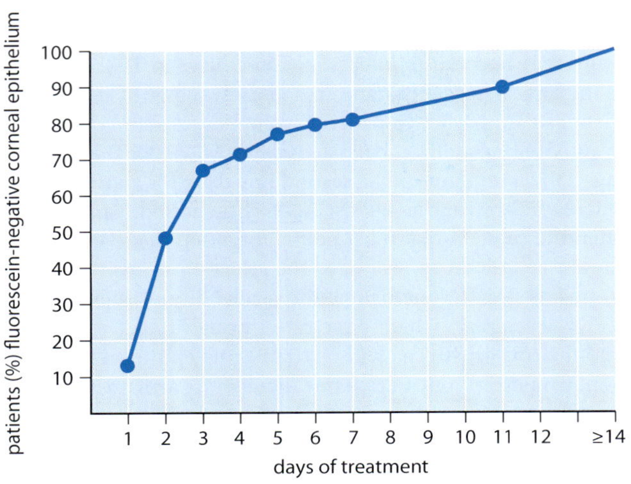


Fig. 2.5 Cumulative healing curve of dendritic keratitis after thermomechanical debridement, no additional antiviral therapy (from: R. Sundmacher, Klin Monatsbl Augenheilkd 169:308–325 (1976))

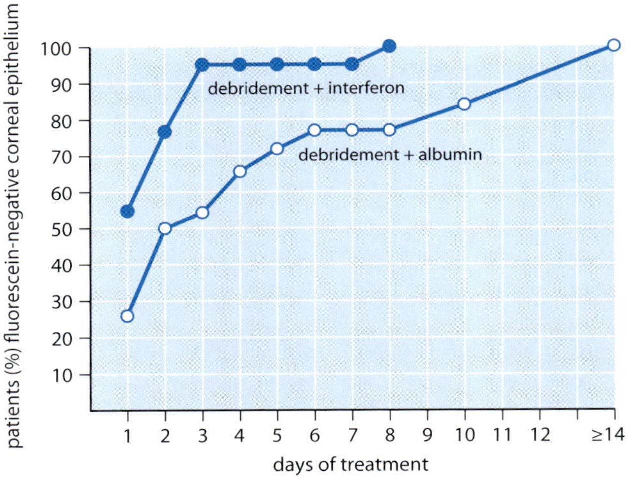


Fig. 2.6 Cumulative healing rates of patients with dendritic keratitis treated with debridement plus interferon or albumin eye drops (from: R. Sundmacher et al., 1976)

tion of other antiviral measures. While zero may be too ambitious, we can indeed approach that goal with a combination therapy of debridement plus either topical antiviral agents or plus topical interferon.

The combination of mwd plus topical *antivirals* has been studied several times, and its value more or less verified. As virtually no adverse side effects need be anticipated, such a combination is at least recommendable for treatment of babies and uncooperative children and adults in whom short anaesthesia is mostly necessary anyway. The dendrites can be mechanically removed and a topical antiviral agent (preferably ACV ointment) applied for the first time. If further topical therapy seems to be impossible, one can thereafter rely on systemic therapy with ACV, which has an equally good effect as topical treatment.

The role of topical *interferon* plus antiviral agents in the treatment of dendritic keratitis will be discussed below. Firstly, it is to be noted that topical interferon is also highly successful in combination with debridement. It eliminates nearly all protracted courses, as shown in a double-blind controlled study (Fig. 2.6).

### 2.2.A.4 The Potential Value of Topical Interferon in Combination with Topical Antiviral Agents

Sufficiently high-titered interferon preparations for successful topical treatment of dendritic keratitis are still not available on the market. German officials licensed a first commercial preparation in the 1980s, but this preparation had to be withdrawn because of patent quarrels with an international pharmaceutical company claiming that they themselves would go to the market with their own preparation, although they never did. After so many years of systematic clinical interferon research, this was bad news for patients and quite some disillusion for clinical researchers.

Meanwhile, with the development of much more efficient production methods for interferon, and a widespread application of systemic interferon for various other severe diseases, it can be hoped that interferon producing companies may again become interested in an ophthalmologic indication – if not for big profit then perhaps for reputation, which also has its own value.

It shall suffice to show in a composite graph how efficient topical interferon enhances not only the average healing rates of dendritic keratitis treated with TFT, but also eliminates all therapeutic failures leading to an as yet unmatched therapeutic success. This success comes only with high interferon titres, and it is further dependent to some degree on the interferon

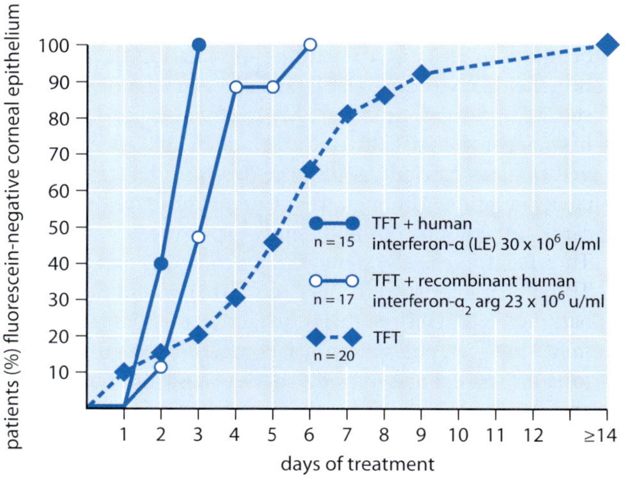


Fig. 2.7 Cumulative healing rates of dendritic keratitis with TFT-monotherapy, and TFT in combination with various topical high-titer interferon preparations (from: Sundmacher (1990))

species used. Combinations of different species have reduced the need for excessively high titres (Fig. 2.7).

## 2.2.B Antiviral Agents Plus Steroids for Deep Viral Disease

Cellular immune reactions against cell-bound viral antigens exert exclusively positive effects in pure epithelial disaese where loss of cells is quickly substituted by gliding and regeneration, and destroyed cells as well as any inflammatory debris are transported away with tear film. This becomes totally different as soon as herpetic disease affects subepithelial layers of the eye. In deep herpetic disease, cellular immune reactions have a Janus-faced character. On the one hand, they are basically needed to stop viral reproduction and cytolysis. On the other hand, an unlimited invasion of immune cells and inflammatory cells on a battle field, from where there is no way out without inflammatory side effects, must lead to severe functional damage with loss of transparency, loss of substance, and scar formation. Consequently, cellular infiltration must be down-regulated to such an extent that the antiviral potencies are still sufficiently preserved, but any cellular infiltration which is not absolutely necessary for viral inactivation must be suppressed. This is achievable by a flexible, case-adapted steroid regime *in addition* to full antiviral therapy. Figure 2.8 depicts the principles of such a combination therapy for deep herpetic viral disease.

1. The antiviral agent should always be started with a 100% efficiency dose, and invariably kept that high as long as at least medium dosed topical steroids are deemed necessary, a border line which we put at 3 drops id.
2. With lower steroid doses, stepwise reduction of the antiviral agent may be considered. While the steroid should always be tapered out slowly, it remains unclear whether or not tapering of the antiviral agent has an equivalent value. Below half the effective dose of an antiviral agent one would not expect any more much useful efficiency. If this assumption is correct, then tapering out can end at this border line, and no minimal doses of antiviral agents must be given for a prolonged time together with mini doses of steroids, which are often necessary. If the doctor feels that his patient should have an efficient antiviral cover even together with mini doses of steroids, then the doctor should consequently decide for sufficiently high doses of antiviral agents and not just hope that mini doses will also do. They probably will not.
3. The steroids have to be variably dosed, allowing the best balance between *"as low as possible"* and *"as much as necessary"*. Finding the safest and most successful compromise for each individual case and course is a matter of experience and can hardly be systemized. The great variability of cases and courses also explains why controlled therapeutic studies with rigidly prefixed systematic therapy regimes in this disease group can only give limited information regarding which combination therapy might be optimal in individual patients.

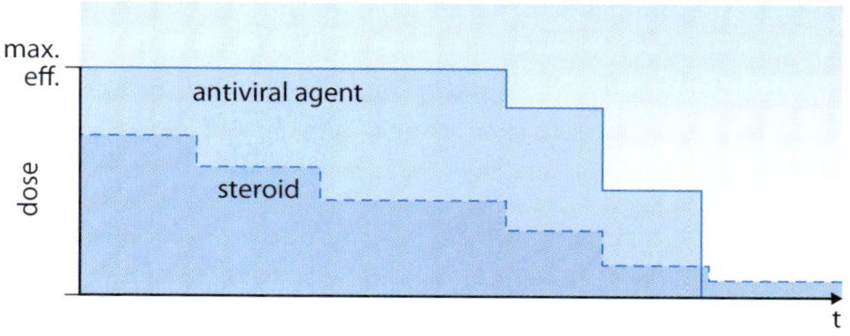


Fig. 2.8 Principles of combination therapy of deep herpetic viral disease (see text)

The following aspects may help in an individualized combination therapy:

- Acyclovir – because of its pharmacokinetic properties and its lack of general toxicity – is currently the best antiviral agent on the market for such a combination therapy, not only as oral medication but also as an ointment.
- If ACV is given orally, which is the preferred pharmaceutical preparation for all cases with iritis, trabeculitis, severe corneal endotheliitis, and for all ulcerating interstitial diseases, then the daily "full" dose is 400 mg 5 qd. For acyclovir ointment, 5 qd is also the normal, sufficient dose.
- With ACV ointment, an accompanying topical steroid should preferably also come from an ointment, and alternatively from a subconjunctival crystalline steroid injection.
- TFT eye drops cannot be recommended for combination therapy of deep viral disease, because their penetration into the corneal stroma is insufficient. If, however, ACV is not available, and TFT is the only antiviral agent at hand, then it fulfils at least the task of protecting the epithelium from dendritic recurrences in the course of necessary steroid treatment.
- Whenever possible, steroid therapy should not exceed moderate levels. Moderate doses are 20–30 mg fluocortolone orally, prednisolone acetate eye drops 1% 3–5 qd, or an injection of a crystalline subconjunctival steroid depot every week or every other week. In severe cases, combinations of these may be necessary. Detailed examples are given in the clinical sections.

## 2.2.C Conservative Resurfacing Measures for Metaherpetic Superficial (Epithelial) Disease

Once a reliable clinical diagnosis of metaherpetic superficial (epithelial) disease has been made (see sec. 2.11), the therapeutic requirements are straight and simple:

1. Refrain from all drugs that may impair epithelial health or regeneration from the limbal stem cells. All antiviral substances and steroids are potentially dangerous.
2. Epithelial regeneration and consolidation should be supported by efficient resurfacing measures, e. g., artificial tears without conservatives, smooth ointments, and therapeutic soft bandage lenses plus liquids without conservatives.

Table 2.3 Recommendable surgical options for cases with deep metaherpetic damage (see Sect. 2.14)

| Deep metaherpetic problems | Therapeutic options |
|---|---|
| Irregular corneal surface from stromal scarring and loss of substance, hard contact lenses unsuccessful | Perforating homo-kp |
| Dense central scars with clear adjacent stroma | Rotational perforating auto-kp |
| Dense scars which can not be rotated | Perforating kp |
| Deep metaherpetic ulcer, vision required, no time pressure | Amnion cover, subsequently elective perforating kp |
| Deep metaherpetic ulcer, vision required, time pressure (e. g., imminent perforation) | Perforating kp à chaud (with no suitable graft at hand: rescue surgery with either amnion, conjunctiva, or cornea, and elective kp thereafter) |
| Deep metaherpetic ulcer or bullous keratopathy, no vision required, or no kp possible | Permanent conjunctival flap |
| Bullous keratopathy vision required | Perforating kp |
| Chronic secondary glaucoma, conservative treatment insufficient | Trabeculectomy |
| Secondary cataract | Cataract surgery with IOL |

3. Surgical measures are not indicated as long as metaherpetic disease manifests itself only as punctate keratopathy or as a shallow epithelial ulcer.

It is certainly better and easier to prophylactically inhibit the development of metaherpetic epithelial disease instead of treating established metaherpetic complications. One should always add dry eye therapy without preservatives when topical antiviral therapy is necessary. This is especially important for cases that have already experienced metaherpetic complications in the course of previous herpes disease.

## 2.2.D Surgical Reconstruction for Metaherpetic Deep Disease

In this therapy group we deal with diseases that have in common chronic damages that can no longer be sufficiently treated by conservative measures alone. Table 2.3 lists the most common surgical methods that have proven to be useful.

## References


Colin J, Chastel C, Renard G, Cantell K (1983) Combination therapy for dendritic keratitis with human leukocyte interferon and acyclovir. Am J Ophthalmol 95: 346–348

Collum LM, Logan P, McAuliffe-Curtin D, Hung SO, Patterson A, Rees PJ (1985) Randomised double-blind trial of acyclovir (Zovirax) and adenine arabinoside in herpes simplex amoeboid corneal ulceration. Br J Ophthalmol 69: 847–850

Collum LM, McGettrick P, Akhtar J, Lavin J, Rees PJ (1986) Oral acyclovir (Zovirax) in herpes simplex dendritic corneal ulceration. Br J Ophthalmol 70: 435–438

Coster DJ, Jones BR, McGill JI (1979) Treatment of amoeboid herpetic ulcers with adenine arabinoside or trifluorothymidine. Br J Ophthalmol 63: 418–421

De Koning EW, van Bijsterveld OP, Cantell K (1982) Combination therapy for dendritic keratitis with human leukocyte interferon and trifluorothymidine. Br J Ophthalmol 66: 509–512

De Koning EW, van Bijsterveld OP, Cantell K (1983) Combination therapy for dendritic keratitis with acyclovir and alpha-interferon. Arch Ophthalmol 101: 1866–1868

Hoh HB, Hurley C, Claoue C, Viswalingham M, Easty DL, Goldschmidt P, Collum LM (1996) Randomised trial of ganciclovir and acyclovir in the treatment of herpes simplex dendritic keratitis: a multicentre study. Br J Ophthalmol 80: 140–143

Jones BR, Coster DJ, Falcon MG, Cantell K (1976) Topical therapy of ulcerative herpetic keratitis with human interferon. Lancet II: 128

La Lau C, Oosterhuis JA, Versteg J, van Rij G, Renardel de Lavalette JG, Craandijk A, Lamers WP, Lamers WP (1982) Acyclovir and trifluorothymidine in herpetic keratitis: a multicentre trial. Br J Ophthalmol 66: 506–508

Maudgal PC, De Clercq E (1991) Bromovinyldeoxyuridine treatment of herpetic keratitis clinically resistant to other antiviral agents. Curr Eye Res 10 Suppl: 193–199

Meurs PJ, van Bijsterveld OP (1985) Berofor Alpha 2 (r-Hu IFN-alpha 2 arg) und Aciclovir in der Behandlung der Herpes-Keratitis-dendritica. Klin Monatsbl Augenheilkd 187: 40–42

Neumann-Haefelin D, Mattes A, Sundmacher R (1981) Trifluorothymidine sensitivity of ocular herpes simplex strains. In: R Sundmacher (ed) Herpetic eye disease. Bergmann, Munich, pp 353–355

Neumann-Haefelin D, Sundmacher R, Frey H. Merk W (1985) Recombinant HuIFN-gamma prevents herpes simplex keratitis in African green monkeys. Demonstration of synergism with recombinant HuIFN-alpha2. Med Microbiol Immunol 174: 81–86

Neumann-Haefelin D, Sundmacher R, Sauter B, Karges HE, Manthey KF (1975) Effect of human leukocyte interferon on vaccinia- and herpes virus-infected cell cultures and monkey corneas. Infect Immun 12: 148–155

Neumann-Haefelin D, Sundmacher R, Skoda R, Cantell K (1977) Comparative evaluation of human leukocyte and fibroblast interferon in the prevention of herpes simplex virus keratitis in a monkey model. Infect Immun 17: 468–470

Poirier RF (1985) Intraocular penetration of vidarabine monophosphate, trifluridine, and acyclovir. In: FC Blodi (ed) Herpes Simplex Infections of the Eye. Contemporary Issues in Ophthalmology vol 1. Churchill Livingstone, NY, pp 101–108

Power WJ, Benedict-Smith A, Hillery M, Brady K, Collum LM (1991) Randomised double-blind trial of bromovinyldeoxyuridine (BVDU) and trifluorothymidine (TFT) in dendritic corneal ulceration. Br J Ophthalmol 75: 649–651

Sundmacher R (1978) Trifluorthymidinprophylaxe bei der Steroidtherapie herpetischer Keratouveitiden. Klin Monatsbl Augenheilk 173: 516–519

Sundmacher R (1982) A general summary of our interferon studies. In: H Shiota, Y Cheng, WH Prusoff (eds): Herpesviruses – clinical, pharmacological and basic aspects. Excerpta Medica Congress Series 571, Amsterdam, pp 308–310

Sundmacher R (1983) Orale Acyclovir-Therapie virologisch nachgewiesener intraokularer Herpes simplex Virus-Infektionen. Klin Monatsbl Augenheilk 183: 246–250

Sundmacher R (1983) Use of nucleoside analogues in the treatment of herpes simplex virus eye diseases. Metab Pediat Syst Ophthalmol 7: 89–94

Sundmacher R (1984) The role of interferon in prophylaxis and treatment of dendritic keratitis. In: FC Blodi (ed): Contemporary issues in ophthalmology, vol 1: herpes simplex infections of the eye. Churchill Livingstone, NY, pp 129–146

Sundmacher R (1985) Therapie der herpetischen Erkrankungen des vorderen Augenabschnitts. Klin Monatsbl Augenheilk 186: 421–423

Sundmacher R (1988) Behandlung viraler Augenerkrankungen. In: OE Lund, TN Waubke (Hrsg): Neuerungen in der ophthalmologischen Diagnose und Therapie. Bücherei des Augenarztes 115: 90–93

Sundmacher R (1996) Therapie der Viruserkrankungen des vorderen Augenabschnittes. In: A Kampik, F Grehn (Hrsg): Das äußere Auge. Bücherei des Augenarztes. Enke, Stuttgart, 137: 121–126

Sundmacher R, Cantell K, Haug P, Neumann-Haefelin D (1978) Interferon Prophylaxe von Dendritica-Rezidiven bei lokaler Steroidtherapie. Ber Dtsch Ophthalmol Ges 75: 569–570

Sundmacher R, Cantell K, Haug P, Neumann-Haefelin D (1978) Role of debridement and interferon in the treatment of dendritic keratitis. Albrecht von Graefes Arch Clin Exp Ophthalmol 207: 77–82

Sundmacher R, Cantell K, Horn C, Neumann-Haefelin D (1979) Kombinationstherapie der Keratitis dendritica mit Trifluorthymidin und Humanleukozyteninterferon. Ber Dtsch Ophthalmol Ges 76: 489–492

Sundmacher R, Cantell K, Mattes A (1984) A combination therapy for dendritic keratitis. High-titer alpha-interferon and trifluorothymidine. Arch Ophthalmol 102: 554–555

Sundmacher R, Cantell K, Neumann-Haefelin D (1978) Combination therapy of dendritic keratitis with trifluorothymidine and interferon. Lancet II: 687

Sundmacher R, Cantell K, Neumann-Haefelin D (1981) Evaluation of interferon in ocular viral diseases. In: E De Maeyer, G Galasso, H Schellekens (eds): The biology of the interferon system. Elsevier, Amsterdam, pp 343–350

Sundmacher R, Cantell K, Skoda R, Hallermann C, Neumann-Haefelin D (1987) Human leukocyte and fibroblast interferon in a combination therapy of dendritic keratitis. Albrecht von Graefes Arch Clin Exp Ophthalmol 208: 229–233

Sundmacher R, Mattes A, Neumann-Haefelin D, Adolf G, Kruss B (1987) The potency of interferon-alpha 2 and interferon-gamma in a combination therapy of dendritic keratitis. A controlled clinical study. Current Eye Res 6: 273–276

Sundmacher R, Neumann-Haefelin D, Cantell K (1976) Interferon treatment of dendritic keratitis. Lancet I: 1406–1407

Sundmacher R, Neumann-Haefelin D, Cantell K (1976) Successful treatment of dendritic keratitis with human leukocyte interferon. A controlled clinical study. Albrecht von Graefes Arch Clin Exp Ophthalmol 201: 39–45

Sundmacher R, Neumann-Haefelin D, Cantell K (1981) Therapy and prophylaxis of dendritic keratitis with topical human interferon. In: R Sundmacher (ed): Herpetic eye disease. Bergmann, Munich, pp 401–407

Sundmacher R, Neumann-Haefelin D, Cantell K (1982) The clinical value of interferon in ocular viral disease. In: K Munk, H Kirchner (eds): Interferon – properties, mode of action, production, and clinical application. Karger, Basel, pp 191–196

Sundmacher R, Neumann-Haefelin D, Manthey KF, Müller O (1976) Interferon in treatment of dendritic keratitis in humans. A preliminary report. J Infect Dis 133 (Suppl) A160–A164

Sundmacher R, Neumann-Haefelin D, Mattes A, Merk W, Adolf G, Cantell K (1985) Human leukocyte interferon plus trifluorothymidine versus recombinant alpha 2 arg interferon plus trifluorothymidine for therapy of dendritic keratitis. A controlled clinical study. In: PC Maudgal, L Missotten (eds): Herpetic Eye Diseases. Doc Ophthalmol Proc Ser 44. Dr W Junk Publ, Dordrecht, 359–366

Sundmacher R, Neumann-Haefelin D, Shresta B (1975) Die Wirkung von Human-Leukozyten-Interferon (HIF) auf experimentelle Viruskeratitiden bei Affen. Albrecht von Graefes Arch Clin Exp Ophthalmol 195: 263–270

Tullo AB, Shimeld C, Blyth WA, Hill TJ, Easty DL (1983) Ocular infection with herpes simplex virus in non immune and immune mice. Arch Ophthalmol 101: 961–964

Van Bijsterveld OP, Meurs PJ, de Clercq E, Maudgal PC (1989) Bromovinyldeoxyuridine and interferon treatment in ulcerative herpetic keratitis: a double masked study. Br J Ophthalmol 73: 604–607

Weber U, Sundmacher R (1988) Die systemische Acyclovirtherapie herpetischer Sekundärglaukome. Fortschr Ophthalmol 85: 85–87

Wilhelmus KR (2000) The treatment of herpes simplex virus epithelial keratitis. Trans Am Ophthalmol Soc 98: 505–532

Yao YF, Inonue Y, Kase T, Uchihori Y, Mori Y, Ohashi Y (1996) Clinical characteristics of acyclovir-resistant herpetic keratitis and experimental studies of isolates. Albrecht von Graefes Arch Clin Exp Ophthalmol 234 Suppl 1: S126–S132

# HSV Blepharitis

Section

2.3

## Core Messages

- HSV blepharitis mostly heals without therapy. Only clinically manifest primary infection, eczema herpeticum, and AIDS patients must be systemically treated.
- The different forms of HSV blepharitis are prognostically important. They allow one to predict the development or non-appearance of complicating anterior segment eye disease.

HSV blepharitis is rarely a therapeutic problem. It usually heals spontaneously and completely without leaving any lid pathology. Nonetheless, doctors tend to liberally prescribe topical antiviral agents (e.g., ACV ointment) for HSV blisters. If this is done to psychologically calm down unjustified anxieties of the patient, it may be justified. However, cellular antiviral immunity is normally so effective in the dermis, and spontaneous healing is so quick that topical antiviral agents can hardly speed up the spontaneous healing course so much that a significant therapeutic effect is reached. This is certainly the case when therapy starts after blisters have already fully developed. It may be, though, that ACV ointment does have a beneficial effect if already intensively applied in the symptomatic preclinical stage when the patient feels that a recurrence may possibly develop. As many patients believe that this is the case with them, they insist on this prophylactic application of topical antiviral ointments. Whether or not they are right is difficult do decide. Scientific evidence is lacking. As long as the applied ointments do no harm, however, we face no real problem with this open question.

There are only three indications to treat monosymptomatic HSV blepharitis. First, in primary HSV infection (see Sect. 2.12), second, in the special situation of atopic patients with eczema herpeticum, and, third, if severe immune incompetence is the problem, e.g., in AIDS patients. The recommended therapy is then systemic ACV.

When HSV blepharitis is present with other HSV disease in the anterior segment of the eye, therapy will always be determined exclusively by the requirements of these other HSV diseases. No special therapeutic attention need to be paid to HSV blepharitis, which heals anyway. Accordingly, literature dealing with HSV blepharitis exists only as far as the differential diagnosis to ophthalmic zoster is concerned.

Diagnostically, attention should be paid to the special form of *intermarginal HSV blepharitis*, which is often unknown to ophthalmologists because of its inconspicuous appearance. Its typical form is pathognomonic for HSV disease. Prognostically, it is important to be able to diagnose monosymptomatic intermarginal HSV blepharitis, because it alerts to the possibility of other more dangerous forms of HSV disease in the ipsilateral eye during future recurrences.

Herpetic canalicular obstruction – a topic also associated with the lids – may sometimes become clinically important, especially after severe HSV primary infection with necrotizing inflammation of the canalicular mucosa. As the proper diagnosis must mostly be suspected from associated other visible HSV disease rather than by the canaliculitis itself, HSV disease of the lacrimal system is not shown in the picture part of this atlas. Efficient therapy has to be systemic ACV due to pharmacokinetic reasons.

The different clinical forms of HSV blepharitis can help us to answer two diagnostic questions:

1. Are we dealing with ordinary recurrent disease or with clinically manifest primary disease?
2. Must additional anterior segment disease be expected in the course of this blepharitis attack, or can we feel reasonably safe that no such complication is imminent?

## Detailed analysis of Fig 2.9

***Clinic:*** Grouped, fully developed, well-demarcated vesicles with yellowish contents on a circumscribed erythematous ground (Fig. 2.9). Some vesicles already dry with crusts. Some slightly dilated conjunctival vessels. No other anterior segment disease.

***Diagnosis:*** Typical picture of endogenously recurrent HSV blepharitis with well-established cellular immunity, and without other complicating HSV disease of the anterior segment. Whether or not a very slight HSV conjunctivitis co-exists is therapeutically irrelevant as long as no other anterior segment HSV disease exists. If the virus had spread to other tissues of the anterior segment and if it had caused recurrent disease there, this should already have been visible at this time in the course of the blepharitis. Therefore, we can feel reasonably certain that no such complication is imminent with this recurrence.

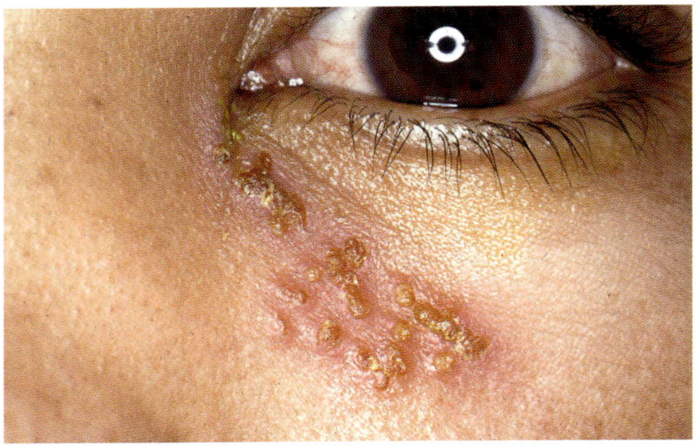

Fig. 2.9 Recurrent HSV blepharitis in a 12-year-old girl

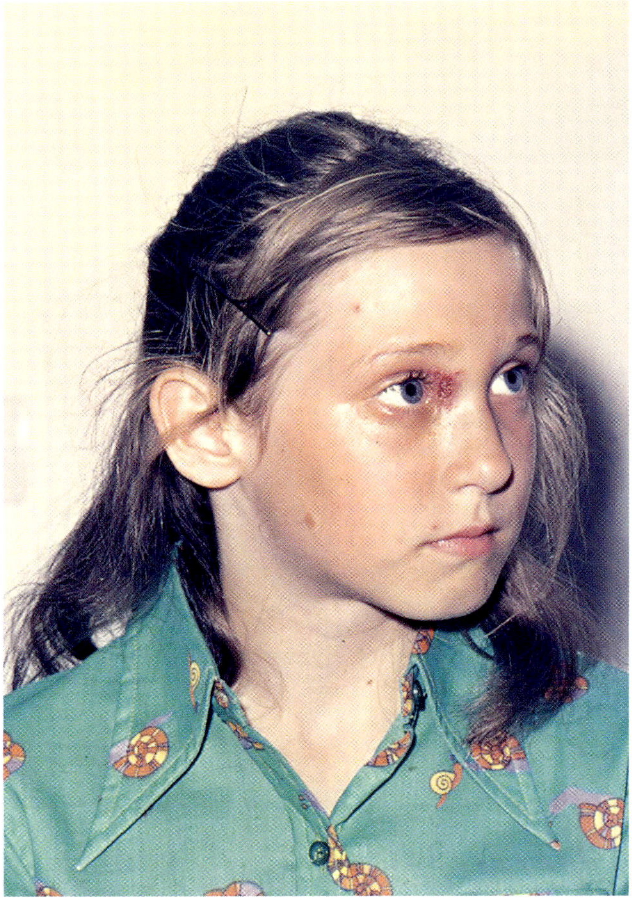

Fig. 2.10 Recurrent HSV blepharitis of the inner lid angle in a 10-year-old girl

Exogenous HSV particles from the skin lesions can easily contaminate the intact corneoconjunctival surface. However, they will not cause superinfection as long as they are not forced into the tissue by rubbing or other injuries.

***Differential diagnosis:*** Primary HSV blepharitis looks different, see Sect. 2.12

***Therapy:*** No rubbing, no antiviral therapy necessary. If rubbing cannot be excluded: topical antiviral agents into the cul-de-sac until crusts have fallen off (TFT eye drops or ACV ointment 5 qd)

## Detailed analysis of Fig 2.10

***Clinic:*** Later in the course of spontaneous healing (Fig. 2.10) with more crusting than in Fig. 2.9. Both eyes white, no inflammation. No signs of previous ocular disease on either side.

***Diagnosis:*** See Fig. 2.9. This picture is shown to specifically illustrate that HSV disease of the anterior segment of the eye, together with HSV blepharitis, normally arises from simultaneous endogenous spreading of the virus to the ocular sites and *not* from surface superinfection. Even massive HSV surface contamination, which has certainly taken place early in the course of this recurrence, does not lead to superinfection or new disease in the conjunctiva or cornea, as long as the surface remains intact and HSV is not "forced" by some trauma into the subepithelial spaces.

***Differential diagnosis:*** None.

***Therapy:*** Unnecessary, no rubbing.

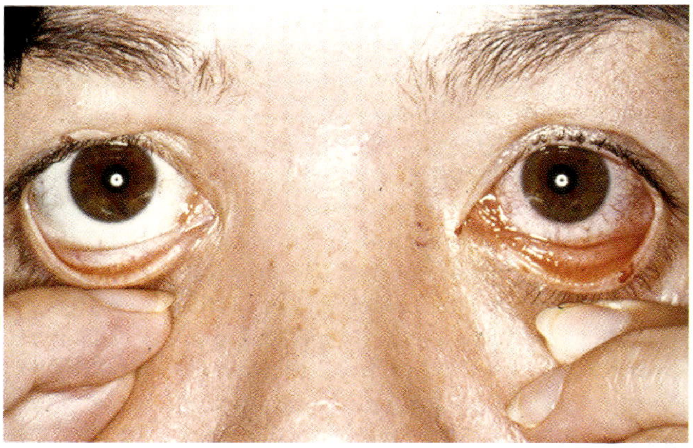

Fig. 2.11 Recurrent intermarginal HSV blepharitis and conjunctivitis in a 22-year-old female (Bengale-Rose)

## Detailed analysis of Fig 2.11

***Clinic:*** Acute serous conjunctivitis on the left side (Fig. 2.11). Some small follicles near the inferior tarsus bilaterally, presumably with no specific disease significance. Well-circumscribed epithelial lesion of the left lower lid margin with some exudate on it. It can easily be overlooked without staining. No additional ocular disease nor any sequelae of previous HSV attacks.

***Diagnosis:*** The HSV etiology of the serous conjunctivitis would clinically remain completely obscure without the finding of the circumscribed epithelial lesion on the lid margin. It will quickly heal spontaneously. Intermarginal blepharitis of this type is *pathognomonic for HSV disease.* HSV intermarginal blepharitis and conjunctivitis, both heal without therapy. Thus, the importance of identifying HSV intermarginal blepharitis is to alert to the potential risk of HSV disease elsewhere in the ipsi-lateral eye, with the need to scrupulously scrutiny the eye for other endogenous HSV recurrence, either in the course of the present or any subsequent

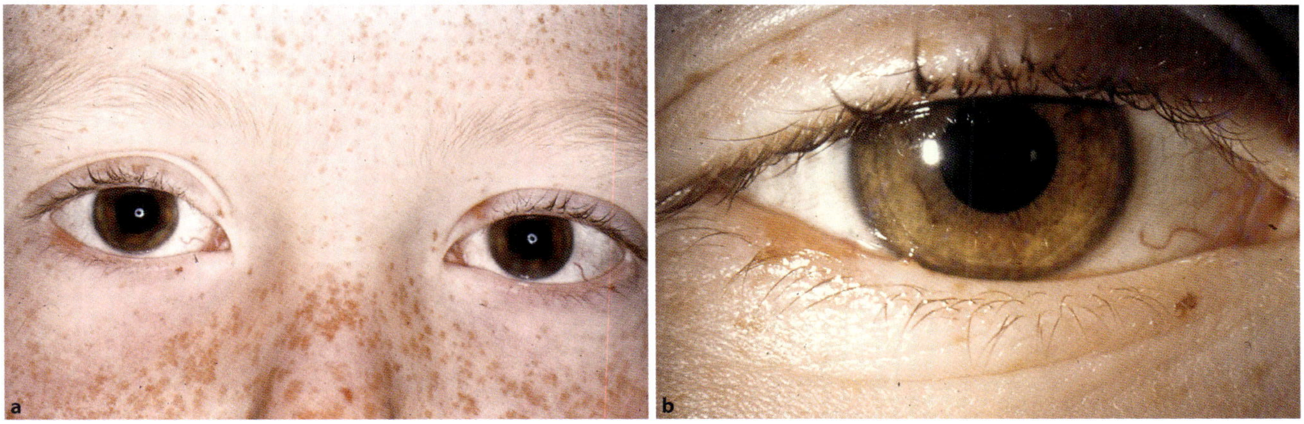


Fig. 2.12a,b Recurrent intermarginal HSV blepharitis on the right side in a 12-year-old girl (unstained)

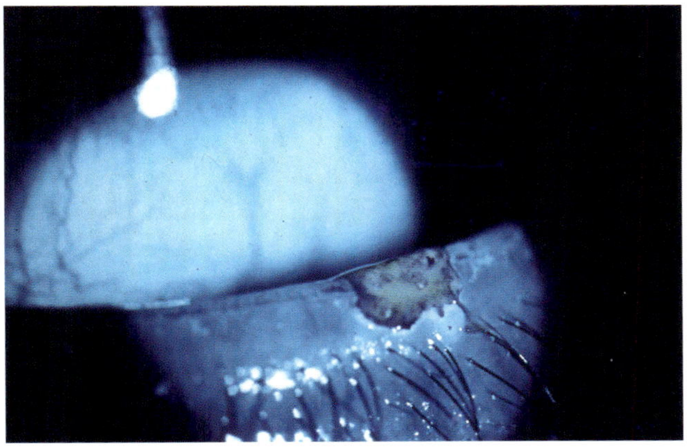

Fig. 2.13 Recurrent intermarginal HSV blepharitis. Staining helps in detecting the otherwise often inconspicuous lesions (fluorescein)

inflammations. Caution should be used because, as HSV conjunctivitis and intermarginal blepharitis are still in an early phase of the recurrence in this case, it cannot yet be excluded that other anterior segment disease will still develop.

***Differential diagnosis:*** Primary intermarginal HSV blepharitis looks different (see Sect. 2.12).

***Therapy:*** If daily controls are possible, then no antiviral therapy is necessary unless other HSV disease occurs. If no controls are possible, systemic full antiviral therapy is advisable for a week. This covers all potential risks, including that of late-developing intraocular herpes (400 mg ACV 5 qd).

## Detailed analysis of Fig 2.12

***Clinic:*** The case in Fig. 2.12 illustrates how little attention is attracted from an unstained HSV intermarginal blepharitis when observed from some distance, especially when both eyes appear equally white and unsuspicious (a). Only a close look discloses the pathognomonic features of a well-demarcated HSV lesion with some exudate on top (b).

***Diagnosis:*** Recurrent intermarginal HSV blepharitis, see Figs. 2.11 and 2.13.

***Differential diagnosis:*** None. *Primary* clinically manifest HSV intermarginal blepharitis looks different and would at least be accompanied by considerable conjunctivitis.

***Therapy:*** None. No rubbing.

## Detailed analysis of Fig 2.14

***Clinic:*** Both lids in Fig. 2.14 are severely affected by umbilicated herpes vesicles in different stages of development with purulent exudate sticking the lid margins together. After opening the lids, both eyes were surprisingly white without inflammation (not shown).

***Diagnosis:*** Eczema herpeticum. This may develop when HSV – either from an endogenous recurrence or from an exogenous source – infects eczematous skin. Distribution of the vesicles reflects the actual main foci of eczema, often in the lid area. In this case, the white and unaffected eyes are another example of the fact that established anti-herpetic immunity is efficient in prevention of superinfection of intact corneoscleral surfaces even in case of massive HSV contamination. Unlike dermis, with its multiple eczematous alterations, the corneoconjunctival surface in such atopic patients may still be intact and can then resist HSV superinfections as long as no severe atopic keratoconjunctivitis leads to breaks in the epithelial lining.

***Differential diagnosis:*** Bacterial rashes on eczematous skin areas may look similar, and clinical differential diagnosis may sometimes be difficult even for an experienced dermatologist. Laboratory help with identification of the infecting agent(s) is then needed.

***Therapy:*** Basic therapy is by maximally dosed systemic antiviral agents (initially 800 mg ACV 5 qd (or ACV infusion therapy), reduced to 400 mg ACV 5 qd after clear onset of healing for 2 more weeks). This normally gives excellent results in spite of the often severe cases. Any potential concomitant eye disease is also efficiently treated with such a systemic therapy, and decision on further therapeutic measures, which may be advisable later on – e.g., additional topical steroids for deep eye disease – can be made once the lids can be opened again spontaneously and the examination of the eyes is again possible.

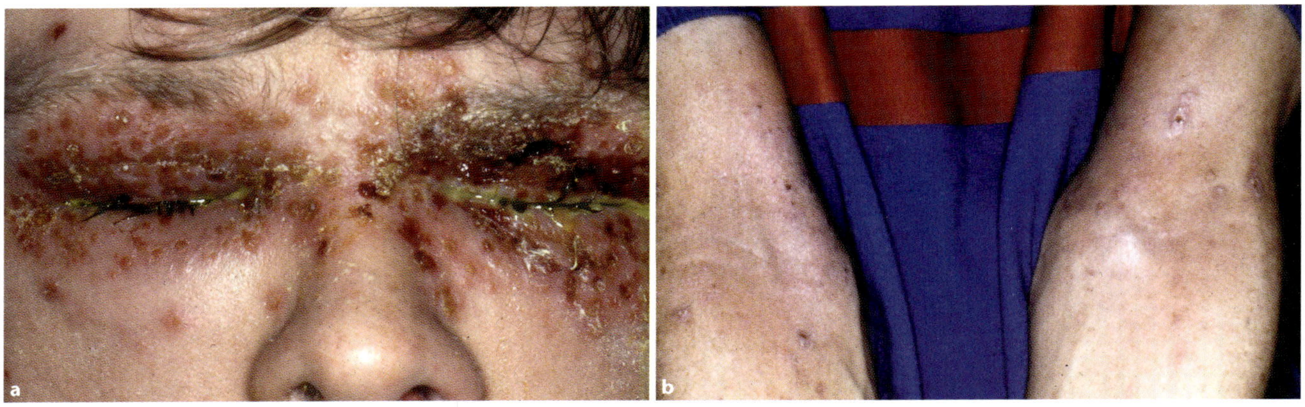

Fig. 2.14 Eczema herpeticum with severe bilateral HSV blepharitis in a young man with endogenous eczema (**a**). Typical aspect of both arms' flexor sides (**b**)

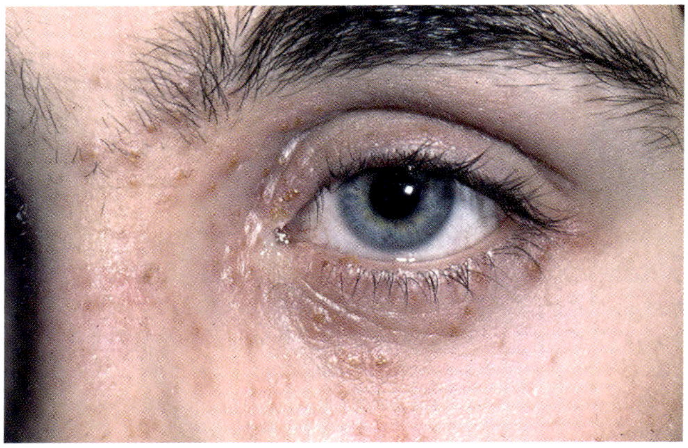

Fig. 2.15 Mild form of eczema herpeticum. A close look at the umbilicated vesicles is needed in order to clinically confirm HSV etiology. In this case, HSV etiology was proven by PCR. The eye was primarily unaffected, and it remained unaffected with systemic ACV therapy

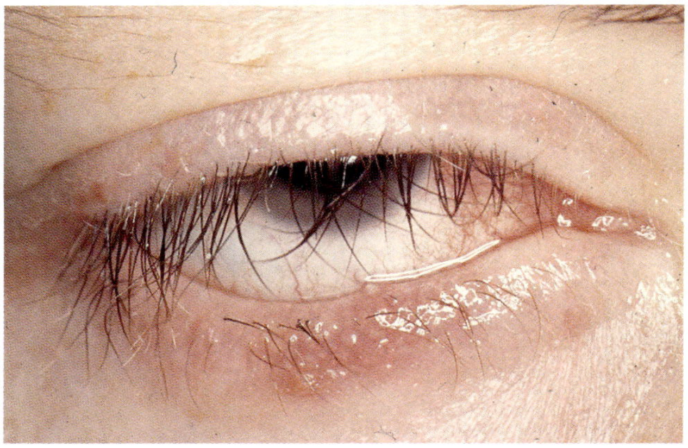

Fig. 2.16 *Differential diagnosis*: Chronic staphylococcal folliculitis with loss of lashes in a young female with seborrhoic dysfunction and associated chronic blepharoconjunctivitis. The infective pustules lack umbilication, and loss of lashes is never a typical sign of HSV blepharitis

## References


Coster DJ, Welham RAN (1979) Herpetic canalicular obstruction. Brit J Ophthalmol 63: 259–262

De Koning EWJ, van Bijsterveld OP (1983) Herpes simplex virus canaliculitis. Ophthalmologica 186: 173–176

Easty D, Entwistle C, Funk A, Witcher J (1975) Herpes simplex keratitis and keratoconus in atopic patients. Trans Ophthalmol Soc UK 95: 267

Egerer I, Stary A (1980) Erosive ulcerative herpes simplex blepharitis. Arch Ophthalmol 98: 1760–1763

Forrest WM, Kaufman HE (1976) Zosteriform herpes simplex. Am J Ophthalmol 81: 86–88

Harris GJ, Hyndiuk RA, Fox MJ, Taugher PJ (1981) Herpetic canalicular obstruction. Arch Ophthalmol 99: 282–283

Harris GJ, Myers WG (1985) Herpetic canalicular obstruction. In: FC Blodi (ed) Herpes Simplex Infections of the Eye. Contemporary Issues in Ophthalmology vol 1. Churchill Livingstone, NY, pp 47–55

Jakobiec FA, Dobli Srinivassan B, Gamboa ET (1979) Recurrent angular blepharitis in an adult. Am J Ophthalmol 88: 744–747

Kalman CM, Laskin OL (1986) Herpes zoster and zosteriform herpes simplex virus infections in immunocompetent adults. Am J Med 81: 775–778

Margolis TP, Ostler HB (1990) Treatment of ocular disease in eczema herpeticum. Am J Ophthalmol 110: 274–279

Prabripataloong T, Margolis TP, Lietman TM, Wong IG, Mather R, Gritz DC (2006) Atopic disease and herpes simplex eye disease: a population-based case-cohort study. Am J Ophthalmol 142: 745–749

Yamamoto S, Shimomura Y, Kinoshita S, Tano Y (1994) Differentiating zosteriform herpes simplex from ophthalmic zoster. Arch Ophthalmol 112: 1515–1516

# HSV Conjunctivitis

Section

2.4

## Core Messages

- Acute HSV conjunctivitis without diagnostically helpful concomitant HSV disease elsewhere cannot be clinically differentiated from non-herpetic types of conjunctivitis, above all not from adenovirus conjunctivitis.
- A rashly prescribed and uncontrolled therapy of any conjunctivitis of unknown origin with topical steroids may induce recurrent HSV keratitis.

In this section, we will address only monosymptomatic recurrent or persistent HSV conjunctivitis. Conjunctivitis in the course of clinically manifest primary infection is presented in Sect. 2.12.

"Collateral" conjunctivitis accompanies all HSV diseases of the cornea, sclera, iris, and trabecular meshwork. Whether this type of conjunctivitis represents a true collateral inflammation without HSV replication in the conjunctiva or whether HSV also multiplies in the conjunctiva, is of no practical interest. The other HSV diseases must be treated intensively regardless, and, if this is done properly, virus production in the conjunctiva is always efficiently co-treated anyway.

The real problem is faced when HSV conjunctivitis presents monosymptomatically, with no diagnostically helpful herpes signs elsewhere. In this situation, no reliable clinical differential diagnosis can be made between HSV disease and disease of other origin, especially of adenovirus origin. More than 4% of cases with presumed adenovirus conjunctivitis turned out to be caused by HSV. If these had been treated with topical steroids, as many doctors still advise for any type of presumed adenovirus conjunctivitis, then every 25th patient would have been put at risk of developing recurrent HSV keratitis or other severe forms of anterior segment HSV disease in a previously unaffected eye.

Recurrent monosymptomatic HSV conjunctivitis may indeed be considered unproblematic as long as only conjunctivitis recurs and the disease does not involve other tissues of the eye. Although conjunctival virus production may be significant in these patients for a short while, the natural and immunologic defence mechanisms seem to be sufficiently effective in limiting recurrent HSV disease to the conjunctiva and in inhibiting further spread to the eye. Thus, the monosymptomatic conjunctival recurrences regularly heal quickly and spontaneously, and they do not need any special therapy. Most patients with this benign type of HSV recurrences are never identified, because the clinical signs are far from being pathognomonic for HSV disease. Although HSV conjunctivitis presents mostly unilaterally, this does not really help to differentiate it from adenovirus conjunctivitis, which characteristically also begins and sometimes remains unilateral. The fact that HSV conjunctivitis on average coincides with smaller follicular reaction than is seen after adenovirus infection, is of no practical help either. As long as there are no reliable, quick, and, above all, affordable laboratory tests for routine differential diagnosis of HSV and adenovirus conjunctivitis, doctors should be very reluctant to prescribe topical steroids for conjunctivitis of unproven origin, especially if no close ophthalmological controls are possible thereafter.

Recurring episcleritis is another diagnostic trap that must be mentioned. Unilaterally recurring HSV conjunctivitis may be mistaken for recurring episcleritis and then also be treated with steroids. This does not occur if the circumscribed topographic character of serous episcleritis is adequately considered. Also, there is no approved indication for steroid treatment of episcleritis anyway.

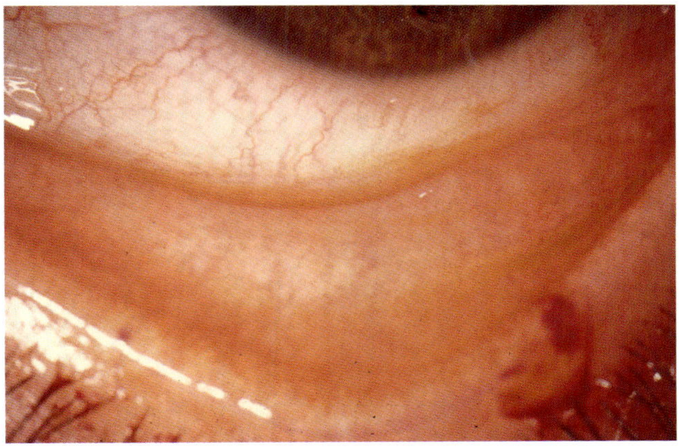

Fig. 2.17 Serous recurrent HSV conjunctivitis and intermarginal blepharitis in a 30-year-old woman (Bengale-Rose)

As an exception from the rule, HSV is rarely not eliminated from the conjunctiva after HSV infection. Instead, it persists in the conjunctiva for months, and it presumably only then leads to a prominent chronic follicular conjunctivitis, which is usually unilateral (see Fig. 2.18). It may require systemic ACV treatment for definite healing.

## Detailed analysis of Fig 2.17

***Clinic:*** Moderately dilated conjunctival vessels in Fig. 2.17 with sparse tiny follicles and some serous exudate in the inferior fornix: clinical etiologic diagnosis is not possible from the aspect of conjunctivitis alone. A circumscribed intermarginal epithelial disease area (Bengale-Rose), however, represents pathognomonic intermarginal HSV blepharitis (see Sect. 2.3). No other parts of the eye are diseased.
***Diagnosis:*** The easily overlooked pathognomonic intermarginal HSV blepharitis is of central importance, as it proves that the conjunctivitis is also of HSV origin. As HSV blepharitis does not ever induce nonviral "collateral" conjunctivitis, it is also apparent that the serous conjunctivitis in this patient is caused by a real viral recurrence with HSV replication in the conjunctiva. As no other tissues of the eye are diseased, and blepharitis and conjunctivitis do not need antiviral therapy for complete healing, no therapy is mandatory as long as the rest of the eye stays uninvolved.
***Differential diagnosis:*** None.
***Therapy:*** No therapy is mandatory as long as frequent controls are possible. It is most important to consequently avoid steroids. If close controls are impossible, 400 mg ACV 3–5 qd orally for about a week should effectively inhibit the potential risk of developing HSV disease elsewhere in the eye.

## Detailed analysis of Fig 2.18

***Clinic:*** Strictly left-sided, dense, medium-sized follicles in the inferior cul-de-sac (Fig. 2.18), some also on the tarsal plate. Bulbar conjunctiva and superior cul-de-sac are normal. No other eye tissues diseased.
***Diagnosis:*** Very rarely, HSV seems to persist in the conjunctiva, leading to a chronic follicular reaction, as has also been reported for adenoviruses. Theoretically, not only peripheral virus persistence, but also frequently recurring endogenous shedding of HSV, may lead to such a clinical picture.
***Differential diagnosis:*** Molluscum contagiosum conjunctivitis (search for molluscum tumor near lid margin), chlamydial conjunctivitis (develops much larger follicles, and upper cul-de-sac is regularly involved), chronic drug intolerance (history), persistent adenovirus conjunctivitis (laboratory).
***Therapy:*** Most likely heals spontaneously after months. To promote healing, *systemic* ACV must be recommended, 400 mg ACV 5 qd for 3–6 weeks as required.

## References


Brown DC, Nesburn AB, Nauheim JS, Pavan-Langston D, Kaufman HE (1968) Recurrent herpes simplex conjunctivitis. Arch Ophthalmol 79: 733–735

Darougar S, Hunter PA, Viswalingham M, Gibson GA, Jones BR (1978) Acute follicular conjunctivitis and keratoconjunctivitis due to herpes simplex virus in London. Br J Ophthalmol 62: 843–849

Easty DL, Tullo AB, Shimeld C, Hill TJ, Blyth WA (1985) The influence of prednisolone on external eye disease, virus proliferation and latent infection in an animal model of herpes simplex keratitis. In: PC Maudgal, L Missotten (eds.): Herpetic Eye Disease. W Junk, Dordrecht, pp 95–97

Kaye SB, Madan N, Dowd TC, Hart CA, Mc Carthy K, Patterson A (1990) Ocular shedding of herpes simplex virus. Br J Ophthalmol 74: 114–116

Maggs DJ, Chang E, Nasisse MP, Mitchel WJ (1998) persistence of herpes simplex virus type 1 DNA in chronic conjunctival and eyelid lesions of mice. J Virol 72: 9166–9172

Nauheim JS (1969) Recurrent herpes simplex conjunctival ulceration. Arch Ophthalmol 81: 592–595

Sundmacher R (1986) Viruskonjunktivitis. Fortschr Ophthalmol 83: 257–262


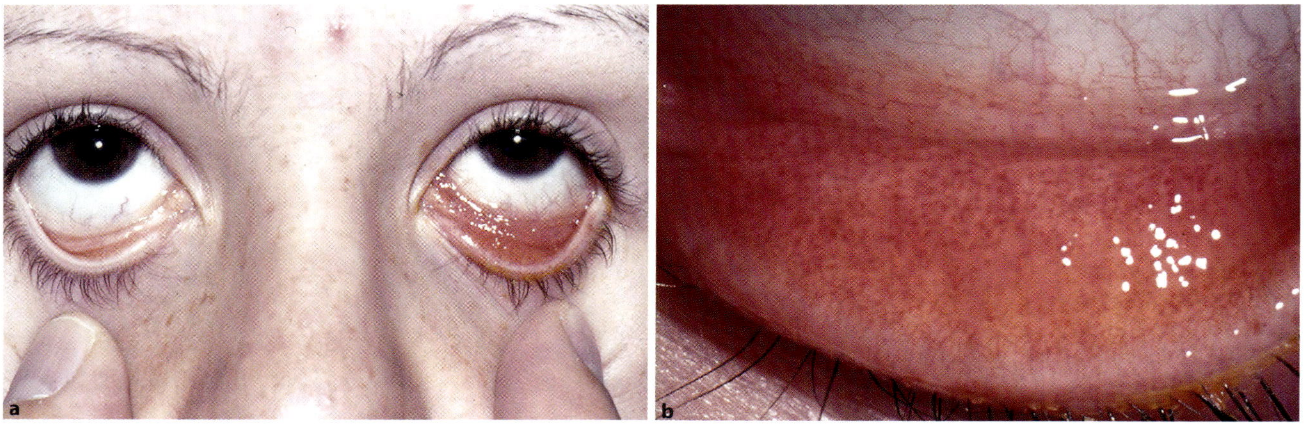

Fig. 2.18a,b Follicular HSV conjunctivitis in a 25-year-old woman; HSV isolated from the cul-de-sac

Sundmacher R, Hillenkamp J, Reinhard T (2001) Therapie und Prophylaxe der Adenovirus-Keratokonjunktivitis. Ophthalmologe 98: 991–1009

Thiel MA, Bossart W, Bernauer W (1998) Clinical evaluation of impression cytology for the diagnosis of superficial viral eye diseases. Klin Monatsbl Augenheilkd 212: 388–391

Uchio E, Takeuchi S, Itoh N, Matsuura N, Ohno S, Aoki K (2000) Clinical and epidemiological features of acute follicular conjunctivitis with special reference to that caused by herpes simplex virus type 1. Br J Ophthalmol 84: 968–972

Wishart PK, James C, Wishart MS, Darougar S (1984) Prevalence of acute conjunctivitis caused by chlamydia, adenovirus, and herpes simplex virus in an ophthalmic casualty department. Br J Ophthalmol 68: 653–655

# Epithelial HSV Keratitis

Section

2.5

## Core Messages

- Untreated dendritic HSV keratitis exhibits pathognomonic biomicroscopic features, which are important for differential diagnosis.
- Other forms of epithelial HSV keratitis (punctate k., stellate k., geographic k.) are clinically less characteristic.
- Therapy is with topical antiviral agents.
- Differential diagnosis comprises the various forms of non-viral pseudodendrites, metaherpetic epithelial disease (see Sect. 2.11), map-dot-fingerprint dystrophies, epithelial adenovirus keratitis, and some rare diseases, such as Thygeson`s punctate keratitis and tyrosinemia.

Dendritic keratitis is the most known form of viral keratitis. It is still a widespread belief that the appearance of a dendritic lesion in the corneal epithelium will allow a reliable diagnosis of HSV disease. This is an incorrect simplification.

A fully developed epithelial dendritic lesion of HSV etiology shows four biomicroscopic criteria, of which *only two are pathognomonic*:

1. The lesion is branched, i.e., dendritic.
2. The branches exhibit a central line of epithelial decomposition.
3. The branches are bordered by a *reticulate band of punctate epithelial microdestruction.*
4. The branches terminate in *end-bulbs* surrounded by the same reticulate microdestruction pattern as is found along the branches themselves.

From these four criteria, only criteria 3 and 4 are pathognomonic. Criteria 1 and 2 are not. The latter can also be found in a large variety of other pathologic situations, most frequently including non-viral pseudodendrites (see differential diagnosis).

The development of a recurrent HSV dendrite can be described as follows: The basal epithelial layer of the cornea is a densely served termination area for the sensory nerves of V/1. The topographical distribution of neurons which transport and shed virus determines in which *area* HSV can cause disease. The distribution of the neurons does not exactly determine the microscopic aspect of the HSV dendritic figure. The latter is mostly the result of the two competing processes: epithelial destruction and epithelial regeneration. On one hand, viral cell destruction results in epithelial loss ranging from punctate to areal defects. On the other hand, healthy epithelium slides in from all sides in curved fronts from the periphery of the cornea towards the center to close such defects. The relative efficiencies of these two competitive processes are different in the course of the disease. Dendritic figures have a different biomicroscopic appearance depending on their stage of development. A branching, dendritic appearance alone is insufficient to prove HSV etiology. A close biomicroscopic look at the borders of the branches is required. In the developing and in the fully developed phases of HSV dendritic keratitis, a typical *reticulate microdestruction pattern of the epithelium* is found (Fig. 2.19).

The second pathognomonic sign, which, however, does not always fully develop, is the development of the end-bulbs of HSV dendritic branches (Fig. 2.20), also surrounded by the pathognomonic microdestruction pattern (Fig. 2.21).

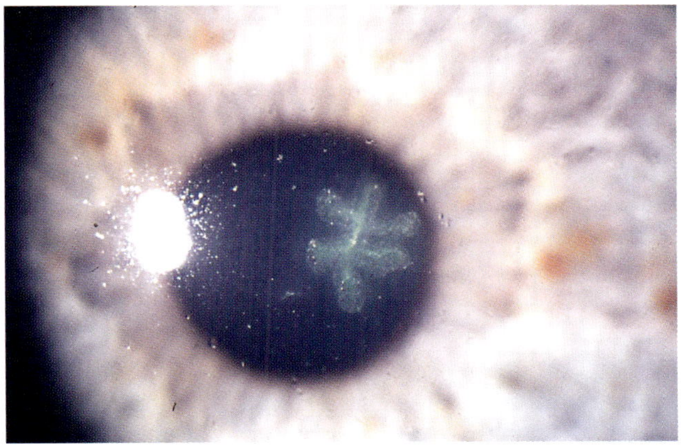

Fig. 2.19 Small, fully developed dendritic lesion at the peak of viral cytolysis exhibiting all pathognomonic biomicroscopic criteria for HSV etiology, above all an impressive microdestruction pattern along the borders (fluorescein, washed out quickly)

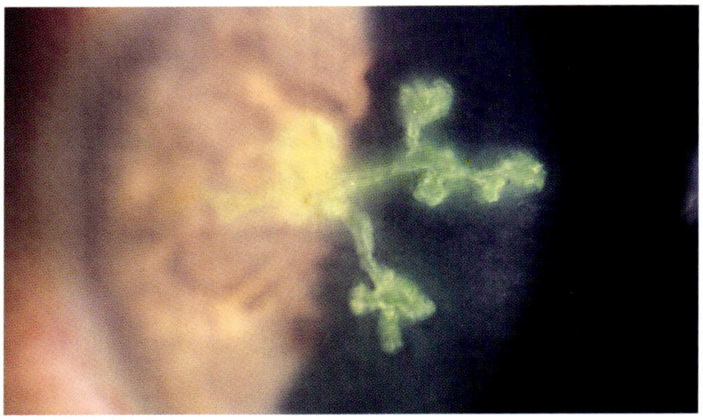

Fig. 2.20 Large HSV dendritic lesion with prominent end-bulbs pathognomonic for HSV etiology (fluorescein)

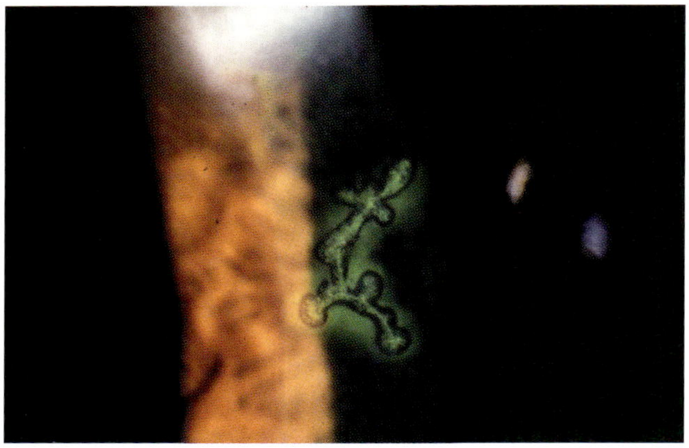

Fig. 2.21 HSV dendrite elevated above the surrounding epithelial surface (fluorescein)

With progressive healing, the dendritic figure shrinks to a fluoresceine-negative "closure line" with often still residual branching. At this stage of disease, viral cytolysis has long been overcome by regeneration, and "microdestruction patterns" have long gone. An ophthalmologist who sees the patient for the first time may then have difficulties when making a biomicroscopic differential diagnosis between HSV disease and similar looking non-herpetic diseases, above all pseudodendritic keratitis. Examples are presented in the picture section.

Differential diagnosis of punctate, stellate, and geographic HSV keratitis may be more difficult, because the pathognomonic biomicroscopy of HSV dendritic keratitis may be partially or totally absent. The reader is also referred to the picture section.

## Detailed analysis of Fig 2.19

*Clinic:* After applying fluorescein, the dye was quickly washed out from the ocular surface in order to inhibit leakage into the epithelium of the dendrite and the adjacent stroma, which would have obscured the biomicroscopic details (Fig. 2.19). After this correctly performed fluorescein staining, the typical contour of a herpetic dendrite with rounded end bulbs and a central decomposition furrow can be seen, but, above all, broad *reticulate bands of punctate epithelial microdestructions* surrounding the dendrite are seen as well.

***Diagnosis:*** Recurrent dendritic keratitis in the stage of fully developed viral cytolysis.

***Differential diagnosis:*** None. All four pathognomonic features of HSV dendrite are present, above all the two pathognomonic ones, microdestruction pattern, and end-bulbs.

***Therapy:*** Topical antiviral agents. TFT eye drops or ACV ointment 5 qd, plus adjuvant artificial tears for about 3–4 days beyond the point of "fluoresceine-negative closure". Thereafter, dry eye care alone is normally sufficient. Prolonged antiviral therapy should be avoided, because it may unnecessarily compromise epithelial regeneration.

## Analysis of Fig 2.20

In Fig. 2.20, fluorescein was not washed out after application. The outlines of the figure with central decompositions areas and impressive pathognomonic end-bulbs are clearly visible. The *reticulate bands of punctate epithelial microdestruction*, however, are mostly obscured by too much dye. The broad central decomposition lines show that this efflorescence is older and more advanced than that in Fig. 2.19.

## Analysis of Fig 2.21

Figure 2.21 also shows all four signs of a typical HSV dendrite. Especially impressive are the well-developed end bulbs. In addition, it is observed that the efflorescence with its swollen cells sticks out of the surrounding normal epithelial surface like an island in the sea.

## Analysis of Fig 2.22

Figure 2.22 was chosen to demonstrate that details of microscopic corneal pathology can also be detected without staining. In this case, central decomposition furrows, *reticulate bands of punctate epithelial microdestruction*, and even some *end-bulbs* can be seen in an area of previous disease (a). The visibility of subtle details without staining is strongly dependent on the observation angle. Thus, the isolated intrapupillary HSV branch could here be easily overlooked without systematic screening. Careful investigation of the cornea *before* staining should be a routine procedure. This allows detection of smallest abnormalities and the appreciation of details otherwise quickly obscured by dye. Further, if suspicious lesions are seen without staining, this alerts to the use short-term application of fluorescein in order to allow optimal conditions for biomicroscopic differential diagnosis.

## Detailed analysis of Fig 2.23

*Clinic:* The pterygium head with its prominent vessels attracts so much attention that it may distract from detecting the multi-branched dendritic figure in front with some end bulbs and broad central decomposition areas bordered by gray lining (Fig. 2.23). Immediately in front of the prominent pterygium, a larger decomposition area has developed and is surrounded by extended areas of thickened white epithelium.

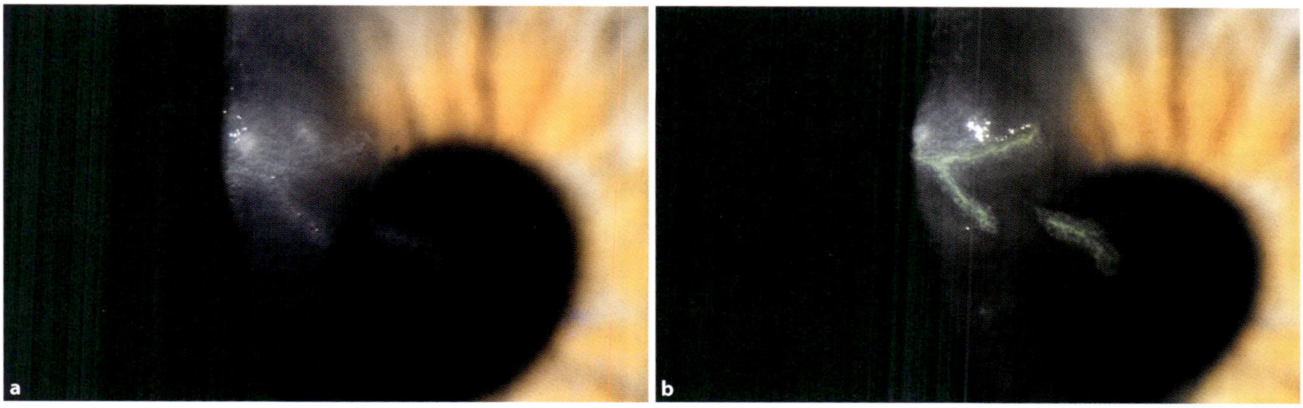

Fig. 2.22 **a** Two branches of an early HSV dendrite lie in the area of previous disease. Intrapupillary, an additional isolated branch is visible (unstained). **b** Fluorescein short-term staining

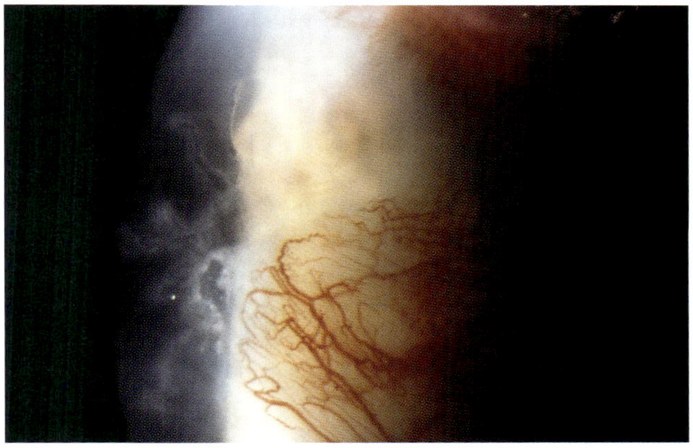

Fig. 2.23 Multi-branched older HSV dendrite in front of a pterygium head (unstained)

Some unspecific dry eye ointment can then be given in addition to ACV. If only TFT eye drops are available with their higher epitheliotoxic potential, one must combine these with artificial tears plus some ointment at night. If epithelial regeneration is very much impeded, it may be safer to rely on the antiviral effect of *systemic* ACV therapy (400 mg 5 qd for about a week) and to reserve topical therapy exclusively for efficient epithelial protection.

## Analysis of Fig 2.24

Fluorescein leaks into the cornea through pathologic gaps in the normally water-tight cell-cell occlusions of the outer epithelial layer, and it quickly stains the intercellular fluid green, thus obscuring pathologic details. Bengal rose, on the contrary, does not stain fluids, but diseased and dead cells and cell material only. Therefore, Bengal rose need not be removed from the cornea after staining. It shows the real extent of the diseased epithelial area (Fig. 2.24).

***Diagnosis:*** Older untreated dendritic keratitis, still virally active, with large viral decomposition areas as well as epithelial linings consisting of thickened regenerative epithelium. It seems to have difficulties to efficiently close the virally induced cell losses. This is especially evident immediately in front of the pterygium head, where the prominence interferes with the build-up of a stable tear film. The regenerative epithelium in this area is repeatedly broken down. This may finally lead to a persisting metaherpetic epithelial ulcer (see Sect. 2.11).
***Differential diagnosis:*** None (two typical signs and one pathognomonic sign are present).
***Therapy:*** It is important to treat not only with topical antiviral agents but to do everything possible to inhibit the development of a metaherpetic epithelial healing disorder (see Sect. 2.11). Additional epithelial protection therapy is absolutely necessary. If ACV-ointment is available, it should be used instead of TFT, because of its lower epitheliotoxic potential and because the ointment base by itself gives some of the required surface protection.

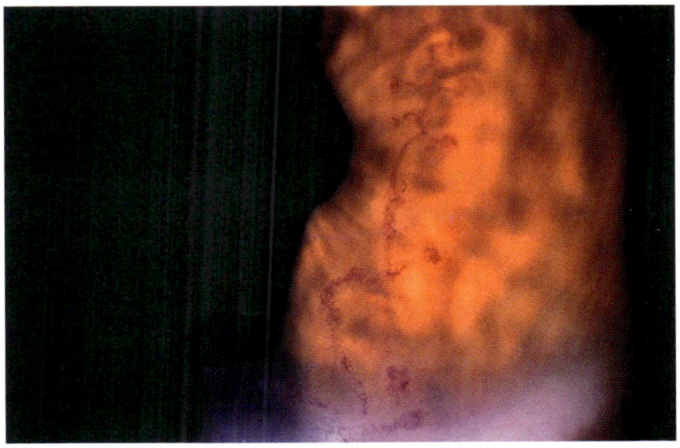

Fig. 2.24 Multi-branched HSV dendritic figure with especially impressive staining of large end-bulbs hanging like grapes on their stalks (Bengal rose)

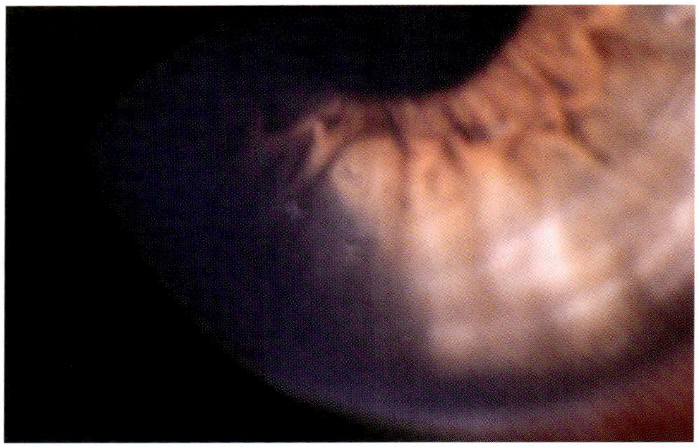

Fig. 2.25 Stellate and punctate HSV keratitis (unstained)

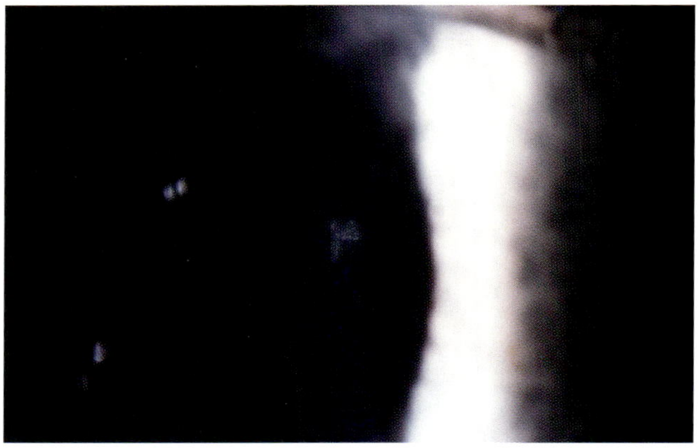

Fig. 2.26 Recurrent HSV stellate keratitis (fluorescein short-term staining)

## Detailed analysis of Fig 2.25

***Clinic:*** Three star-shaped mini-dendrites with mini-branches each seem to show a reticulate destruction pattern as well as some evolving budding. However, this is by no means convincing biomicroscopic evidence for HSV etiology as in Figs. 2.19 to 2.23. A fourth punctate efflorescence at 6 o'clock has no HSV characteristics whatsoever. While the aspect of the three stellates makes HSV etiology probable, another observation renders it fairly safe: In spite of massive bulbar injection (right lower border of Fig. 2.25), the stellates lie within totally normal surrounding epithelium like islands in a quiet sea. This "island in a quiet sea" aspect is an important characteristic for HSV stellates and punctates when compared with the very similar adenovirus ones which lie "in a rough sea" (Fig. 2.39).
***Diagnosis:*** Recurrent stellate and punctate HSV keratitis.
***Differential diagnosis:*** Acute epithelial adenovirus keratoconjunctivitis (Fig. 2.39), VZV punctates and stellates (Figs. 3.10 and 3.11).
***Therapy:*** Topical antiherpetic agents (TFT or ACV 5 qd).

## Analysis of Fig 2.26

The stellate efflorescence, or mini-dendrite, in Fig. 2.26 clearly exhibits the reticulate microdestruction pattern pathognomonic for HSV cytolysis in its early stages.

## Detailed analysis of Fig 2.27

***Clinic:*** Scattered all over the cornea, about 30 efflorescences at different stages of development are seen in Fig. 2.27, the majority of which shows branching and budding sufficiently pathognomonic for HSV etiology. There is very little injection of the conjunctiva.
***Diagnosis:*** Recurrent HSV keratitis in an atopic patient with endogenous eczema. The large number of efflorescences without adequate conjunctival injection must raise the suspicion of concomitant steroid therapy. That was indeed the case. The atopic patient was treated with systemic steroids for his endogenous eczema.
***Differential diagnosis:*** None.
***Therapy:*** If steroids can be totally withdrawn from this patient, topical antiviral therapy (ACV or TFT 5 qd) will suffice. If steroids have to be continued, however, a combined topical plus systemic antiviral therapy (ACV 400 mg 5 qd) is necessary to inhibit progression to geographic types of herpes keratitis.

## Detailed analysis of Fig 2.28

***Clinic:*** Large branching efflorescence extending from the limbal area towards the corneal center (Fig. 2.28). Ulceration is widest at the limbus with smooth, rounded borders, and no obvious characteristics for HSV etiology in that part, although a close look after fluorescein *short-term staining* (not done here) may have revealed single areas of typical microdestruction pattern somewhere in the borders of the geographic ulcer. This peripheral part is historically described as geographic keratitis. It never seems develop spontaneously, but it is typical for the enlargement of an HSV dendrite under steroid therapy. Towards the corneal center, the outlines of the dendrite become more and more characteristic for an HSV etiology. These are the parts of the dendritic figure, which have developed only recently.
***Diagnosis:*** Geographic HSV keratitis as a complication of topical and/or systemic steroid therapy.
***Differential diagnosis:*** None.
***Therapy:*** Withdraw steroids immediately, if possible. Then, topical antiviral therapy will suffice. If steroids have to be continued for general reasons, maximal topical plus systemic antiviral treatment is necessary.

## Analysis of Fig 2.29

Inflammatory injection of the conjunctiva may be so suppressed by steroids that development of HSV dendritic keratitis and its insidious enlargement to geographic keratitis passes unnoticed by the patient until his vision becomes affected. This is especially dangerous, if the patient has never experienced herpetic disease before and is unaware of this risk. A major threat comes from steroid treated monosymptomatic HSV conjunctivitis (Fig. 2.29) for which no reliable clinical differential diagnosis exists. Therefore,

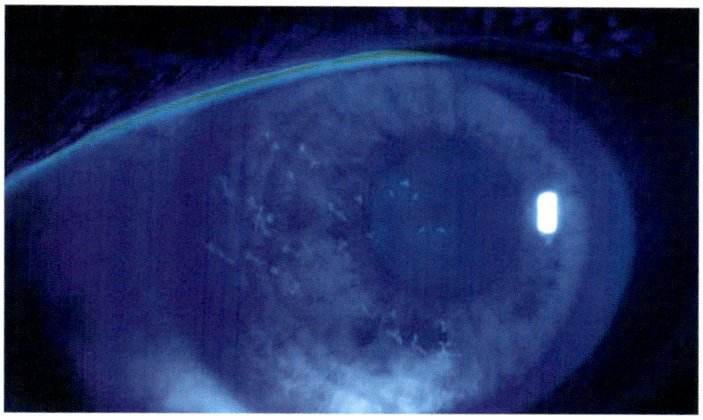

Fig. 2.27 Numerous HSV efflorescences at different stages of early development, atopic patient (fluorescein, blue light)

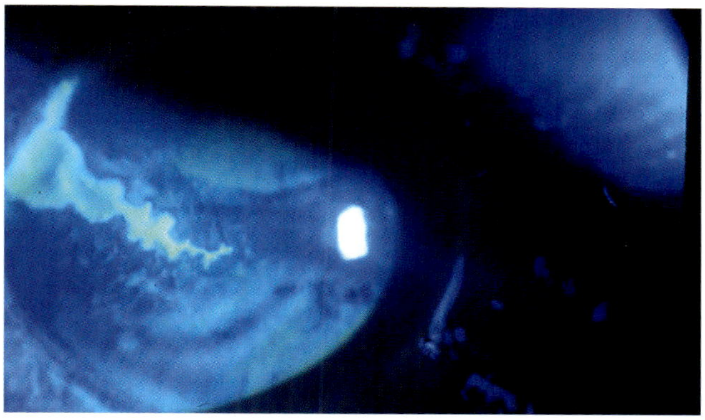

Fig. 2.28 Geographic HSV keratitis, which developed as a complication of concomitant steroid therapy (fluorescein, blue light)

steroid therapy of any conjunctivitis of unknown origin is especially dangerous if no close ophthalmological follow-up can be arranged (see Sect. 2.4).

## Detailed analysis of Fig 2.30

***Clinic:*** The residual branches extending from the old geographic areas of the left part of the efflorescence have mostly lost their end bulbs (Fig. 2.30). They have changed into *end spikes*, indicating that regeneration has overcome destruction, and healing was finally at hand. Then, however, HSV disease evidently relapsed with development of two new HSV efflorescences: a very typical one with classical microdestruction pattern extending from the right part of the old geographic area, and a second isolated linear one in the middle of the picture with less visible microdestructions.
***Diagnosis:*** The patient had experienced several epithelial as well as stromal HSV recurrences. After the last attack, which improved under ophthalmological control, the patient carried on to treat himself with a monotherapy of topical steroids "as needed" without further consulting his doctor. When he finally had to seek medical advice because his vision was continuously deteriorating, a large geographic keratitis was detected, overlying stromal scars and infiltrations. The patient was treated with a combination of antiviral agents plus steroids as indicated, and the keratitis slowly improved. He then continued with the treatment course, "ran out" of his antivirals, and went on with steroids as usual. Consequently, healing of the old geographic areas could not continue, and new dendrites had a chance to flare up.
***Differential diagnosis:*** None.
***Therapy:*** To improve compliance of the patient is at least as important as proper therapeutic measures. The therapeutic basis is an intensive long-term regime of topical plus systemic antiviral therapy (ACV). Steroids should be avoided for some time unless deep corneal infiltrations make additional steroid therapy immediately necessary. If so, cautiously dosed subconjunctival injections of crystalline (depot) steroids are a helpful option. Generally, the same principles should be followed as for interstitial ulcerating HSV keratitis (see Sect. 2.6).

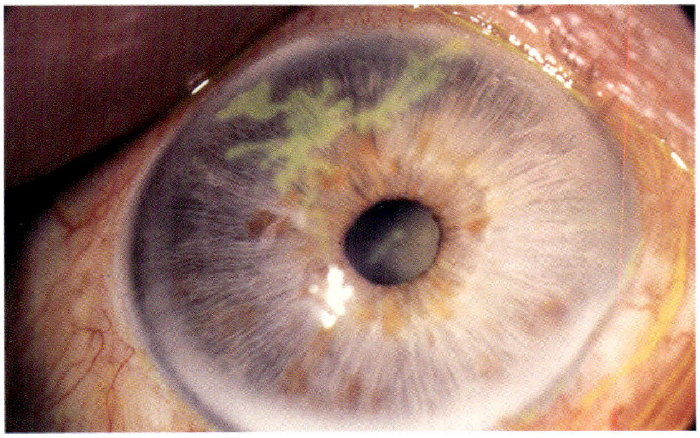

Fig. 2.29 Geographic HSV keratitis that has developed unexpectedly under topical steroid therapy for conjunctivitis (fluorescein)

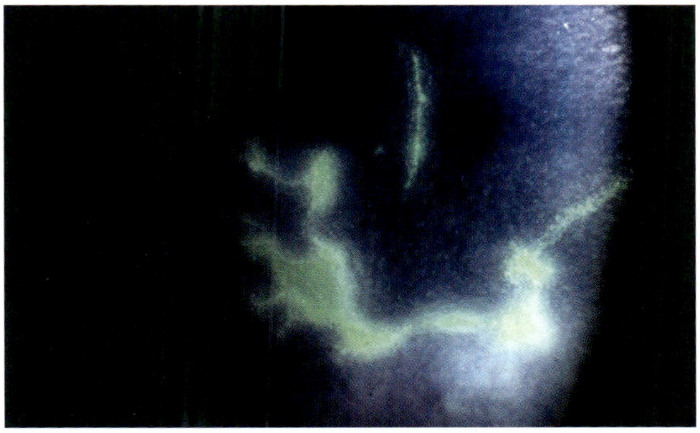

Fig. 2.30 Insufficiently treated HSV disease as documented in the cornea: longstanding geographic HSV keratitis with recent development of two new dendritic branches (fluorescein, blue light)

## Detailed analysis of Fig 2.31

***Clinic:*** Large area of geographic keratitis of presumed HSV origin but without unequivocal pathognomonic biomicroscopic findings (Fig. 2.31). Only slight reduction of vision (incipient steroid cataract), only moderate bulbar injection because the patient was on a low dose of systemic steroids for his endogenous eczema. No major complaints. No HSV history.

***Diagnosis:*** HSV was isolated and the suspected HSV etiology thus proven.

***Differential diagnosis:*** Patients with endogenous eczema may exhibit various kinds of non-viral atopic corneal epithelial complications, varying from punctate keratopathies to epithelial ulcers of different sizes and shapes.

***Therapy:*** With severe endogenous eczema, it is safest to start immediately with a combination therapy of topical (5 qd) plus systemic ACV (400 mg ACV 5 qd). Under this antiviral cover, the virological proof of the diagnosis can be awaited. Second, whenever possible, eczema therapy should be switched from steroids to non-steroidal agents. I have had excellent experiences with oral cyclosporine A, which can be given to many patients with great success for a limited time period, provided proper medical controls are feasible.

## Analysis of Fig 2.32

The pseudodendrites in Fig. 2.32 can in fact not be mistaken for viral ones. Only one out of the four criteria of HSV dendritic keratitis is present, this being the branching of the lesion. The pseudodendrite lacks the other three characteristics:

1. There is *no central line of epithelial decomposition*.
2. There is *no reticulate band of epithelial microdestruction* along the borders of the lesion.
3. The branches do *not terminate in end-bulbs*.

The pseudodendrite is composed of epithelial closure lines consisting completely of gray pathologic epithelium shoved together by the regenerative movements and forces. Even if epithelial regeneration is basically sufficient, the epithelial surface cannot normalize in the areas of the pseudodendrites as long as these especially stressed areas lack the necessary protection by a sufficiently normal tear film. Therefore, therapy is simple, although by no means easy: Care for a stable, sufficiently protective tear film, and all pseudodendrites will fade away quickly. Erroneous treatment with topical antiviral agents, however, will deteriorate the situation of the epithelium and potentially lead to even more pseudodendritic complications.

There is another clue for the non-herpetic etiology: the pseudodendrites are surrounded by diffusely and severely compromised epithelium, giving a granular appearance in the picture. To the left of the pseudodendrite, similar small lesions can be seen within diffuse superficial punctate keratopathy. HSV keratitis can, of course, also arise in eyes with severe sicca syndrome. In this case, however, we see nothing but sicca signs, and no sign for a viral etiology.

## Analysis of Fig 2.33

This efflorescence in Fig. 2.33 is a good example for two features characteristic for all pseudodendrites:

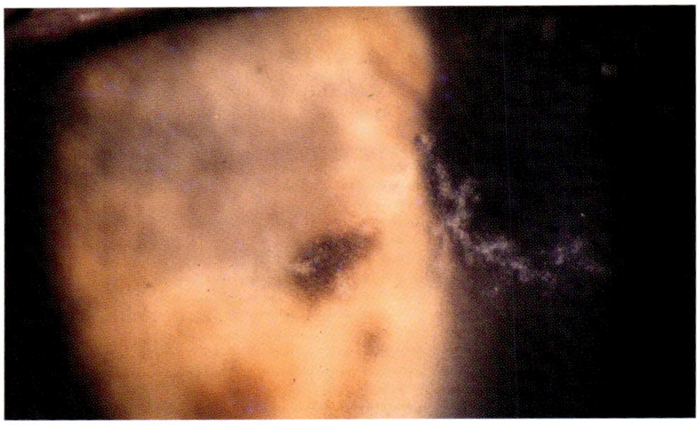

Fig. 2.32 Differential Diagnosis: Pseudodendrites in a severe sicca syndrome

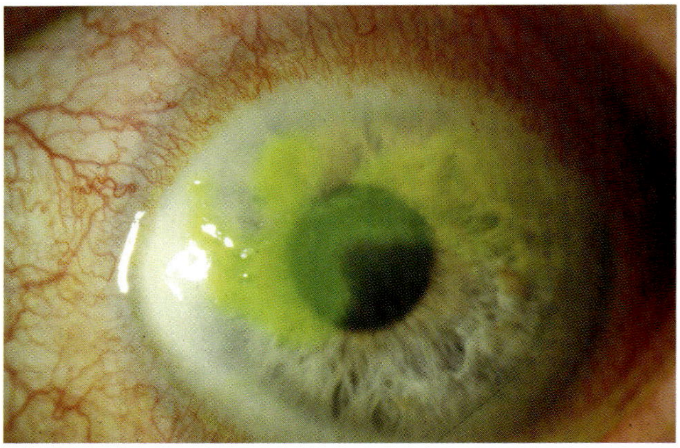

Fig. 2.31 Geographic HSV keratitis in a patient with steroid-treated endogenous eczema (fluorescein)

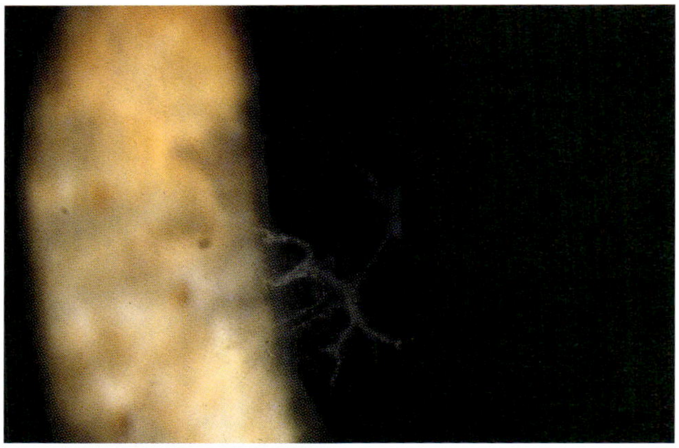

Fig. 2.33 Differential diagnosis: Pseudodendrite in a cornea with chronically compromised epithelial regeneration

1. The branches consist in all parts of equally-looking grey pathologic epithelium. There is no structural difference between the center and the borders of a branch, not even in the broadest branches.
2. The ends of branches tend to "spike".

## Analysis of Fig 2.34

The precise etiology of the lesion in Fig. 2.34, which arose in a "quiet" eye some months after otherwise uneventful ophthalmic zoster, is still disputable (see Sect. 3.8, Fig. 3.38). From the point of practical therapy, it belongs to the pseudodendrites. It is shown here because at a quick glance it seems to be a typical HSV dendrite with end bulbs, but it is *not*: This pseudodendrite is exclusively composed of prominent homogenous crests of grey, pathologic epithelium, with some light reflexes on the convexly elevated branches, which give a shiny appearance. They seem to be partly composed of pathologic mucous. Whether or not VZV plays a role in the initiation of such "metazosteric" lesions, must be further investigated and is interesting from a pathophysiological point of view. From a practical therapeutic point of view, however, this open question is unimportant. These late pseudodendrites after zoster heal with efficient dry eye therapy only, with or without additional mucosolvents. No antiviral therapy is ever needed.

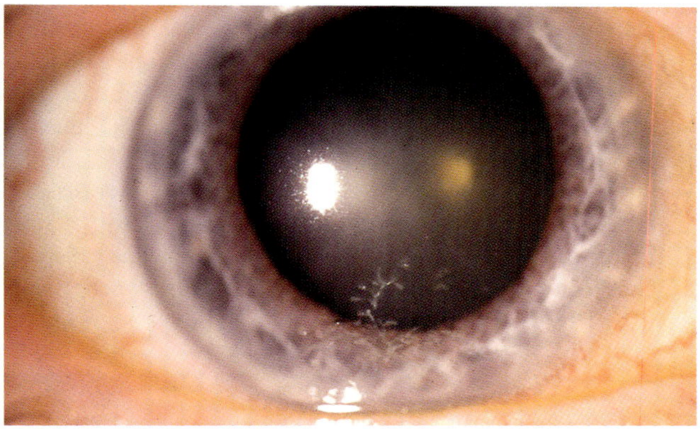

Fig. 2.34 Differential diagnosis: Late pseudodendrite after ophthalmic zoster

## Analysis of Fig 2.35

The pseudodendrite in Fig. 2.35 lies within an area of diffusely and severely altered epithelium (punctate keratopathy), typical of Sjögrens syndrome. Rounded red flecks represent more extended areas of epithelial disease and death, and must not be mistaken for end bulbs. There is another important sign for non-viral etiology of this pseudodendrite: severe punctate keratopathy and elongated dendritic figures were *exactly the same in both eyes* with the dendrites´ position exactly symmetric on the lateral sides of each cornea (not shown here). Such a perfect symmetric bilateral set-up can never be of viral origin. The pseudodendrites disappeared after bilateral occlusion of the lower lacrimal puncti plus adequate dry eye therapy.

## Analysis of Fig 2.36

In this case, Bengal rose staining in Fig. 2.36 does not really help with differential diagnosis of the dendritic lesion. For differential diagnosis, fluorescein short-term staining would have been better. However, Bengal rose uniquely reveals how diffusely, not only the corneal, but also the conjunctival epithelium is compromised in Sjögrens with large conjunctival areas colored red (out of focus).

## Analysis of Fig 2.37

The long pseudodendrite in Fig. 2.37 within bullous epithelium follows the contour of the lower limbus and is uniformly made up of grey epithelial cells. The short branches form regularly arranged arcades. Both peculiarities are uncharacteristic for HSV dendrites, but typical for pseudodendrites in bullous keratopathies.

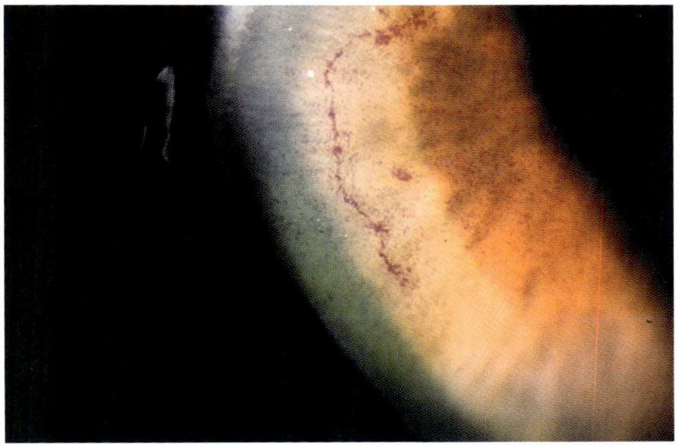

Fig. 2.35 Differential diagnosis: Pseudodendrite in Sjögrens syndrome (Bengal rose)

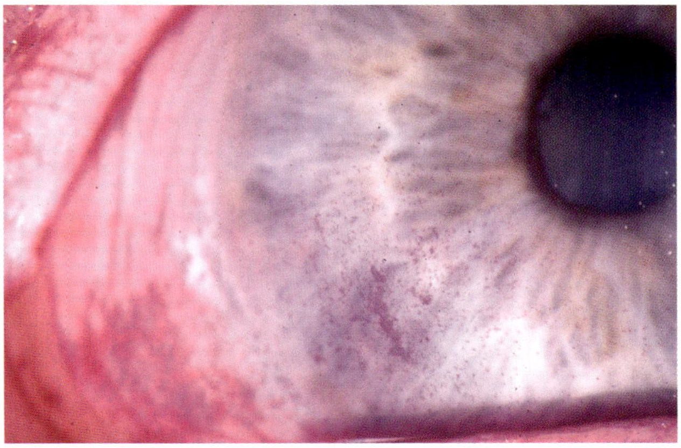

Fig. 2.36 Differential diagnosis: Pseudodendrite in Sjögrens syndrome (Bengal rose)

## Analysis of Fig 2.38

Map-dot-fingerprint (mdf) dystrophies such as that in Fig. 2.38 are often mistaken for HSV dendritic keratitis. Admittedly, biomicroscopic findings in various stages of mdf dystrophies share some similarities with HSV dendritic keratitis, but too little to explain this frequent confusion. The main reason is certainly the chronically recurrent nature of these epithelial dystrophies.

A close biomicroscopic investigation of a mdf dystrophy as in Fig. 2.38 will quickly reveal that no borderlines with epithelial micro-destruction pattern are present, as in HSV epithelial disease. Instead, we find the pathologic intraepithelial basement products of various kinds, and circumscribed micro-separations of the epithelium from its basal membrane, rendering this disease recurrently symptomatic. Partially separated epithelial sheets form micro-bullae, which stain only faintly and irregularly with fluorescein as long as the epithelial roof of the micro-bulla is mostly intact. After (recurrent) erosion, however, with disruption of the epithelial sheet, fluorescein diffusely stains all fluid pools. Both micro-bullae and frank erosion normally heal quickly with any surface-protecting measures and also without. No subsequent subepithelial scarring is ever observed if healing is brought about quickly enough after each attack.

There are many more criteria for differential diagnosis between HSV epithelial disease and mdf dystrophies:

- Mdf patients typically report to have suffered from very frequent attacks of dendritic keratitis, often every 3 weeks. HSV disease does not recur after healing at such a frequency.
- According to its bilateral dystrophic nature, asymptomatic mdf changes can often be found also in the partner eye, which then facilitates mdf diagnosis.
- If mdf disease goes on for months and years, the frequency of attacks often increases, and often progression from unilateral to bilateral disease is observed. Bilateral HSV disease, on the contrary, is rather rare.
- Mdf patients report that *each attack is very painful*. This is definitely not the case with HSV disease. Therefore, questioning regarding pain is the most important.
- Testing corneal sensitivity is also helpful in these cases: After numerous HSV recurrences, sensitivity should be found to be reduced. After mdf recurrences, sensitivity stays always normal, irrespectively of the number of previous attacks.
- Mdf patients report that the affected corneal area normally heals within only some (3–4) days with which topical therapy ever. This is much too quick for an average healing of an HSV dendrite, which may take about 7 days with antiviral therapy and a number of weeks without.
- If the patient insists to have had numerous recurrences, and the ophthalmologist cannot find residual subepithelial scars compatible with such a frequently recurring herpes disease, then this is also very typical for mdf dystrophies, which characteristically heal without scars.

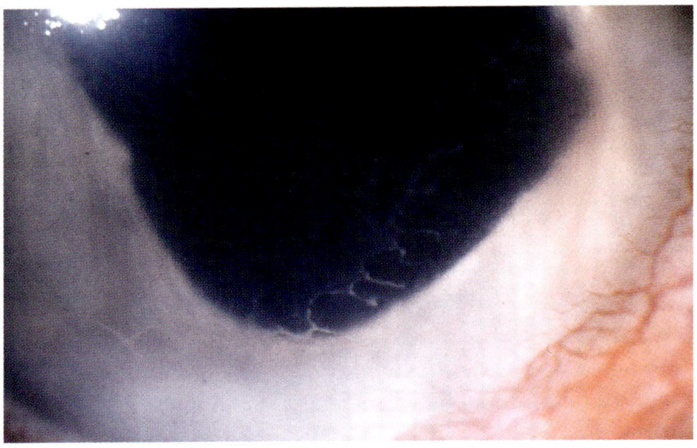

Fig. 2.37 Differential diagnosis: Pseudodendrite in aphakic bullous keratopathy

## Analysis of Fig 2.39

Adenoviruses (ADV) always infect the corneal epithelium exogenously. If infection is severe, a diffuse punctate keratitis results

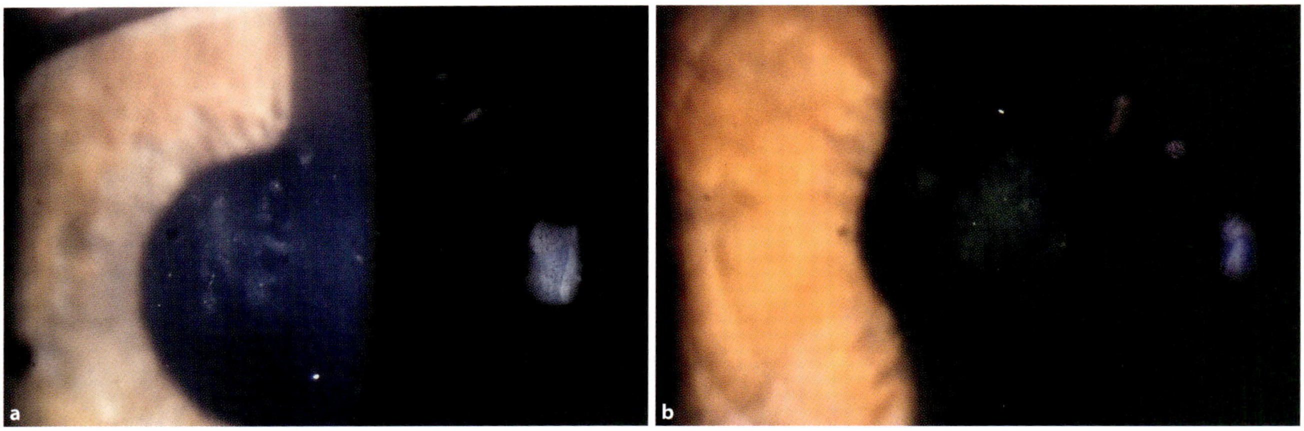


Fig. 2.38 Differential diagnosis: Map-dot-fingerprint dystrophies with recurrent erosions (two patients, unstained (**a**), fluorescein (**b**))

with varying formations of cytolytic foci. Some of these foci may spread to *stellate lesions*, which in the beginning are impossible to differentiate from HSV stellate efflorescences. While HSV stellates typically have an appearance of islands in a quiet sea (i.e., the surrounding epithelium appears widely normal, as in Fig. 2.25), ADV stellates appear like islands in a rough sea (Fig. 2.39): The surrounding epithelium is diffusely affected by punctate and aggregated cytolytic lesions as a consequence of the exogenic ADV attack. Another image may be helpful for differential diagnosis: fluorescein stained severe exogenous corneal ADV infections give an appearance of a *night sky densely crowded with single stars and star constellations of all sizes* (Fig. 2.39). Such a picture is practically never encountered with recurrent HSV epithelial infection. The differential diagnosis of severe ADV infection with severe *primary* HSV infection may rarely be difficult. The reason is evident: In this situation, HSV also causes *exogenous* infection. However, HSV limbitis mostly allows a safe differential diagnosis (see Fig. 2.112).

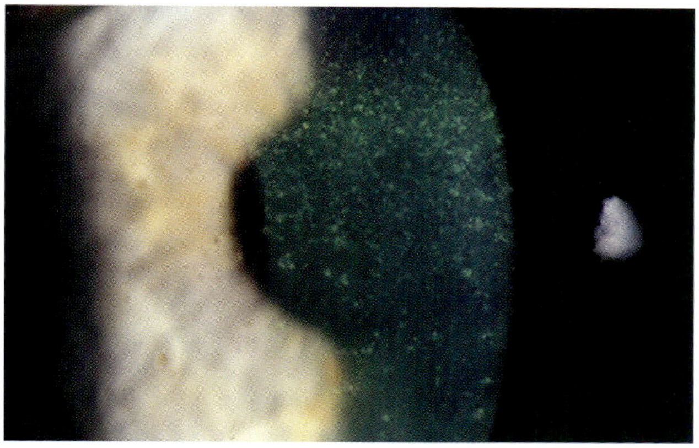

Fig. 2.39 Differential diagnosis: Epithelial adenovirus keratitis with stellate efflorescences (fluorescein)

## Analysis of Fig 2.40

Ophthalmologists not familiar with Thygeson's punctate keratitis (Fig 2.40) regularly diagnose it as some frequently recurring bilateral coarse punctate HSV keratitis. While the etiology of Thygeson´s keratitis is still unknown, the frequently recurring painful attacks symptomatically have much in common with map-dot-fingerprint micro-erosions. Consequently, the arguments for differential diagnosis are similar in both diseases. Additionally, for Thygeson´s disease, it is typical that the efflorescences do not only fade away spontaneously after some days, but their disappearance can also reliably be accelerated by topical steroids. However, steroids do not have any influence on the recurrence rate. In Thygeson´s disease, even more regularly than in mdf dystrophies, the single attacks heal without traces, even after many years of recurrences. All this makes differential diagnosis to epithelial HSV disease principally easy.

## Analysis of Fig 2.41

Tyrosinemia, a recessively inherited systemic dystrophy, is chosen as a last example for differential diagnosis (Fig. 2.41). The kids are conspicuous because of their aversion to light and because of frequent tearing and complaints from bilateral erosive central pseudodendrites. These may have some similarity with healing HSV dendrites. However, their chronic persistence in perfect symmetry in both corneal centers is not compatible with HSV etiology. If additionally circumscribed hyperkeratoses are found on the foot plates, the clinical diagnosis of tyrosinemia becomes probable and must be proven in the laboratory. The diagnosis is important, because an early consequently established diet is the only chance for these children to develop normally.

More clinical conditions with similar bilateral dystrophic corneal pseudodendrites which are *not* caused by tyrosinemia exist. To date, their biochemical background remains unknown.

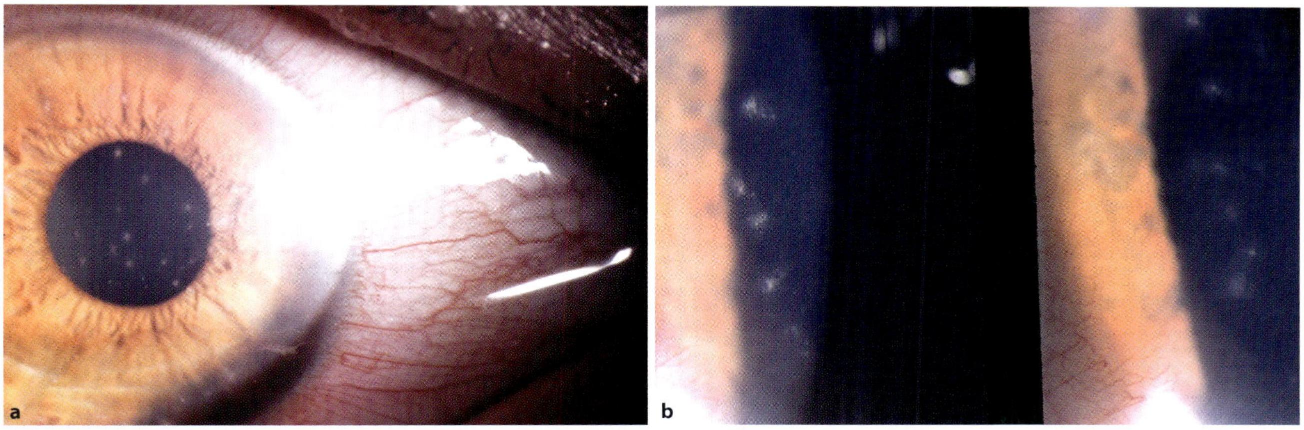



Fig. 2.40a,b Differential diagnosis: Thygeson´s punctate keratitis. **a** Strictly intraepithelial coarse punctate efflorescences consisting of "degenerated" epithelium. **b** Each efflorescence has a limited life cycle, after which it fades away without a trace

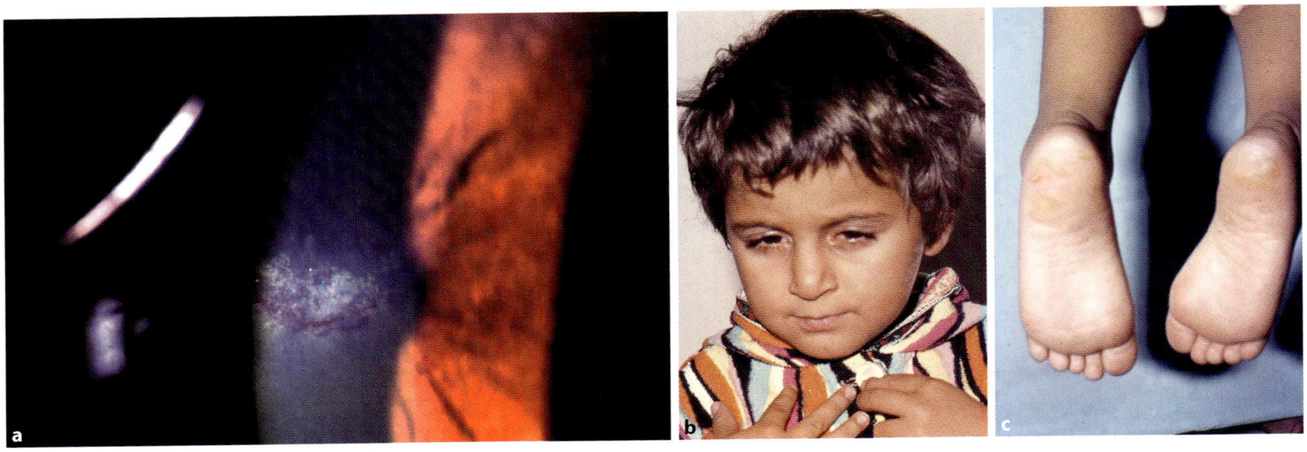

Fig. 2.41a–c Differential diagnosis: Central corneal pseudodendrites in tyrosinemia (Richner–Hanhart syndrome). **a** Micro-erosive chronic central corneal pseudodendrite. **b** Chronic aversion to light. **c** Hyperkeratoses on the foot plates

## References


Carter C, Easty DL (1981) The influence of antiviral immunity in epithelial herpetic keratitis. In: R. Sundmacher (ed): Herpetic Eye Diseases. Bergmann, Munich, pp 111–116

Collum LM, Logan P, McAuliffe-Curtin D, Hung SO, Patterson A, Rees PJ (1985) Randomised double-blind trial of acyclovir (Zovirax) and adenine arabinoside in herpes simplex amoeboid corneal ulceration. Br J Ophthalmol 69: 847–850

Connell PP, O´Reilly J, Coughlan S, Collum LM, Power WJ (2007) The role of common viral ocular pathogens in Thygeson´s superficial punctate keratitis. Br J Ophthalmol 91: 1038–1041

Coster DJ, Jones BR; Falcon MG (1977) Role of debridement in the treatment of herpetic keratitis. Trans Ophthalmol Soc UK 97: 314–317

Coster DJ, Jones BR, McGill JI (1979) Treatment of amoeboid herpetic ulcers with adenine arabinoside or trifluorothymidine. Br J Ophthalmol 63: 418–421

Easty DL, Tullo AB, Shimeld C, Hill TJ, Blyth WA (1985) The influence of prednisolone on external eye disease, virus proliferation and latent infection in an animal model of herpes simplex keratitis. In: PC Maudgal, L Missotten (eds.): Herpetic Eye Disease. W Junk, Dordrecht, pp 95–97

Herpetic Eye Disease Study Group (1997) A controlled trial of oral acyclovir for the prevention of stromal Keratitis or iritis in patients with herpes simplex virus epithelial keratitis. Arch Ophthalmol 115: 703–712

Müller LJ, Vrensen GFJM, Pels L, Nunes Cardozo B, Willekens B (1997) Architecture of human corneal nerves. Invest Ophthalmol Vis Sci 38: 985–994

Neumann-Haefelin D, Mattes A, Sundmacher R (1981) Trifluorothymidine sensitivity of ocular herpes simplex virus strains. In: R Sundmacher (ed) Herpetic Eye Diseases. Bergmann, Munich, pp 353–355

Reinhard T, Roggendorf M, Fengler I, Sundmacher R (2004) PCR for varicella zoster genome in corneal epithelial cells of patients with Thygesons superficial punctate Keratitis. Eye 18: 304–305

Sundmacher R (1977) Bilaterale Pseudokeratitis dendritica (Richner-Hanhart-Syndrom). Klin Monatsbl Augenheilk 170: 84–88

Sundmacher R, Hillenkamp J, Reinhard T (2001) Therapie und Prophylaxe der Adenovirus-Keratokonjunktivitis. Ophthalmologe 98: 991–1009

Sundmacher R, Press M, Neumann-Haefelin D, Riede U (1977) Keratitis superficialis punctata Thygeson. Klin Monatsbl Augenheilk 170: 908–916

Tabery HM (1998) Early epithelial changes in recurrent herpes simplex virus keratitis. Acta Ophthalmol Scand 76: 349–352

Tullo AB, Shimeld C, Blyth WA, Hill TJ, Easty DL (1983) Ocular infection with herpes simplex virus in non immune and immune mice. Arch Ophthalmol 101: 961–964

Wilhelmus KR (2000) The treatment of herpes simplex virus epithelial keratitis. Trans Am Ophthalmol Soc 98: 505–532

Wilhelmus KR, Coster DH, Jones BR (1981) Acyclovir and debridement in the treatment of ulcerative herpetic keratitis. Am J Ophthalmol 91: 323–327

# Interstitial and Ulcerating HSV Keratitis

Section

2.6

## Core Messages

- In this type of deep HSV disease, viral cytolysis and cellular immune-destructions work together. Both are always to be treated simultaneously with antiviral agents as the basic therapy, plus steroids for the necessary down-regulation of immune-destruction.
- Non-steroidal immunosuppressive agents may be an alternative if steroid therapy appears to be too risky.
- *Differential diagnosis 1:* Inflammation in the anterior chamber is generally much lower with interstitial HSV keratitis, when compared to bacterial or mycotic infections.
- *Differential diagnosis 2:* Hypopyon is never a sign of HSV infection itself. If present in a herpes eye, it indicates bacterial or mycotic superinfection.
- *Differential diagnosis 3:* In amebic keratitis, pain is the most important symptom.

Interstitial keratitis is almost never the first clinical manifestation of HSV disease. Dendritic keratitis has typically been observed before. This facilitates the assignment of subsequent recurrent stromal disease to HSV etiology. If a typical HSV dendrite has not been identified before, the diagnosis of interstitial HSV keratitis may become more difficult, because the density and shape of interstitial infiltrations are not always such to make a differential diagnosis possible. Differential diagnosis is often helped, however, by the fact that inflammation in the anterior chamber is generally much lower with corneal HSV infections as compared with bacterial or mycotic ones. Especially hypoyon is never brought about by HSV infection alone. If it arises in a herpes eye, it indicates bacterial or mycotic superinfection. For differential diagnosis of amebic keratitis, which, like herpes, arouses very little anterior chamber reaction, pain is the one most important differentiating symptom. Interstitial keratitis by VZV or adenoviruses may sometimes be impossible to differentiate from HSV disease on a morphological basis only. In these cases, the history and the course of the disease will often give diagnostic help. Laboratory confirmation of a causative infectious agent, viral or other, must of course be sought whenever necessary and possible. The difficulties with laboratory confirmation of infectious eye diseases must not be underestimated, however, and a good knowledge of the various aspects of clinical differential diagnosis remains the basis of successful and, above all, quick therapy.

The longer recurrent HSV disease has gone on in a patient and the more recurrences his eye had to suffer, the greater the incidence of stromal keratitis. Concomitantly, the incidence of dendritic keratitis decreases. The reasons for this striking change in disease character have not been well investigated to my knowledge. It seems, though, that several mechanisms play a role: a change in the stromal target cell composition, an increasing stimulation of the natural and immunologic defence mechanisms of the host, and also an increasing tendency for HSV to establish peripherally persistent infections in the corneal stroma.

The most easily accessible target cells for HSV recurrences change in the long run. While in the beginning, corneal epithelial cells are far more easily infected by HSV than keratocytes in their normal stromal surrounding, this situation changes once HSV has finally succeeded to also establish infection in keratocytes. Thereafter, the stroma is invaded by various inflammatory, immunologic, and regenerative cell populations. These create a target cell milieu which becomes increasingly attractive not only for normal lytic HSV infection but probably also for very slow HSV replication with very little cell lysis but constant stimulation of immune reactions, a status that I call peripheral persistence.

Whether such peripherally persistent HSV infection is the main reason for chronic persistent keratitis and whether additional pathogenetic impact comes from frequent endogenous HSV shedding, could not be investigated to date. However, the necessary therapeutic measures are evident without knowing the exact pathophysiologic background: First, HSV replication has to be suppressed as efficiently as possible by antiviral therapy. Second, the cell infiltrations have to be removed from the stroma as quickly as possible. For this task, steroids are the drug of choice. The quick reduction of infiltrates is above all necessary to keep or restore the functional clarity of the cornea.

A change in stromal target cell composition does not explain why the incidence of dendritic keratitis concomitantly goes down. A reason may be an increasing stimulation of the natural and immunologic defence mechanisms of the host. They remain still insufficient to beat stromal disease quickly, especially when it comes to persistent slow disease. However, their efficiency to primarily inhibit endogenous re-infection of the epithelium seems to increase on an average.

On the whole, therapy of interstitial and ulcerating HSV keratitis is much more difficult than that of any other herpetic eye disease. In dendritic keratitis, we can observe a reliable healing endpoint, and we can then be relatively sure that the virus has practically gone, at least for this recurrence. With stromal types of HSV disease, such confidence can never be expected. It has long been found that "quiet" herpes corneas are not at all quiet and still contain inflammatory cells as well as HSV, in which status ever. This reflects our current inability to clinically judge what is pathophysiologically actually going on in the corneal stroma.

Nonetheless, we need practical rules for practical handling of this difficult disease group. I have found the following rules and advice helpful:

1. The earlier a "clinical recurrence" arises a new after cessation of therapy, the more probably we deal with peripheral persistence of insufficiently treated HSV disease. "Clinical recurrences" that follow each other after only a couple of weeks are most probably brought about by peripheral persistence and not primarily by endoneurally recurring disease, although the latter may additionally occur.
2. For safety, a sufficiently long therapy of interstitial HSV keratitis is necessary. Therapy which is a number of months long is safer than therapy which is a few weeks long.
3. The effects of antiviral therapy – unlike with dendritic keratitis – *cannot* directly be observed when treating interstitial HSV keratitis. The severity and acuity of interstitial keratitis are exclusively determined by the reactive inflammatory and immunologic infiltrates.
4. Any biomicroscopically seen improvement and "clearance" are brought about by the steroid therapy. The efficiency of the basic antiviral therapy, which determines the lasting success of treatment, cannot be judged as long as steroids are given.
5. Consequently, the "moment of truth" does not come before the last drop of steroid has been tapered, and not before some weeks have elapsed thereafter. With every month that the cornea remains "quiet", the probability increases that the combination therapy of antiviral agent plus steroids was sufficient to eradicate (persistent) HSV infection from the cornea.
6. Controlling herpes patients frequently enough *after* cessation of therapy is therefore more important than controlling them while still under combination therapy.
7. In spite of correct and sufficiently long combination therapy, some patients never become totally free from peripherally persisting HSV, because the efficiency of antiviral agents goes down considerably if viral replication is reduced to a minimum. The target enzymes are then no longer sufficiently available. In such cases, a minimally dosed unlimited steroid therapy, which keeps the cornea symptomatically "quiet" (e.g., 1 drop qd or every other day) is a justifiable compromise, which will keep functioning longer than would be the case after total withdrawal of steroids with frequently recurring infiltrations.
8. If topical and/or systemic steroids cannot be given, nonsteroidal immunosuppressive agents may be an alternative, e.g., cyclosporine A. These drugs also have topical and systemic side effects, but they are different from those of the steroids and may be preferable to steroids in special situations for a limited time period, e.g., in severe diabetes, or with associated severe dry eye syndromes.
9. In *ulcerating interstitial HSV keratitis*, lysing inflammatory cells cause the stroma to melt away. This may rapidly lead to descemetocele and perforation. Normal *topical* steroid therapy would further aggravate epithelial regeneration problems and must be avoided as long as the deep ulcer has not been closed by new epithelium. Systemic steroids at low to moderate doses, together with cautiously dosed injections of subconjunctival crystalline steroid depots, are a valuable alternative to topical therapy. They create a constant steroid level in the cornea which suppresses destructive infiltrations while still allowing for sufficient epithelial regeneration.

## Detailed analysis of Fig 2.42

***Clinic:*** Subepithelial dense infiltrates, like imprints of an immediately preceding dendritic keratitis at the same site of the cornea (Fig. 2.42).

***Diagnosis:*** Superficial interstitial HSV keratitis arising topographically exactly below preceding HSV dendrites. The epithelial viral disease seems to have "burned" down into the superficial stroma. It is more likely, however, that the viruses were set free at the same time from the same nerve trunks intra-epithelially and subepithelially, the former leading *quickly* to dendritic keratitis, and the latter, with a few days delay, leading to infection of the *less permissive* keratocytes with circumscribed dense immune infiltrates thereafter.

***Differential diagnosis:*** None, if the HSV dendrites were unequivocally verified earlier. The plump "dendritic" shape of the stromal infiltrates is also a relatively reliable sign for HSV etiology, but not invariably a safe one.

***Therapy:*** Topical antiviral-steroid combination, e.g., ACV ointment

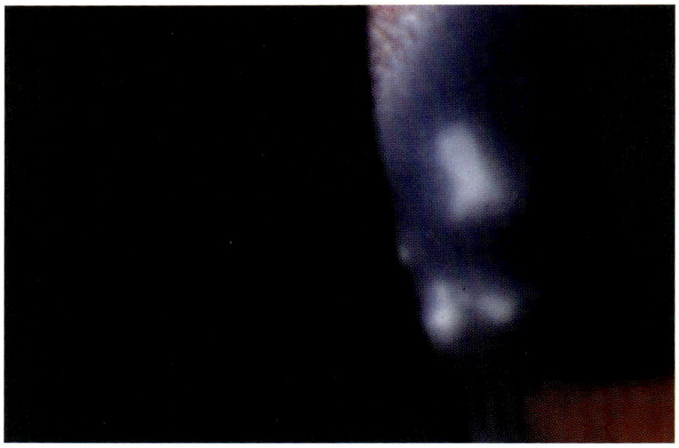

Fig. 2.42 Superficial interstitial HSV keratitis after immediately preceding dendritic keratitis in the same location

5 qd plus steroid ointment 2–3 qd. TFT eye drops 5 qd plus steroid eye drops 2–3 qd are also an option, though a minor one, because TFT in this combination can only prophylactically inhibit new HSV dendrites. It cannot efficiently treat subepithelial HSV infection of the keratocytes. Therefore, if only TFT is available, topical steroids should be dosed even more cautiously. A better alternative would then be to give systemic ACV plus topical steroids.

## Analysis of Fig 2.43

Figure 2.43 demonstrates that the "dendritic" shape of subepithelial HSV infiltrates, like those in Fig. 2.42, is preserved for a long time and serves as a relatively reliable indication for HSV etiology. Therapeutically, nothing needs to be done, if the patient is off therapy already. The remaining subtle infiltrates will fade away spontaneously with time, e.g., within a year, provided no new endogenous recurrence occurs. If quicker "clearance" of the scars is required, then a normal antiviral-steroid combination therapy (see Fig. 2.42) must be given for at a least a few months rather than only for a couple of weeks. Because patients' compliance with combination therapy decreases with clearing scars, premature self-determined abrupt termination of treatment may be more disadvantageous in the end than refraining from therapy all together.

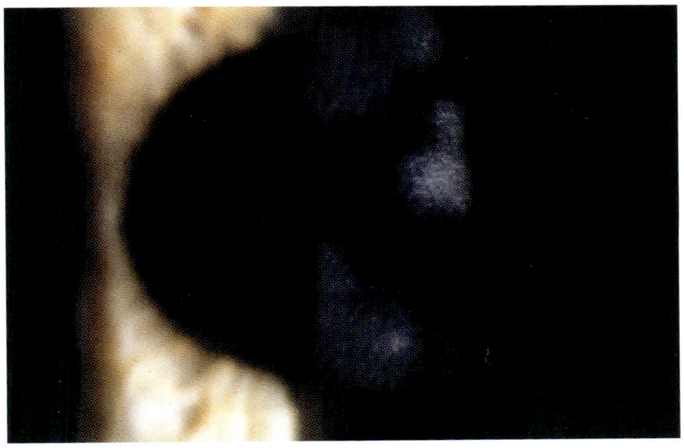

Fig. 2.43 Faint scars with some residual infiltrates after superficial interstitial HSV keratitis (stromal "imprints" of dendrites)

## Detailed analysis of Fig 2.44

***Clinic:*** Fluffy new infiltrations shown in Fig. 2.44 have arisen at three sites in the cornea a couple of weeks after topical therapy of a previous HSV interstitial keratitis was finished. The scars of previous herpes diseases extend far into the pupillary area.

***Diagnosis:*** Flaring-up of an insufficiently treated interstitial keratitis with HSV still present in the stroma at the time when further therapy was deemed unnecessary. Treatment was stopped too early.

***Differential diagnosis:*** None.

***Therapy:*** Resume combined topical antiviral-steroid therapy following the principles outlined in Sect. 2.2 and Fig. 2.42. The re-instituted treatment should be given considerably longer than previously.

## Detailed analysis of Fig 2.45

***Clinic:*** Infiltrations form two relatively dense balls with fluffy outlines involving the whole stromal thickness (Fig. 2.45). A typical HSV dendritic keratitis was documented in the course of previous herpes disease. This time, the epithelium is normal. The interstitial keratitis is the first deep herpetic disease documented for this patient. There are only sparse cells in the aqueous humor. The iris seems to be unharmed. Several small precipitates are grouped on the central endothelium. There is no frank corneal edema.

***Diagnosis:*** Fully developed interstitial HSV keratitis plus beginning topographically associated HSV endotheliitis (Sect. 2.7). Without immediate therapeutic intervention, the disease will progress to typical disciform HSV keratitis (Sect. 2.7).

***Differential diagnosis:*** None.

***Therapy:*** Start with combined topical antiviral-steroid therapy as outlined in Fig. 2.42. If the endotheliitic component deteriorates in spite of topical treatment and disease deteriorates to disciform keratitis, additional systemic combined therapy is advisable.

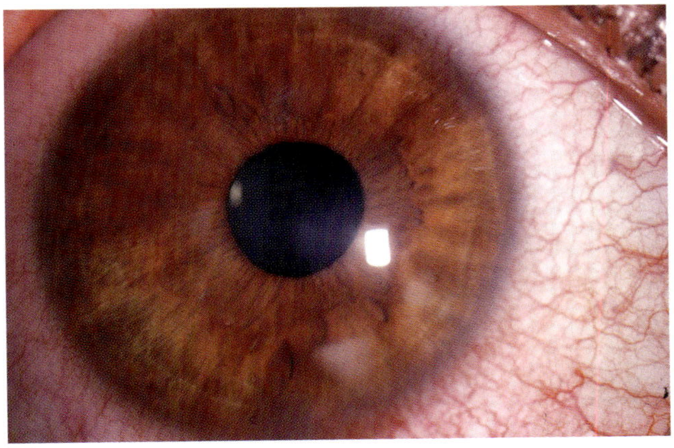

Fig. 2.44 Fluffy new infiltrations in a faintly scarred herpes cornea

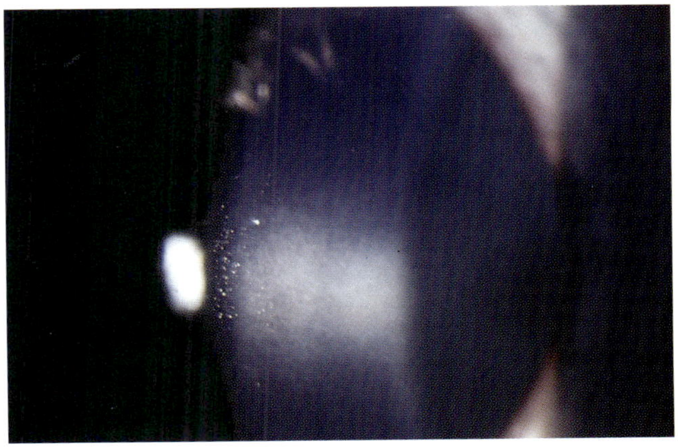

Fig. 2.45 Interstitial HSV keratitis plus beginning endotheliitis

## Analysis of Fig 2.46

Contrary to Fig. 2.45, in Fig. 2.46, the endothelial precipitates are of clearly different sizes – minor gray ones and large slightly pigmented ones. The distribution of precipitates also follows two principles – triangular-iritic as well as independence of aqueous gravity flow. Finally, some deep striae and epithelial edema (visible at the right side) are signs of frank corneal edema caused by endothelial decompensation. Altogether, interstitial HSV keratitis is here associated with additional HSV endotheliitis (see Sect. 2.8) and HSV iritis (see Sect. 2.9).

## Detailed analysis of Fig 2.47

*Clinic:* Large parts of the peripheral cornea are diffusely, though faintly, scarred, in addition to most of the pupillary area (Fig. 2.47). Some dense infiltrates are so white, providing a "purulent" aspect. The anterior chamber exhibits no remarkable inflammation. Also, virtually no precipitates can be made out. No corneal edema. Several deep vessels reach the area of most obvious stromal destruction on the left.

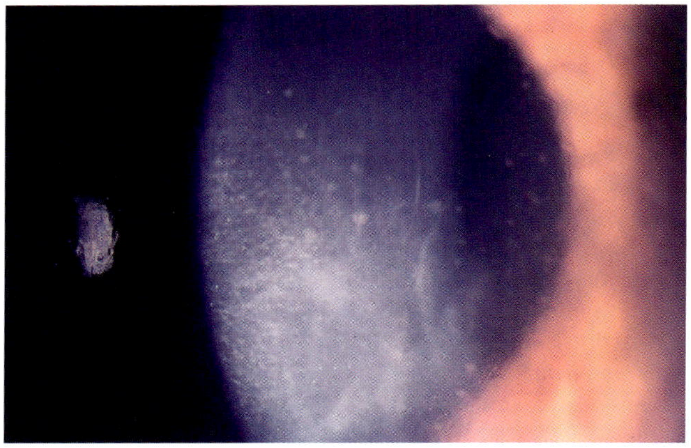

Fig. 2.46 Interstitial HSV keratitis plus scattered endothelial precipitates

*Diagnosis:* Recurrent multifocal interstitial HSV keratitis in a vascularized and scarred herpes cornea that has already experienced some recurrences of deep herpetic disease. This not only increases the risk of persistent peripheral HSV disease, it must also be suspected that additionally a granulomatous reaction against Descemets (and possibly Bowmans) is operative in creating and intensifying the extremely dense infiltrates.

*Differential diagnosis:* None. History and corneal findings are sufficiently characteristic for HSV etiology. No bacterial or mycotic (super)infection has to be suspected, in spite of the dense infiltrations. The "clean" anterior chamber would not support such a suspicion.

*Therapy:* Normal long-term combination therapy with topical antivirals plus steroids suffices. If the clinical suspicion of granulomatous reaction against Descemets is correct, the infiltrates will be even more refractive than they are anyway in "normal" interstitial HSV keratitis. Therefore, therapy has to be much longer and requires even more patience than usually. As granulomatous reaction is presumably a secondary inflammatory reaction independent of a continuing presence of HSV, it may be necessary to carry on with small amounts of steroids for a long time until the cornea becomes "quiet". Each definite withdrawal of steroids may be followed by prompt flare-up of stromal infiltrates.

## Analysis of Fig 2.48

The dense white interstitial infiltration-ball in Fig. 2.48 can be regarded as a maximal variant of the small dense white infiltrations in Fig. 2.47. In Fig. 2.48. The impression of a "purulent" lesion is even more suggestive because of its large dimension. However, as the aqueous humor is practically normal, true purulent infiltration cannot exist and bacterial and mycotic etiologies become improbable. Inflammatory cells liberate lytic enzymes as confirmed by the small "clearing" area supra-centrally. Subsequent ulceration with descemetocele and perforation are therefore threatening if no efficient therapy is immediately started. In this patient, long-term topical combination therapy over many months inhibited progression to ulceration and finally led to permanently quiet scars. Loss of stromal substance with resulting corneal irregularity caused functional loss, of course.

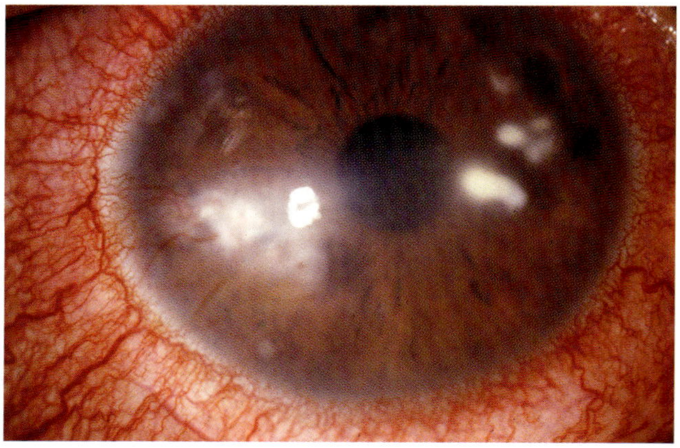

Fig. 2.47 Multiple separate foci of unusually dense interstitial HSV keratitis in a partially vascularized and scarred herpes cornea

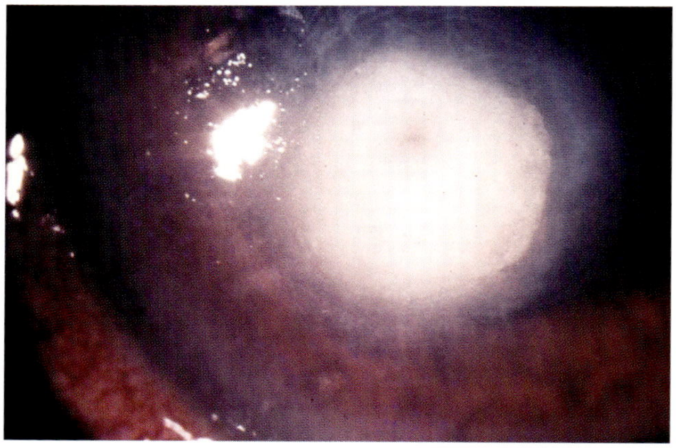

Fig. 2.48 Unusually dense interstitial HSV keratitis, probably complicated by granulomatous reaction against Descemets

## Detailed analysis of Fig 2.49

***Clinic:*** Large vascular trunks, which split up in medium and fine vessels, invade a diffusely and densely infiltrated stroma aiming at the main points of infiltration (Fig. 2.49). Parts of the cornea are colored salmon red by the vascular fans.

***Diagnosis:*** Healing phase with aggressive vascular resorption of infiltrates in severe HSV interstitial keratitis.

***Differential diagnosis:*** None, if the HSV nature of disease has been verified before. Principally, such aggressive vascular resorption is more typical for bacterial, mycotic, or mixed severe infections of the cornea – and classifically for syphillitic keratitis, of course. However, occasionally, such severe vascularization is also observed with HSV disease. There is no characteristic type of vascular ingrowth in corneal herpes. Ingrowth may be massive or may be totally lacking in very similarly looking clinical conditions. It would be important to know more about the biochemical differences that cause such different behavior in the individual cases.

***Therapy:*** Once vessels have started to grow into a densely infiltrated inflammatory battlefield, they can hardly be stopped, not even by maximally enforced steroid therapy, which has its own risks. The normal topical combination regime of antiviral agents plus steroids should suffice and is safer. Administered long enough, the amount of infiltrates is gradually reduced, and this reduction also automatically reduces the vascular-attractive signals. The vessels either turn to ghost vessels or at least shrink so much that they no longer present functionally important optic obstacles. Therefore, such a massive vascularization is no reason for nervousness. Simply, reduce the infiltrates, and the vessels will regress concomitantly.

## Analysis of Fig 2.50

Figure 2.50 gives an example of a slowly progressing vascular front in an only moderately infiltrated interstitial HSV keratitis. If normal topical combination therapy is consequent and long enough, the vessels will halt in the present topical situation. Thereafter, they will shrink or obliterate and present no functional problem.

## Analysis of Fig 2.51

Courses with spontaneous healing offer two aspects. First, spontaneous healing does not regularly lead to catastrophic results. Spontaneous healing of the severe limbus-adjacent herpetic infiltrations in Fig. 2.51 has lead to a dense para-pupillary vascularized corneal scar. As this scar is not functionally incapacitating, the results of spontaneous healing are still compatible with useful function. This is not so bad. Some therapists would be content to see such a treatment result. Second, we are reminded that iatrogenic success can generally only be claimed for those results that are more successful than the results of spontaneous healing. Comparing the para-limbal 3 o'clock region in Fig. 2.51a with the spontaneous healing result in Fig. 2.51b suggests that proper therapy would not invariably have led to a better result. That is different with the dense infiltration area para-pupillary at 4 o'clock in Fig. 2.51a. It would have certainly benefited from correct and timely treatment with topical antivirals plus steroids. Less subsequent corneal distortion and functional impairment would have developed than after spontaneous healing.

***Differential diagnosis:*** Formally, the limbus-adjacent vascularized scar in Fig. 2.51 with its rounded border towards the pupil has some similarity with chronic interstitial demarcating immune keratitis, as described in Sect. 3.5 (Figs. 3.23 to 3.27). The latter is suspected to be caused by VZV. Its pathologic processes are much slower than those in HSV disease, and vascularization is accordingly much lower.

## Analysis of Fig 2.52

Figure 2.52 outlines one of the main risks of steroid monotherapy of deep herpetic eye disease, especially of interstitial HSV keratitis. This patient with chronic flaring-up of interstitial HSV keratitis was correctly put on a long-term topical combination therapy with antiviral agents plus steroids. On a holiday trip, the patient ran out of antiviral drugs and carried on with steroids only, which he himself dosed "as needed". A steroid associated geographic keratitis developed (see Sect. 2.5), which the patient did not notice himself because of too dense infiltrations. It was only detected when he finally saw his doctor again after 6 weeks. Still small and

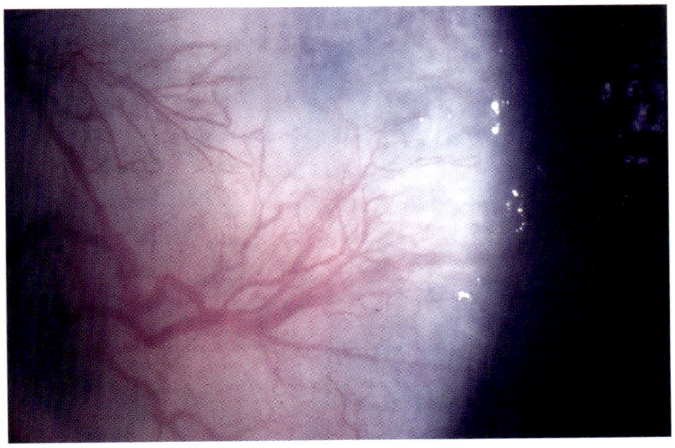

Fig. 2.49 Aggressive stromal vascularization in interstitial HSV keratitis

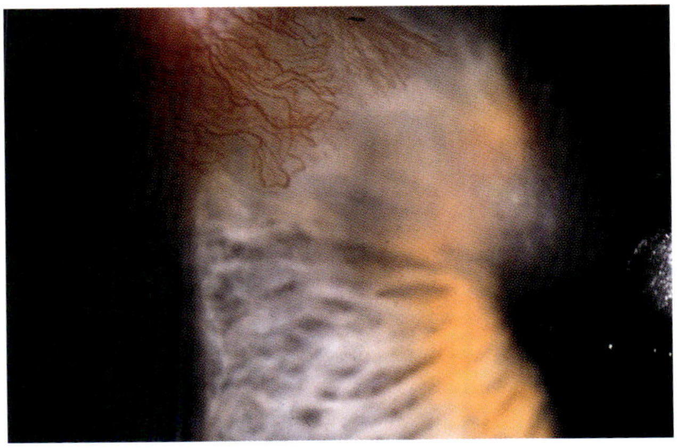

Fig. 2.50 Vascular front in moderately infiltrated interstitial HSV keratitis

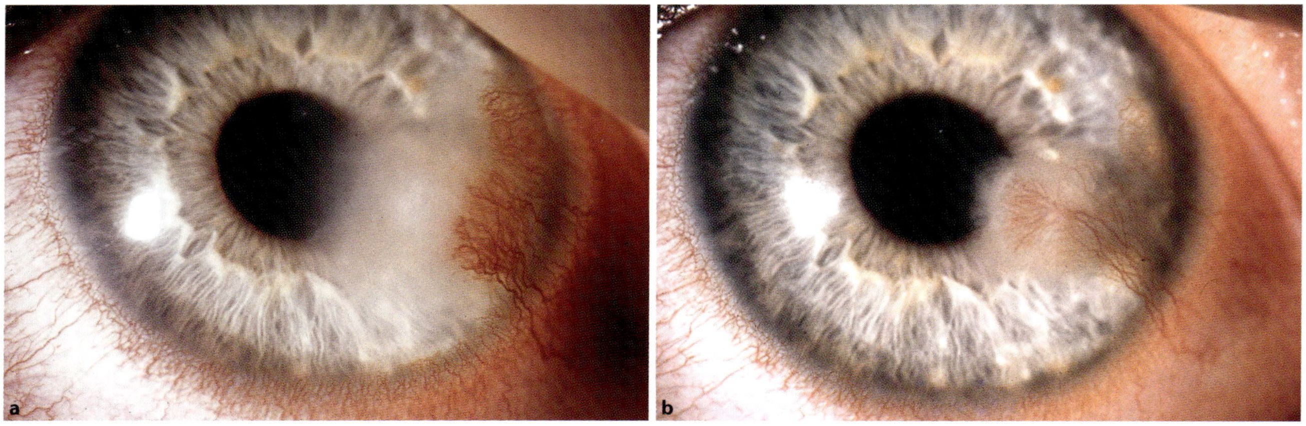

Fig. 2.51 Spontaneous healing of a dense limbus-adjacent infiltration in HSV interstitial keratitis (time interval between **a** and **b**: 2 months)

comprising the superficial epithelium only (which can be taken from the diffuse Bengale-Rose stain), this complication was manageable without severe additional damage. With ongoing steroid self-treatment, however, much more severe ulceration would certainly have occurred (see Fig. 2.53). For therapy in this case it suffices to resume full dose topical antiviral therapy and to leave off the steroids until the geographic lesion has been resurfaced by epithelium. This should quickly be the case. Thereafter, steroids are slowly added again as required by the interstitial process.

## Analysis of Fig 2.53

The patient in Fig. 2.53 had a comparable history to the patient in Fig. 2.52. In Fig. 2.53, however, non-compliance led to an even longer steroid monotherapy, and, consequently, much more extended geographic ulcerations which partly already extend into the stroma. At some sites of the geographic outlines, where the diseased epithelium is colored deeply red, the pathognomonic budding contours of epithelial HSV efflorescences are appreciable even at this low magnification (see Sect. 2.5). For therapy, see Fig. 2.52.

## Detailed analysis of Fig 2.54

***Clinic:*** Dense disseminated interstitial infiltrations and a large ulceration at 6 o'clock (still mostly epithelial), together with massive injection of the conjunctiva, show that this eye in Fig. 2.54 is at high risk of rapid further deterioration in spite of some previous therapeutic efforts (hyphema as sequelae of subconjunctival injections). Especially noteworthy are several epithelial buddings at the otherwise straight geographic outlines, and an additional small dendrite para-limbally at 3 o'clock.

***Diagnosis and history:*** Severe interstitial HSV keratitis with complicated large geographic epithelial keratitis. The biomicroscopic details document an impressive sequence of insufficient or failing therapy: A severe interstitial HSV keratitis was "treated" by the patient himself with topical steroid monotherapy, leading to the complication of geographic keratitis. Once this was noticed, topical steroids were substituted by subconjunctival injections of a crystalline steroid (which is a correct option), plus topical antivirals (ACV ointment every 2 hrs). The geographic lesion began to heal slowly, as shown by the straightened outlines and by a deeply indenting epithelial regeneration front (upper left). Then

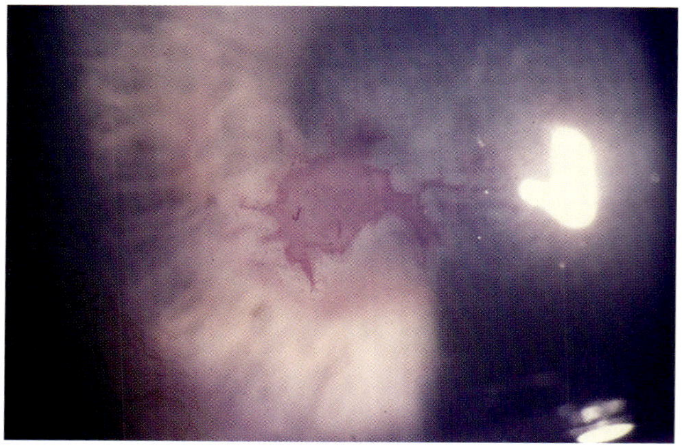

Fig. 2.52 Small geographic HSV keratitis as a complication of steroid-monotherapy of interstitial HSV keratitis (Bengal-Rose)

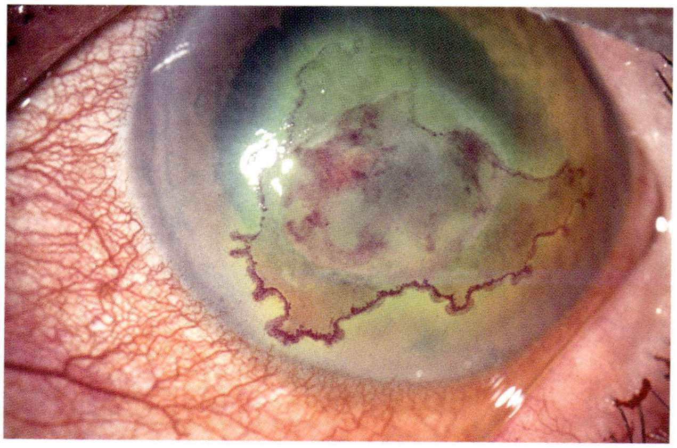

Fig. 2.53 Large geographic HSV keratitis as a complication of steroid-monotherapy of interstitial HSV keratitis (fluorescein and Bengal-Rose)

the patient must have felt that with diminishing infiltrations and slowly reappearing vision, the disturbing application of ointment so often per day was no longer necessary. The indispensable antiviral therapy was no longer correctly applied, which led to quick reappearance of new epithelial HSV lesions at the geographic outlines (new buddings), and it additionally led to a new separated HSV dendrite para-limbally at 3 o'clock.

***Differential diagnosis:*** None.

***Therapy:*** The first task must be improvement of patient's compliance. If otherwise impossible, such patients must be treated for a while in the hospital under strict control. Treatment consists of intensive systemic and topical antiviral therapy (ACV 800 mg 5 qd, ACV ointment every 2 hrs) plus moderately dosed systemic steroids and subconjunctival injections of small amounts of crystalline steroids, as outlined in Sect. 2.2. After epithelial closure of the ulcer, topical steroid therapy can be cautiously resumed as needed, and antiviral therapy can be reduced to topical application alone (5 qd). If the patient's compliance with the application of topical antiviral agents remains unreliable, a prolonged course with systemic antivirals (ACV 400 mg 4–5 qd) over a number of months is often the more successful therapeutic option.

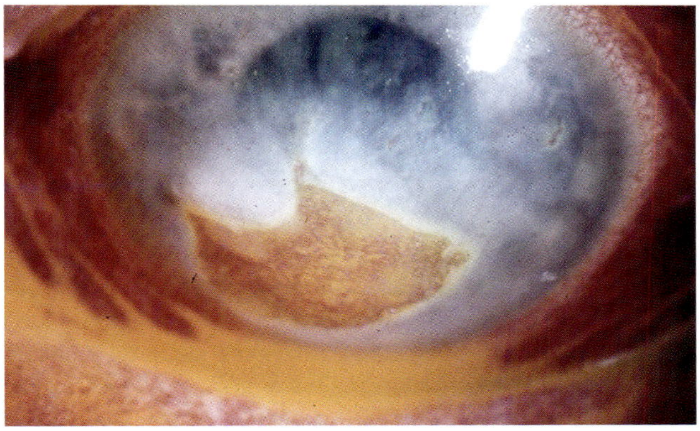

Fig. 2.54 Documentation of insufficient therapy in severe interstitial HSV keratitis (fluorescein and Bengal-Rose)

## Detailed analysis of Fig 2.55

***Clinic:*** Moderately deep oval stromal ulcer immediately adjacent to the limbus, painless (Fig. 2.55). Relatively sparse infiltration. Severe adjacent vascular reaction, still without significant transgression of the limbus. Anterior chamber normal.

***Diagnosis:*** Ulcerating interstitial HSV keratitis.

***Differential diagnosis:*** A previously verified HSV dendritic keratitis allows the diagnosis of ulcerating interstitial HSV keratitis. But also without such knowledge, an HSV etiology is strongly suggested by the absence of notable inflammation in the anterior chamber. A non-viral marginal ulcer usually has a limbus-parallel configuration and not a centrally directed one, as in this case.

***Therapy:*** Topical combination therapy with antiviral agents (preferably ACV ointment 5 qd) plus steroids (subconjunctival crystalline steroid injection to begin with, later switched to low-dosed topical steroids) will quickly result in healing.

## Detailed analysis of Fig 2.56

***Clinic:*** The density of the ball-shaped infiltrates in Fig. 2.56 resembles that in Fig. 2.47. In spite of this massive infiltration, the anterior chamber appears to be relatively normal. The lower part of the infiltration area is deeply ulcerated, but still without signs of imminent perforation. The deep corneal stroma and the pre-Descemet area are especially densely infiltrated. This may indicate the additional development of granulomatous reaction against Descemets.

***Differential diagnosis:*** As this is a known herpes eye, HSV etiology is definite. Bacterial and/or mycotic infections with such infiltrations would cause a greater anterior chamber reaction. Amebic stromal infection looks very different (see Fig. 2.65).

***Therapy:*** Because of the amount of infiltration and destruction, and because perforation must in any case at any cost be prohibited, maximal systemic plus topic combination therapy is necessary, with subconjunctival crystalline depots being repeatedly injected, until the ulcer has been recovered by epithelium (see Sect. 2.2).

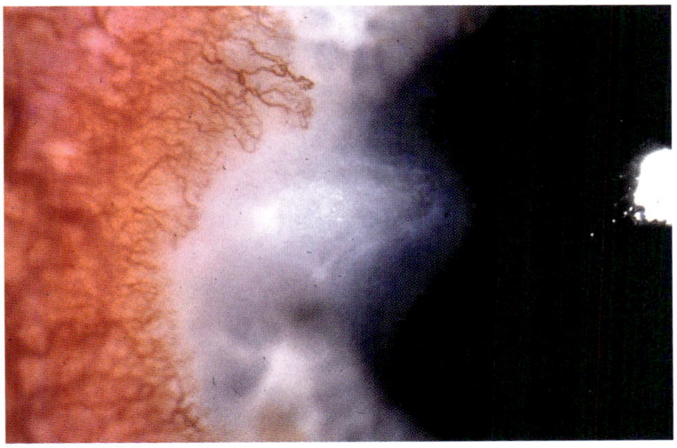

Fig. 2.55 Ulcerating interstitial HSV keratitis adjacent to the limbus

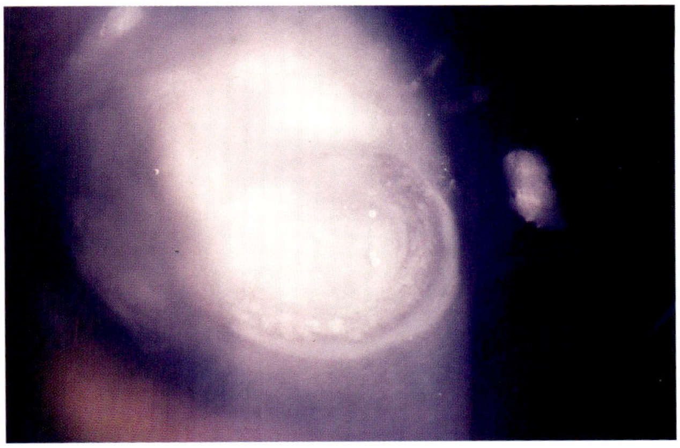

Fig. 2.56 Central interstitial ulcerating HSV keratitis with massive white infiltrates

## Detailed analysis of Fig 2.57

***Clinic:*** Massive diffuse white infiltrates adjacent to the limbus with correspondingly massive deep vascular ingrowth give a salmon-red appearance (Fig. 2.57). The upper part of the infiltration area is already invaded by vessels, and is deeply ulcerated with progressive evolvement of a descemetocele. The rest of the cornea and the anterior chamber are nearly unaffected.

***Diagnosis:*** Ulcerating interstitial HSV keratitis progressing to descemetocele with massive vascular ingrowth. Comparing the types of infiltration and the types of vascular reaction in Figs. 2.55 to 2.60 reveals striking differences in type and intensity of vascularisation. The causes of this are not always evident in the individual cases.

***Differential diagnosis:*** None from history and the biomicroscopic findings.

***Therapy:*** See Fig. 2.56.

## Analysis of Fig 2.58

Figure 2.58 demonstrates a constellation which is quite typical for ulcerating interstitial HSV keratitis, although by no means pathognomonic: subcentral circumscribed infiltrations seem to proceed to ulceration more often than infiltrations at other sites. Once an epithelial defect has formed, the stroma may so rapidly lyse, that a descemetocele develops within short time, e. g., after 10 days already. This has not been the case in Fig. 2.58. The vascular fan approaching the infiltration shows that vascular ingrowth must have gone on for some time already. The approaching vessels could not inhibit the melting process. It may even be that paracentral vessel fans of this kind, which do not grow into the infiltration area, even enhance ulceration by enforced leukocyte migration from the vessels into the ulcer, where they augment the lytic process by their freed enzymes. It is conspicuous that with metaherpetic paracentral epithelial erosions, the same constellation can be observed of vessel fans and not healing epithelial ulcers (see Sect. 2.11). If this speculation is correct, it might be helpful, if such vessels are therapeutically obliterated early enough. Once such a large descemetocele has developed, however, conservative therapy is no longer an option. One could seek resort in intermediate tectonic surgical measures, but an immediate definite surgical solution, i. e., perforating keratoplasty *à chaud*, would certainly be the best option (see Sect. 2.14).

## Detailed analysis of Fig 2.59

***Clinic:*** The infiltration area beneath the shallow large ulcer in Fig. 2.59 is composed of five round subcenters densely packed together like cobblestones. The lowest one, at 5 o'clock, has an especially white appearance, somehow "compact" and "chalky", which may be a sign of granulomatous reaction against Descemets. While the intensive conjunctival and episcleral injections reflect the severity of this chronic keratitis, the aqueous humor is stunningly free of inflammatory cells.

***Diagnosis:*** Chronically ulcerating interstitial HSV keratitis in an eye with multiple previous typical herpes recurrences. The chronicity and relative therapy resistance, which were observed in this case, are probably due to the presence of granulomatous reactions against Descemets.

***Differential diagnosis:*** None from history and from biomicroscopy. Any bacterial or mycotic infection of this extent would cause notable aqueous humor reactions or even hypopyon. As we deal here with ulcerating HSV keratitis only, and not with concomitant HSV iritis (which would in fact make differential diagnosis more difficult), the normal status of the anterior chamber practically proves HSV etiology. An amebic ulcer would have a different, more horizontal shape and could be further differentiated by its typical pain.

***Therapy:*** Although it is possible to "heal" this severe keratitis by conservative therapy or with assistance of additional intermediate tectonic measures – above all by an amnion cover – conservative therapy will not result in a great success. The suspected granulomatous reactions against Descemets will considerably prolong healing, and after many months of systemic and topical combination therapy, the eye will still be functionally mostly useless because of too much scarring and corneal distortion. Therefore, if the patient desires functional rehabilitation, *quick* keratoplasty à chaud must be advocated, which removes all cellular infiltrations

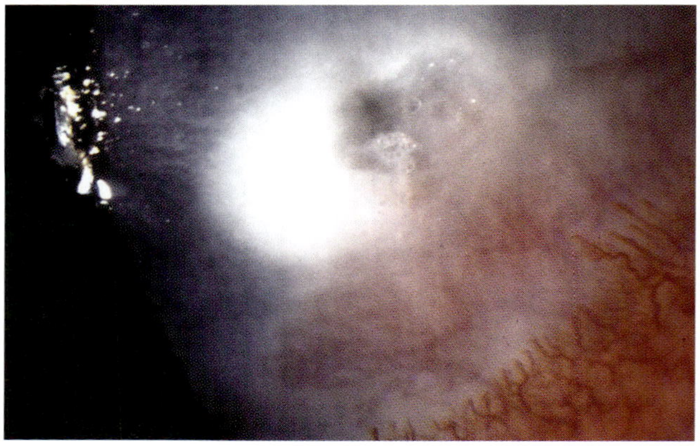

Fig. 2.57 Ulcerating interstitial HSV keratitis progressing to descemetocele with imminent perforation

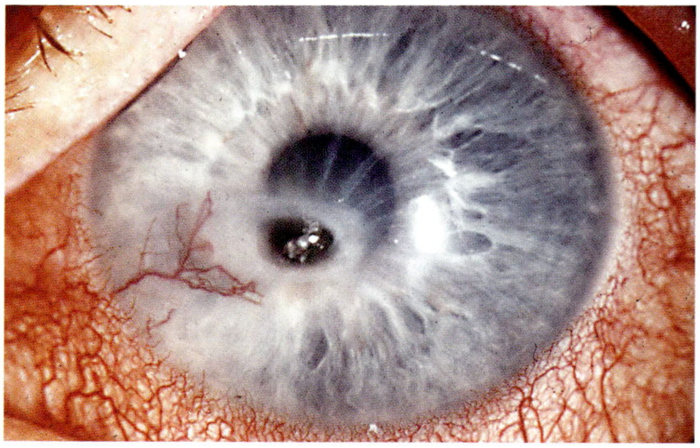

Fig. 2.58 Large descemetocele from ulcerating interstitial HSV keratitis

responsible for chronicity, restores function, and has a good prognosis, provided adequate post-keratoplasty therapy and controls can be organized (see Sect. 2.14).

## Analysis of Fig 2.60

Figure 2.60 was chosen to illustrate how the corneal aspect could appear after "healing" of a chronic ulcerating interstitial keratitis with granulomatous reaction against Descemets, as shown in Fig. 2.59. The ulcer has epithelized. The diffuse infiltrations are somewhat reduced, but large calibre vessels are still present. The granulomatous foci stick out from the surrounding still infiltrated areas like solid yellow-white knobbles. There is no noticeable tendency for them to disappear or shrink any further. The whole area has not really healed but still represents chronically persistent interstitial HSV keratitis plus multiple foci of therapy resistant granulomatous reactions. As such a cornea is functionally worthless and usually still requires a topical long-term steroid therapy to keep it "clinically quiet", the only good therapeutic advice in such cases is perforating keratoplasty.

## Analysis of Fig 2.61

Figure 2.61 shows a scarred herpes cornea. The white triangular area on the right comes from degenerative lipid and possibly also calcium deposition in the stromal scar. The pupillary area is not densely occluded, but the reading ability is already greatly diminished. In such a case, *elective* keratoplasty – ideally with an excellently matched corneal graft – can be advocated to restore function. Although even such quiet appearing corneas are rarely free of all inflammatory cells, and peripheral persistence of HSV must always be suspected, this does not reduce the good prognosis of keratoplasty, provided all necessary therapeutic and prophylactic measures can be taken after surgery. Waiting one or two years for the herpes cornea to become "quiet" before keratoplasty is finally performed, is an outdated rule. It is unnecessary and does not improve prognosis. Statistically, however, it is helpful to use a well HLA matched corneal graft for a better long-term prognosis (i. e., 10–20 years). If organizing that takes some extra time, the waiting time is well invested (see Sect. 2.14).

## Detailed analysis of Fig 2.62

***Clinic:*** Insidious appearance of disseminated nummuli without preceding typical epidemic keratoconjunctivitis is characteristic (Fig. 2.62). Not all nummuli are round or oval, some also "distorted". With the onset of healing, some of them take a shooting target appearance, which seems to be typical.

***Diagnosis:*** "Dimmers keratitis" remains a "morbus dubius". The original description raises too many questions to be absolutely reliable. It is clear, that adenoviruses are not the cause. The only other viruses that may unequivocally be correlated with this clinical picture in selected cases have been herpes simplex viruses. It seems, therefore, that clinical pictures, such as that in Fig. 2.62, must make us suspect HSV etiology, unless proven otherwise. In the case of Fig. 2.62, the herpes diagnosis remained

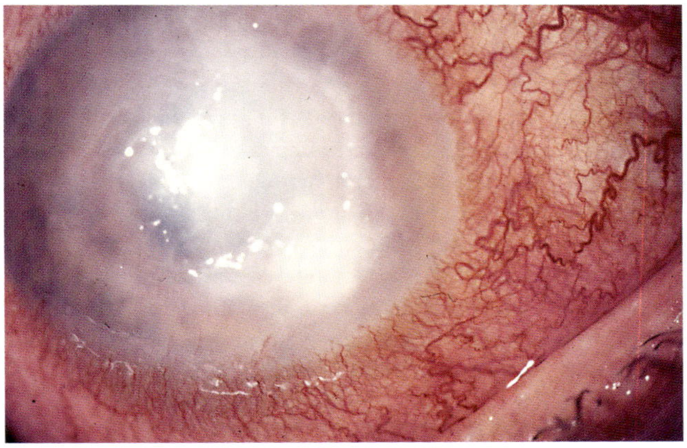

Fig. 2.59 Chronic ulcerating interstitial HSV keratitis with a large shallow ulceration containing presumably granulomatous reactions against Descemets

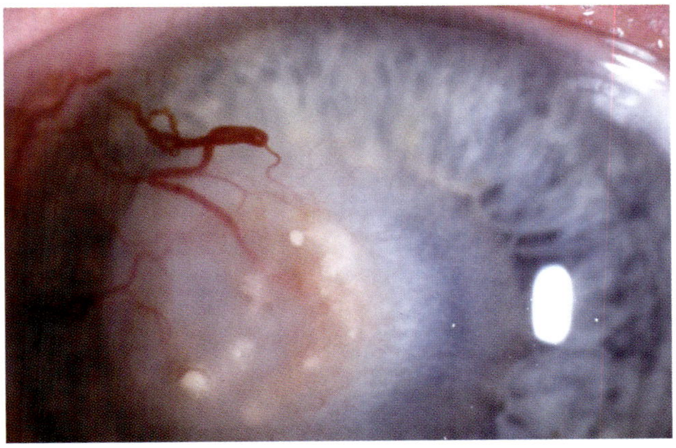

Fig. 2.60 Chronically smouldering, partly vascularized interstitial HSV keratitis with multiple foci of granulomatous reaction against Descemets

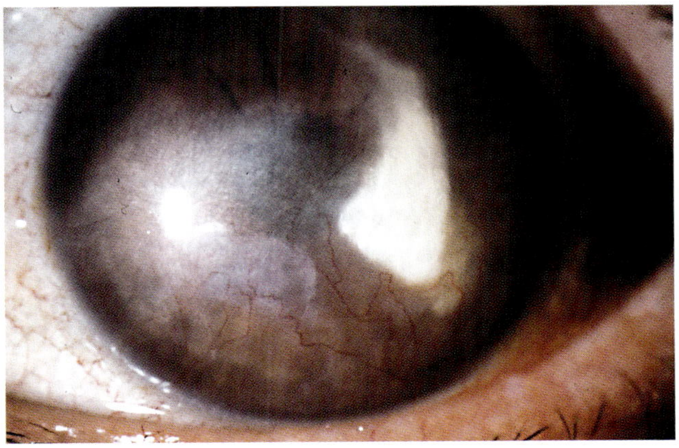

Fig. 2.61 Herpes scars with an area of dense lipid degeneration and residual shrunken corneal vessels after multiple attacks of interstitial HSV keratitis

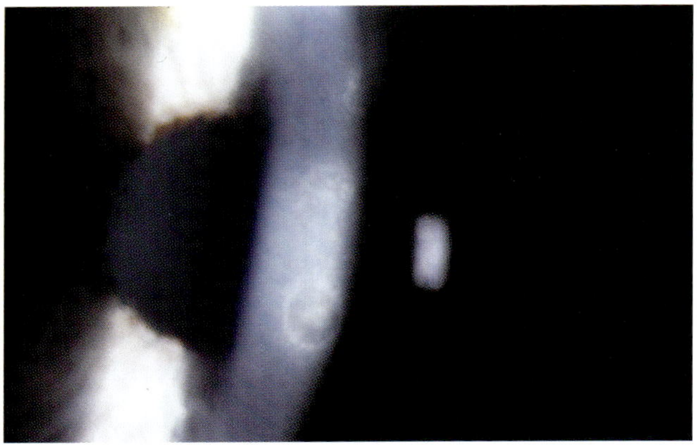

Fig. 2.62 "Dimmers nummular keratitis", a rare variant of interstitial HSV keratitis

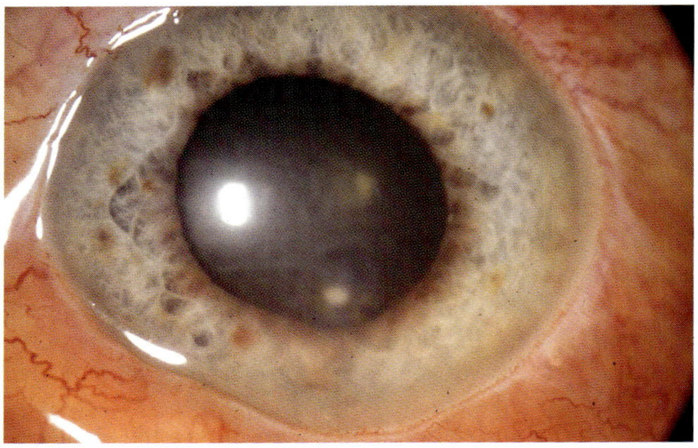

Fig. 2.63 Differential diagnosis: Bacterial keratitis with severe inflammatory reaction of the surrounding tissues

unsettled until the patient for a first time developed a classical dendritic HSV keratitis two years after Dimmers disease. For unkown reasons, the normal sequence of recurrences (first dendritic keratitis, and only thereafter interstitial HSV disease) was reversed in this case.

***Differential diagnosis:*** All diseases which can produce nummuli have to be considered, and above all: adenovirus diseases, VZV diseases, brucellosis, and chronic stromal immune reactions in corneal transplants.

***Therapy:*** Topical combination therapy with antiviral agents and steroids.

## Analysis of Fig 2.63

With the preceding cases, it was repeatedly pointed out that HSV interstitial keratitis – irrespective of how massive the infiltrations may be – does not lead to significant anterior chamber inflammatory reaction, unless such an inflammation comes from concomitant HSV iritis. In Fig. 2.63, this important differential diagnostic sign is underlined from the bacterial side: There is just one minor infiltration paracentrally at 6 o'clock. If this would be herpetic, the surrounding corneal tissues, the aqueous humor, and the conjunctiva would hardly show much reaction. In this case of bacterial infection, however, half of the cornea is severely edematous, as is the whole bulbar conjunctiva, and the aqueous humor shows a dense flare (not to be seen here). That is, in spite of minimal infiltration, we have a maximal "toxic" reaction of the surrounding tissues, and such reactions can never be of HSV origin.

## Analysis of Fig 2.64

The disease course in Fig. 2.64 demonstrates that hypopyon must never be mistaken as a sign of HSV disease. Either we deal primarily with bacterial or/and mycotic infections, or – as in this case – we deal with microbial *superinfection* of a herpes cornea: The *atopic* patient had suffered multiple recurrences of HSV keratitis and trabeculitis with finally chronic secondary glaucoma, which made a goniotrephination necessary (a). Interstitial HSV keratitis never healed completely, and HSV endotheliitis led to endothelial decompensation and corneal edema. This facilitated bacterial superinfection with rapid evolvement of a hypopyon (b). Intensive topical plus systemic antibiotic therapy stopped bacterial infection within a few days (c), and the hypopyon disappeared. As the incapacitated corneal endothelium would not allow a functional clearing of the cornea in spite of all conservative therapeutic efforts, it was decided to immediately perform a keratoplasty *à chaud* plus IOL implantation after surgical pupillary dilatation (d). The transplant could be kept clear without HSV recurrences until the patient's death 10 years later.

## Analysis of Fig 2.65

Amebic corneal infection may be misdiagnosed as herpes keratitis at all stages of development. At every stage, however, there are also relatively typical biomicroscopic signs for amebic etiology and, above all, the patients complain about *severe* pain. Pain is never a sign of HSV disease. Laboratory proof of amebic infection remains to be difficult. Many cases are only detected, therefore, in the course of histopathologic investigation of the excised corneal button after keratoplasty. Even then, less experienced pathologists have to be reminded beforehand of this potential etiology in order not to miss the diagnosis. With a corneal ulcer like that in Fig. 2.65, however, every experienced ophthalmologist would primarily suspect amebic etiology. It is the shape of this often deep central ulcer with the grey appearance of the thickened ulcer margins, together with relatively little infiltration and often together with an additional zone of chronic epithelial ulceration (from 3 to 6 o'clock), which make a difference to ulcerating interstitial HSV keratitis. There is no difference, however, as to a rather restricted inflammatory reaction in the anterior chamber. In this respect, HSV and amebic keratitis are mostly indistinguishable.

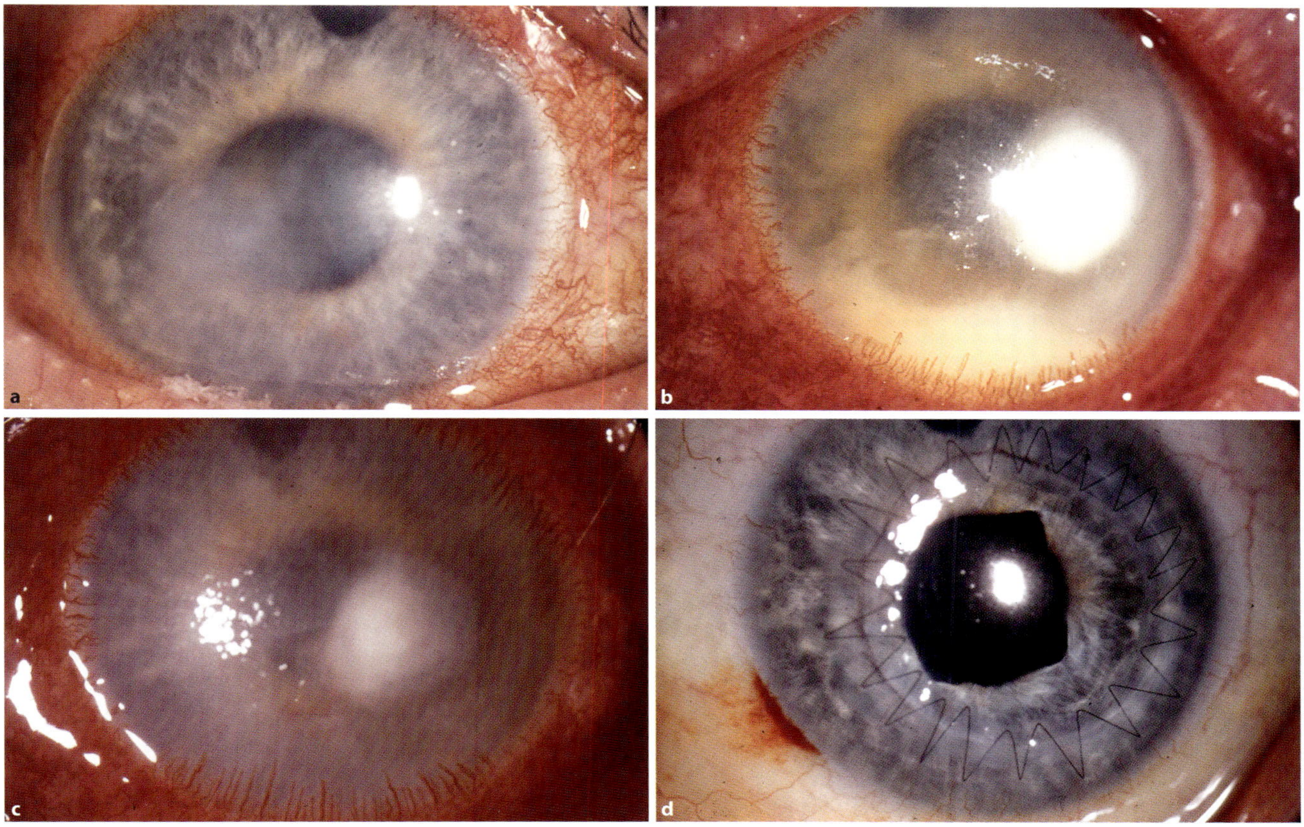

Fig. 2.64a–d Differential diagnosis: Bacterial superinfection in a herpes eye with chronic secondary glaucoma after multiple interstitial and intraocular HSV recurrences (**a** herpes scars, **b** infiltration and hypoypon from superinfection, **c** superinfection successfully treated, **d** three months after triple procedure)

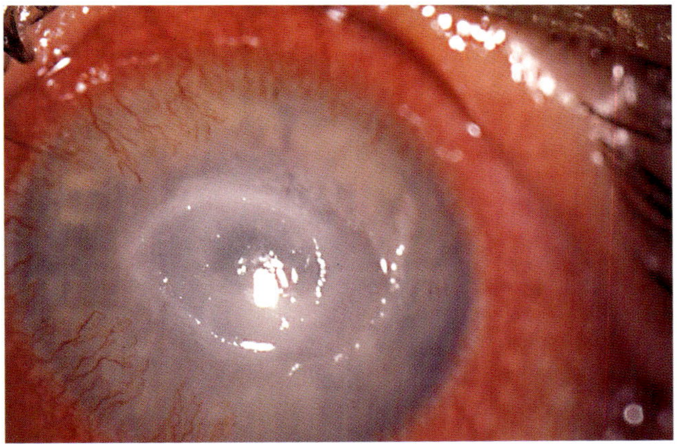

Fig. 2.65 Differential diagnosis: Chronic amebic ulcer

## References


Ahonen R, Vannas A, Mäkitie J (1984) Virus particles and leukocytes in herpes simplex keratitis. Cornea 3: 43–50

Babu JS, Thomas J, Kanagat S, Morrison LA, Knipe DM, Rouse BT (1996) Viral replication is required for induction of ocular immunopathology by herpes simplex virus. J Virol 70: 101–107

Banerjee K, Biswas PS, Kamaragurn U, Schoenberger SP, Rouse BT (2004) Protective and pathological roles of virus-specific and bystander CD8+ T cells in herpetic stromal keratitis. J Immunol 173: 7575–7583

Barney NP, Foster CS (1994) A prospective randomised trial for oral acyclovir after penetrating keratoplasty for herpes simplex keratitis. Cornea 13: 232–236

Brik D, Dunkel E, Pavan-Langston D (1994) Persistent herpes simplex virus in the corneal stroma despite topical and systemic antiviral therapy. Arch Ophthalmol 111: 1883–1896

Coster DJ (1978) Herpetic keratitis and corneal destruction. Trans Ophthalmol Soc UK 98: 372–376

Easty DL, Shimeld C, Claoue CMP, Menage M (1987) Herpes simplex virus isolation in chronic stromal keratitis: human and laboratory studies. Curr Eye Res 6: 69–74

Hendricks RL (1997) An immunologist´s view of herpes simplex keratitis: Thygeson lecture 1996. Cornea 16: 503–506

Hendricks RL, Tumpey TM (1990) Contribution of virus and immune factors to herpes simplex type-1 induced corneal pathology. Invest Ophthalmol Vis Sci 30: 1929–1939

Hendricks RL, Tumpey TM, Finnegan A (1992) IFN gamma and IL-2 are protective in the skin but pathologic in the corneas of HSV-1 infected mice. J Immunol 149: 3023–3008

Herpetic Eye Disease Study Group (1994) A controlled trial of oral acyclovir for herpes simplex stromal keratitis. Ophthalmol 101: 1871–1882

Herpetic Eye Disease Study Group (1994) A controlled trial of topical corticosteroids for herpes simplex stromal keratitis. Ophthalmology 101: 1883–1896

Herpetic Eye Disease Study Group (1996) Risk factors for herpes simplex virus epithelial keratitis recurring during treatment of stromal keratitis or iridocyclitis. Br J Ophthalmol 80: 969–972

Holbach LM, Font RL, Baehr W, Pittler SJ (1991) HSV antigens and HSV DNA in avascular and vascularized lesions of human herpes simplex keratitis. Curr Eye Res 10 Suppl: 63–68

Holbach LM, Font RL, Nauman GOH (1990) Herpes simplex stromal and endothelial keratitis. Granulomatous cell reactions at the level of Descemet´s membrane, the stroma, and Bowman´s layer. Ophthalmology 97: 722–728

Johns KJ, O´Day DM, Head WS, Neff RJ, Elliott JH (1987) Herpes simplex masquerade syndrome: acanthamoeba Keratitis. Curr Eye Res 6: 207–212

Kaye SB, Baker K, Bonshek R, Maseruka H, Grinfeld E, Tullo A, Easty DL, Hart CA (2000) Human herpesviruses in the cornea. Br J Ophthalmol 84: 563–571

Kortüm GF, Seibel W, Völcker HE, Naumann GOH (1981) Zur Klinik der granulomatösen Reaktion gegn Descemetsche Membran. In: R Sundmacher (ed) Herpetic Eye Diseases. Bergmann, Munich, pp 163–166

Mathers WD, Goldberg MA, Sutphin JE, Ditkoff JW, Folberg R (1997) Coexistent Acanthamoeba keratitis and herpetic keratitis. Arch Ophthalmol 115: 714–718

Mauriello JA Jr, McLean IW, Riddle PJ (1995) Granulomatous reaction to Bowman´s layer in herpetic keratitis and band keratopathy. Can J Ophthalmol 30: 203–207

Metcalf JF, Kaufman HE (1976) Herpetic stromal keratitis – Evidence for cell-mediated immunopathogenesis. Am J Ophthalmol 82: 827–834

Metcalf JF, Hamilton DS, Reichert RW (1979) Herpetic keratitis in athymic (nude) mice. Infect Immune 26: 1164–1171

Meyers-Elliott RH, Chitjian PA (1981) Immunopathogenesis of corneal inflammation in herpes simplex virus stromal keratitis: role of the polymorphonuclear leucocyte. Invest Ophthalmol Vis Sci 20: 784–798

Niemialtowski MG, Rouse BT (1992) Predominance of Th1 cells in ocular tissues during herpetic stromal keratitis. J Immunol 149: 3035–3039

Sabbaga EM, Pavan-Langston D, Bean KM, Dunkel EC (1988) Detection of HSV nucleic acid sequences in the cornea during acute and latent ocular disease. Exp Eye Res 47: 545–553

Seitzman GD, Strauss EC, Margolis TP (2006) "Steel wool keratopathy": a clinical sign of chronic inflammation. Cornea 25: 742–744

Shimeld C, Tullo AB, Easty DL, Thomsit J (1982) Isolation of herpes simplex virus from the cornea in chronic stromal keratitis. Brit J Ophthalmol 66: 643–647

Streilein JW, Dana MR, Ksander BR (1997) Immunity causing blindness: five different paths to herpes stromal keratitis. Immunology Today 18: 443–449

Sundmacher R (1978) Trifluorthymidinprophylaxe bei der Steroidtherapie herpetischer Keratouveitiden. Klin Monatsbl Augenheilk 173: 516–519

Teitelbaum CS, Streeten BW, Dawson CR (1987) Histopathology of herpes simplex virus keratouveitis. Curr Eye Res 6: 189–194

Thomas J, Gangappa S, Kanangat S, Rouse BT (1997) On the essential involvement of neutrophils in the immunopathologic disease: Herpetic stromal keratitis. J Immunol 158: 1383–1391

Tullo AB, Easty DL, Hill TJ (1985) Isolation of herpes simplex virus from corneal discs of patients with chronic stromal keratitis. Trans Ophthalmol Soc UK 104: 159

Van Bijsterveld OP, Obster R (1983) Keratitis nummularis Dimmer, Morbus dubius. Klin Monatsbl Augenheilkd 183: 169–172

Wilhelmus KR, Coster DJ, Donovan HC, Falcon MG, Jones BR (1981) Prognosis indicators of herpetic keratitis. Analysis of a five-year observation period after corneal ulceration. Arch Ophthalmol 99: 1578–1582

Wilhelmus KR, Dawson CR, Barron BA, Bacchetti P, Gee L, Jones BR, Kaufman HE, Sugar J, Hyndiuk RA, Laibson PR, Stulting RD, Asbell PA (1996) Risk factors for herpes simplex virus epithelial keratitis recurring during treatment of stromal keratitis or iridocyclitis. Br J Ophthalmol 80: 969–972

Witschel H, Orsoni J (1981) Granulomatous keratitis and its relationship to herpetic disease. In: R Sundmacher (ed) Herpetic Eye Diseases. Bergmann, Munich, pp 167–173

Witschel H, Sundmacher R, Seitz HM (1984) Amebic keratitis. A clinico-histopathologic case report. Klin Monatsbl Augenheilkd 185: 46–49

# HSV Endotheliitis and Disciform Keratitis

Section

2.7

## Core Messages

- HSV infection of corneal endothelial cells leads to endotheliitis with circumscribed areas of edematous endothelium marked by *endotheliitic immune-precipitates*, which specifically adhere to HSV-antigens expressed in infected cells.

- *Iritic precipitates*, on the contrary, have no specific immunologic attraction to endothelial cells. They simply sediment – without any immunologic binding – on those endothelial cells which they touch while floating in the thermal currents of the aqueous, and they cause no cell damage. This leads to a triangular distribution in iritis with the largest precipitates at the base.

- In its beginning, HSV endotheliitis leads only to circumscribed endothelial cell edema. Hydration control of the cornea is then still sufficient. With increasing endothelial dysfunction, the aqueous barrier breaks and frank *corneal* edema evolves. It is topographically confined to the area of endothelial infection and dysfunction.

- *Endotheliitis is often combined with topographically associated interstitial HSV keratitis*, leading to an edematous corneal disc with significant interstitial cellular infiltration. Such a combination of deep HSV "sandwich disease" is traditionally called *disciform keratitis*.

- Persistant interstitital HSV disease in the corneal stroma has no specific biomicroscopic characteristics. This makes therapeutic control extremely difficult. Persistent HSV endotheliitis, on the contrary, is easily identifiable by the immuno-precipitates which mark the persistently infected endothelial cells. We can thus judge whether or not persistent infection in endothelial cells is still a problem. This makes therapy in HSV endotheliitis and disciform keratitis relatively reliable.

The term "endotheliitis" needs some introductory explanation because there may be difficulties in accepting the ending "itis", i.e., inflammation, for disease of an avascular cellular monolayer. How can an avascular monolayer become inflamed if inflammatory vascular reactions – one of the classical criteria of inflammation – cannot directly affect this layer? The explanation is that "endotheliitis" in this special situation is used in the restricted sense as "immune inflammation" or "immune endotheliitis" only. It applies to cellular immune attacks on endothelial cells which are in their outer membranes marked with "foreign" antigens. In the case of HSV endotheliitis, we deal with HSV antigens in the cell membranes. The immune attacks are exerted by immune cells floating in the aqueous humor. As soon as these primed immune cells come into contact with their target receptor in an endothelial cell membrane, they adhere specifically to this marked cell. They start their demolition work and, by their presence, they biomicroscopically mark the infected cells. No direct vascular contribution is needed for such an "immune endotheliitis".

HSV endotheliitis is just one endotheliitis among many others. The "foreign" antigens in the cell membranes vary. However, the basic pathophysiology is the same. Therefore, all types of endotheliitis look clinically similar. Not only HSV, but also VZV and CMV, cause endotheliitis (see Sect. 3.5 and Chap. 4). Also other viruses may infect the endothelium. The most often observed ones are adenoviruses. Another "foreign" antigen situation arises after perforating corneal transplantation. Then, foreign HLA antigens are the target for cellular immune attacks on the transplant endothelium. Autoimmune reactions against the host's own endothelium seem to be another type of endotheliitis, though a rare one. HSV and VZV endotheliitis are normally easy to diagnose.

HSV endotheliitis may develop independently of other associated HSV disease in the anterior segment of the eye, but very rarely so. Most often, it arises in combination with interstitial HSV keratitis, with HSV iritis, and with HSV trabeculitis. As the latter three regularly tend to mask the coexistence of HSV endotheliitis, the endothelium must always be carefully checked for signs of coexisting endotheliitis. If overlooked, acute endotheliitis may rapidly destruct so much of this layer that irreversible metaherpetic bullous keratopathy results (see Sect. 2.11). More often, however, HSV leads to a chronically persistent endothelial infection with frequently recurring circumscribed corneal edema, which finally also leads to irreversible bullous keratopathy.

The most frequent combination of HSV diseases of the eye is that of HSV endotheliitis plus topographically correlated interstitial HSV keratitis. As the diseased area often has a disciform appearance, this disease was historically named disciform keratitis. Moreover, as the coexisting HSV endotheliitis went unnoticed until some decades ago, disciform keratitis is still today considered by some as an exclusively stromal disease. Historic names have their own right and can rarely be altered. It should be common knowledge by now, however, that behind the opaque stromal disc of disciform keratitis, another plane of HSV disease is regularly present and needs special attention. This is HSV endotheliitis.

## Detailed analysis of Fig 2.66

***Clinic:*** Two small linear dendrites lie in the pupillary area (Fig. 2.66). A closer microscopic look possible in this picture would disclose typical features of HSV etiology. Considerable mixed injection. Lower half of the cornea slightly edematous. No endothelial precipitates visible. Aqueous humor almost normal. Intraocular pressure (digitally estimated) suspected to be higher than in the partner eye.

***Diagnosis:*** Dendritic HSV keratitis plus beginning HSV endotheliitis. The classical biomicroscopic features of endotheliitis are still lacking in this early phase, but the diagnosis can already be made with great certainty:

- The mixed injection is too intensive to be caused only by the two small dendrites. Some additional deep disease is, therefore, very probable.
- The circumscribed faint edema visible from 3 over 6 to 7 o'clock in the lower half of the cornea can only have a circumscribed endothelial cause.
- The most probable reason for localized endothelial dysfunction in combination with HSV dendritic keratitis is HSV endotheliitis.
- In the very beginning of HSV endotheliitis, reactive immune attacks are still building up and are not yet biomicroscopically visible. In this early stage, viral cytolysis alone leads to some functional incapacitation of the infected endothelial cells. If destructive enough, it may lead to subtle corneal edema without additional immunologic cell destruction. In this special case, circumscribed corneal edema developed so quickly and massively (not shown here), that the typical endotheliitic precipitates became only visible after the cornea had cleared again under efficient therapy many days later.
- Elevated intraocular pressure, which is regularly associated with intraocular HSV replication and thus may also be a sign of acute HSV endotheliitis, must not be so high as to be easily diagnosed by digital palpation, especially not in the early phase of the disease (see Sect. 2.8).

***Differential diagnosis:*** None.

***Therapy:*** The extended circumscribed edema in this early phase indicates an aggressive course of the endotheliitis and calls for primary use of maximally dosed systemic antiviral therapy together with topical antivirals. As endotheliitic precipitates are not yet visible, it is possible to refrain from steroids in this early phase of endotheliitis and it is possible to treat with antivirals only until the dendrites have disappeared. As soon as this is the case, however, topical steroids must be added starting with 2 drops qd and possibly not exceeding 3 (4) drops qd, while maintaining maximal antiviral treatment until complete healing has occurred. Thereafter, the combination therapy can be gradually tapered out as described in Sect. 2.6.

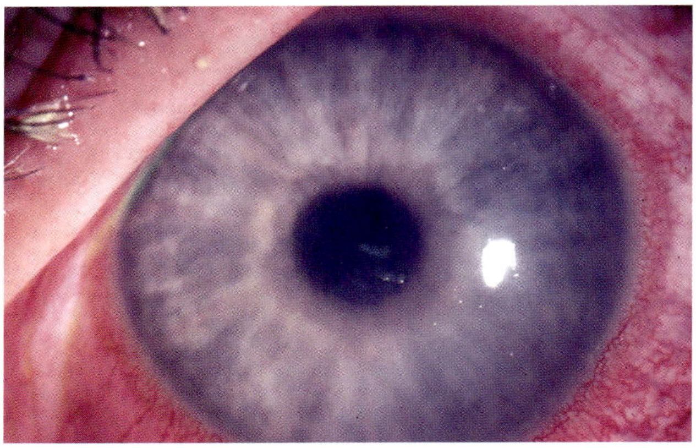

Fig. 2.66 Small HSV dendrites plus beginning HSV endotheliitis (fluorescein)

## Detailed analysis of Fig 2.67

***Clinic:*** Extended multifocal area of corneal edema composed of several rounded areas plus one area touching the limbus on the left (Fig. 2.67). Especially in this latter area, grey small precipitates are visible, and they are strictly confined to the edema. No precipitates are present in areas where the cornea is normal and transparent, especially not in the lower half at 6 o'clock. The corneal stroma is mostly free of cellular infiltrates. Therapeutic mydriasis. Aqueous humor with some cells only. Intraocular pressure 20 mm Hg, compared to 14 mm Hg in the normal partner eye. Minimal mixed injection.

***Diagnosis:*** Extended HSV endotheliitis under combination treatment with antivirals plus steroids.

***Differential diagnosis:*** None. Even if this eye would not have been known as herpes eye, there is practically no differential diagnosis of HSV disease. We deal with the relatively rare case of pure HSV endotheliitis. More frequently, endotheliitis is combined with either interstitial HSV disease (see disciform keratitis), which is not the case here (no interstititial infiltrates). There is also no combination with HSV iritis (iritic precipitates are clearly absent, they should have aggregated on the endothelium at 6 o'clock in a triangular fashion, see Sect. 2.9). Intraocular pressure rise, as found here, is a typical sign for intraocular HSV replication in the anterior segment (see Sect. 2.8), and thus confirms HSV endotheliitis.

***Therapy:*** Combination therapy with systemic plus topical antiviral agents and topical steroids has already shown effectiveness. Most of the injection has already disappeared and the corneal edema begins to disappear. The stage of disease in Fig. 2.67 is about the same as that seen after 10 days of treatment of the early endotheliitis in Fig. 2.66.

## Detailed analysis of Fig 2.68

The ultimate biomicroscopic criterion and marker for corneal endotheliitis is a cellular immune attack on antigens in the cell mem-

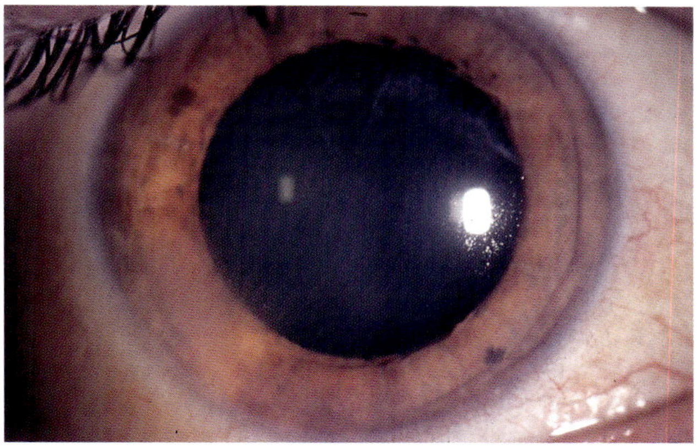

Fig. 2.67 Large area of corneal edema from acute HSV endotheliitis with typically located immune precipitates under combination therapy

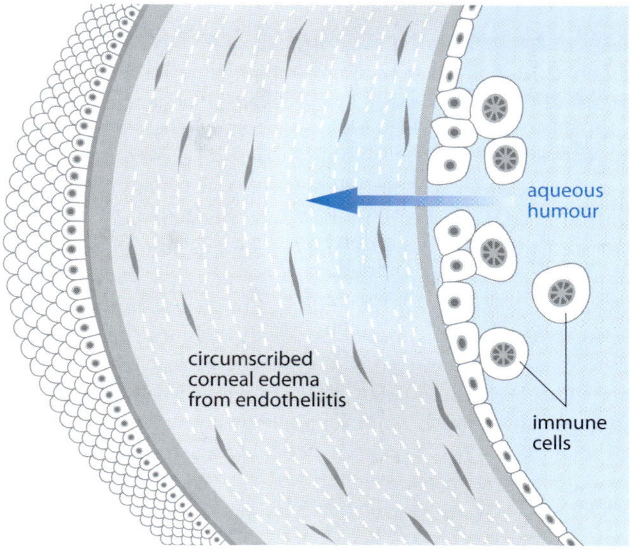


Fig. 2.68 Schematic characteristics of endotheliitis with cellular immune attacks

brane of corneal endothelial cells (Fig. 2.68). In the beginning, this immune attack leads only to endothelial *cell* edema, which is visible with special slit lamp techniques or endothelial microscopes only. In this early stage, the cornea is still transparent. When endothelial cell damage becomes severe and widespread enough, the aqueous humor barrier breaks, and frank *corneal* edema develops. Edema as well as endotheliitic precipitates are always strictly topographically correlated. This is the first important difference from iritic precipitates, which follow physical sedimentation rules without specific attraction to marked cells. The second important difference is the cell-damaging action of endotheliitic precipitates, while iritic precipitates normally lie "innocently" on the endothelium without doing harm. Accordingly, iritic precipitates show no correlation with edema (see Sect. 2.9).

While the foregoing description applies to every endotheliitis (e.g., also for immune reactions against donor antigens), an endotheliitis of viral origin, e.g., an HSV endotheliitis, shows the *additional characteristic* that endothelial dysfunction does not only result from secondary immune attacks but also from *primary viral cytolysis*. This viral effect may be quite variable. In acute aggressive cases like that in Fig. 2.66, viral cytolysis by itself may suffice to cause corneal edema. More often, however, viral cytolysis is only moderate or even only borderline, i.e., development of significant corneal edema more often needs the *potentiating* cell damage by immune attacks. This pathophysiologic background explains the need for full-dose antiviral therapy in order to stop HSV replication and antigen expression as quickly as possible, and it explains also the need for adequately dosed steroids in order to reduce the dangerous immune cytolysis as much as possible.

Theoretically, an endotheliitis can also develop if only *humoral* immune attacks incapacitate the corneal endothelium. In this case, no precipitates would develop, which would serve as a reliable marker for endotheliitis. The clinical appearance of early endotheliitis, as shown in Fig. 2.66, would be a lasting one. To my knowledge, such pure humoral cases have not been identified with certainty, and to date it remains questionable whether or not they exist.

## Analysis of Fig 2.69

Figure 2.69 shows the characteristic correlation of endotheliitic precipitates with corneal edema. The precipitates become visible only at the borders of the edematous area. They cover, of course, the whole backside. An undisturbed look at them is impossible because of too dense corneal edema. The transparency of the diseased corneal area is further reduced by a beginning interstitial invasion of immune cells as a sign of coexistent interstitial HSV keratitis, especially paracentrally at 8 o'clock. The combination of HSV endotheliitis plus interstitial HSV keratitis is historically addressed as disciform keratitis. If the interstitial component is lacking and we deal with endotheliitic edema only, as in the right part of Fig. 2.69, such disease has also been called "disciform edema", which is another historic name.

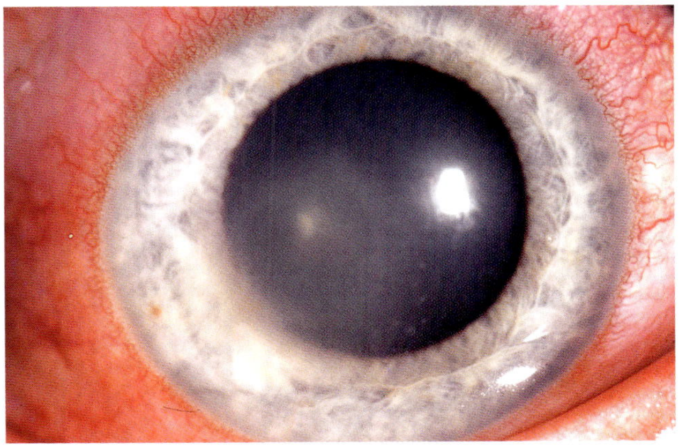

Fig. 2.69 Large multifocal area of HSV endotheliitis, early disciform keratitis

## Analysis of Fig 2.70

Figure 2.70 is the rare document of an acute HSV endotheliitis showing the whole diseased central corneal area covered by endotheliitic precipitates of various sizes. It seems that endotheliitis began subcentrally at 6 o'clock, where the precipitates are largest and most dense. From there, endothelial HSV infection has spread in all directions with the borders between diseased and non-diseased areas marked by a line of fine precipitates similar to Khodadoust's line in endothelial immune reactions after homologous keratoplasty. The large size of precipitates in the disease center indicates that quite some time must have elapsed before therapy finally started. The relatively clear view of most of the still densely packed precipitates after only 5 days of treatment indicates that there is no major additional interstitial infiltration. Accordingly, there is a good chance that consequent therapy will lead to nearly complete clearing of the cornea. Sufficiently many endothelial cells will presumably survive to rebuild a functioning aqueous barrier.

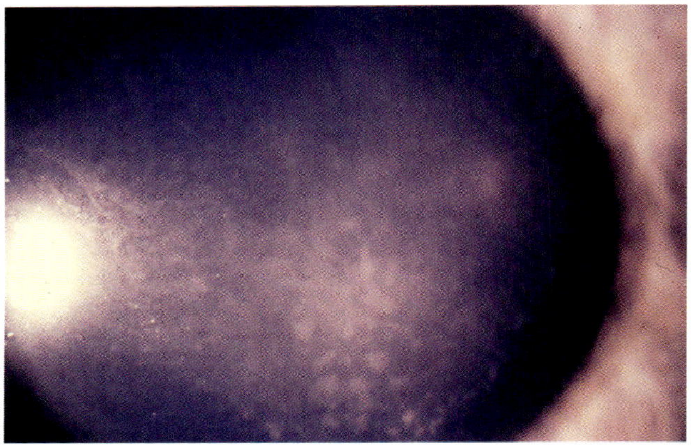

Fig. 2.70 Acute HSV endotheliitis after 5 days of combination treatment

## Analysis of Fig 2.71

The cloudiness of the diseased area in Fig. 2.71 is nearly exclusively caused by corneal edema from HSV endotheliitis. Significant stromal infiltrates are not present. This is prognostically positive, because consequent therapy will restore a mostly clear cornea. Also, it makes therapeutic decisions easy, because we can rely on the disappearance or persistence of endotheliitic precipitates. A recommendable rule is the following: treatment (e.g., ACV ointment 5 qd plus steroid ointment 2–3 qd) has to be maintained at full dose well beyond the date (about 2 weeks longer) when the last precipitate disappeared. Only thereafter, therapy should be tapered out over another 3 weeks. In case just one persisting precipitate is overlooked or ignored and therapy erroneously finished too early, persistent HSV endotheliitis may result with prompt flare-up of inflammation once steroids are withdrawn.

## Analysis of Fig 2.72

Figure 2.72 shows classic disciform HSV keratitis. A swollen, opaque corneal disc is surrounded by clear cornea. The disc is too cloudy to be caused by edema alone. Additionally, infiltrates of still low degree of interstitial HSV keratitis are present. The borders of the discs are marked by clearly visible endotheliitic precipitates. There are no iritic precipitates. The aqueous contains only a few cells. Therapy is the same as outlined above for pure endothelial disease. Also, for this "sandwich disease", the observation of persistence or disappearance of endotheliitic precipitates serves as a reliable indicator for correct adaptation of therapy in the course of healing. The infiltrates of interstitial keratitis will mostly leave a faint disciform scar. The perfect disciform shape of such a lesion may be explained by an initially small infectious focus of infection in the endothelium which spreads without hindrance in all directions until finally halted by immune reactions. Unlike the epithelium, where natural and immunologic defence mechanisms are easily available everywhere, and where epithelial cell regeneration is very effective, endothelium has no quick response regeneration, and natural as well as immunologic defences are not as readily available. This probably explains why in the epithelium we deal with dendritic lesions, while in the endothelial monolayer such dendritic configurations cannot arise because there are no

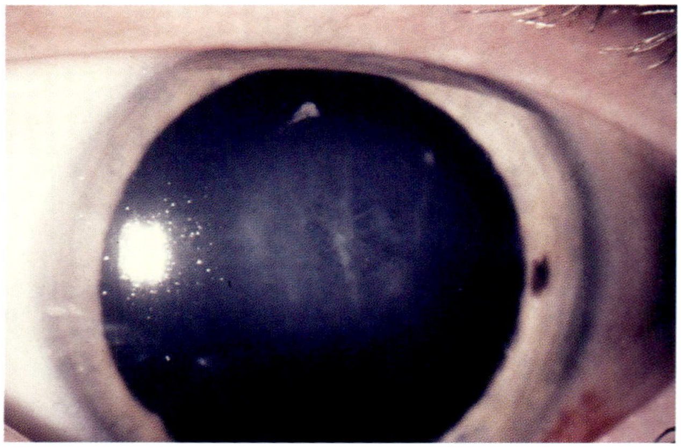

Fig. 2.71 Therapeutically much improved HSV endotheliitis, therapy still needed for a few more weeks

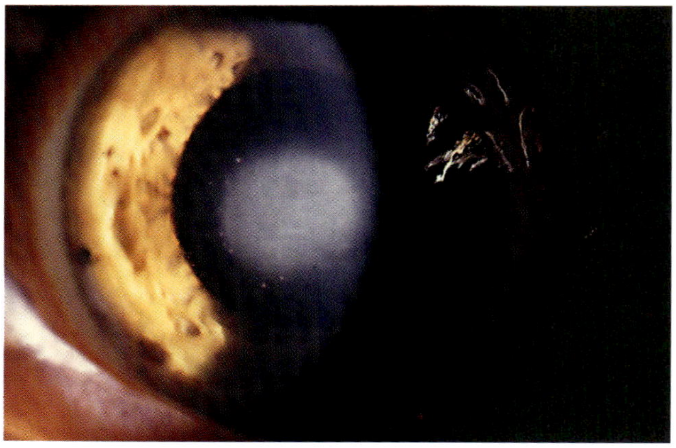

Fig. 2.72 Small diameter disciform HSV keratitis

equivalent modelling regenerative movements of the endothelium. Instead, primarily unhindered infectious expansion in the endothelium leads to a perfect disciform shape.

## Analysis of Fig 2.73

If significant stromal infiltration makes the observation of endotheliitic precipitates difficult, as in Fig. 2.73, it is recommended to maintain full efficiency combination therapy as long as a reduction in disc opacity is observed. This may take weeks or even months. Often, the stromal infiltrates clear so much that the endotheliitic precipitates then become visible for the first time. From then on, they can serve as a reliable indicator for further guidance of therapy.

## Analysis of Fig 2.74

Figure 2.74 shows that the combination of HSV endotheliitis and HSV interstitial keratitis must not always manifest itself in the classical configuration of disciform keratitis. It also occurs in irregular topographic combinations. That may have its explanation in a more diffuse or multifocal endothelial and interstitial infection. Again, biomicroscopically controllable endotheliitic precipitates serve as the best indicator for guidance of therapy.

## Analysis of Fig 2.75

Figure 2.75 is a historic document from the times when no efficient antiviral therapy was available for deep herpetic disease, and steroid monotherapy was the only alternative to no therapy at all. The latter regularly led to prominent disciform scars, often vascularized. Steroid monotherapy, on the contrary, led to symptomatic removal of infiltrating cells and, thus, to an often impressive clearance of the disc. However, this clearance was rarely lasting. One complication of symptomatic steroid monotherapy was HSV persistence in the stroma and endothelium with ever-recurring inflammations after each withdrawal of the steroids. The other frequent complication was dendritic keratitis. With nowadays available combination therapy of full dose antiviral agents plus variably dosed steroids, such developments, as in Fig. 2.75, can no longer occur. If they do, something has gone wrong, if not with therapy design in general, then certainly with the compliance.

## Analysis of Fig 2.76

Figure 2.76 is a historic document of a vascularized dense disciform scar after spontaneous healing of severe disciform keratitis. Similar scars arise, if acute disciform keratitis does not heal, but turns into chronic persistent infection. With access to modern combination therapy and with adequate compliance, such functionally incapacitating scars should become a rare exemption.

## Analysis of Fig 2.77

Figure 2.77 is a reminder that clinically "quiet" corneal herpes scars, such as in Fig. 2.76, are often by no means quiet. Not only do they regularly contain inflammatory cells, they may also contain the herpes simplex virus, in whatever complete or molecular form. Here, virus particles can be seen indicating that in this recipient cornea, which was excised in the course of perforating keratoplasty, there was ongoing HSV replication, presumably in the form

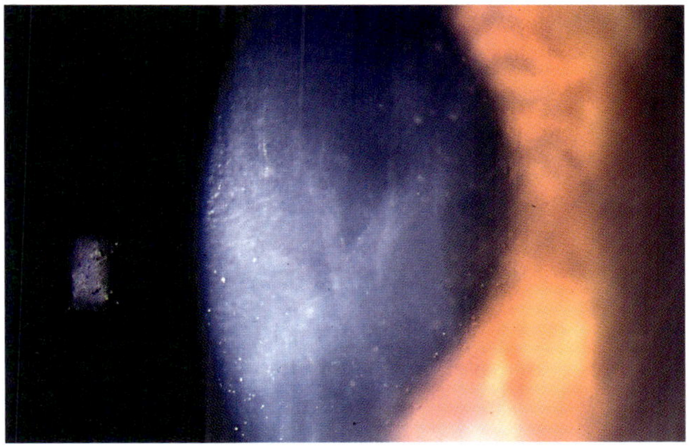

Fig. 2.74 Diffuse interstitial HSV keratitis plus HSV endotheliitis without disciform configuration

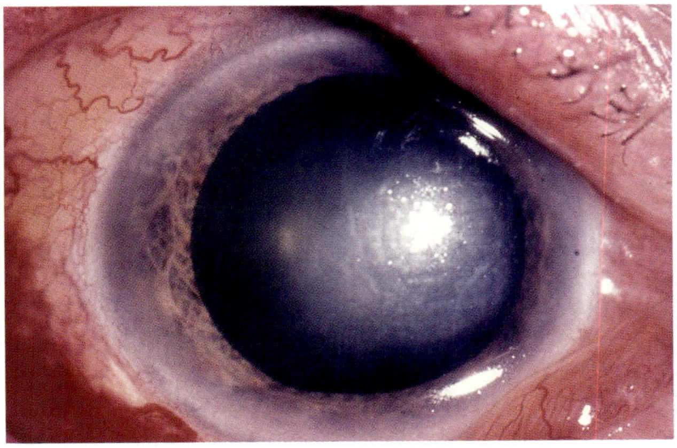

Fig. 2.73 Disciform keratitis with significant stromal infiltration

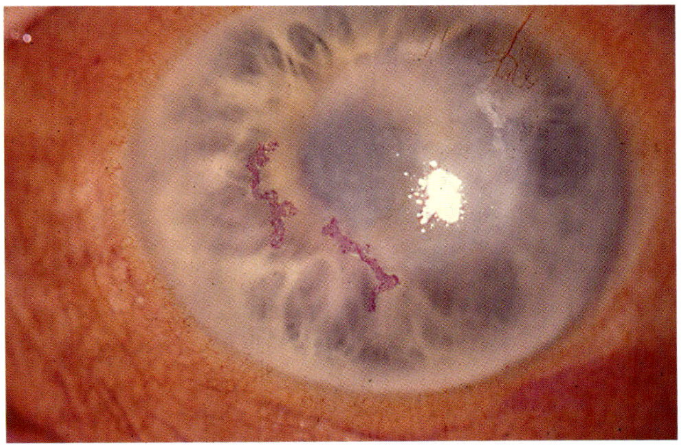

Fig. 2.75 Dendritic keratitis as a complication of steroid monotherapy of disciform keratitis (Bengal rose)

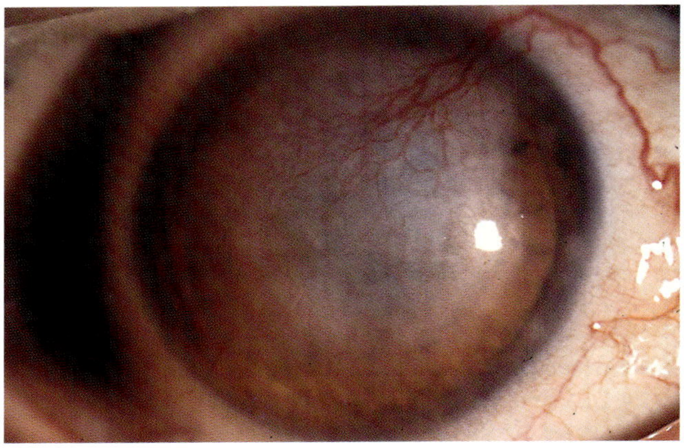

Fig. 2.76 Vascularized scar after multiple recurrences of HSV disciform keratitis

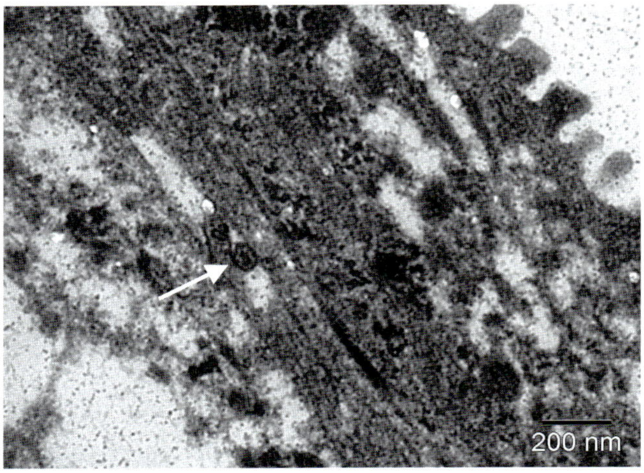


Fig. 2.77 Electron microscopy: HSV particles in the corneal stroma of a case similar to that in Fig. 2.76 (courtesy of Claudia Auw-Hädrich M. D.)

of chronically persistent HSV disease. With keratoplasty, we have a chance to remove circumscribed areas of persisting HSV disease, and with adequate post-surgical therapy, persistent HSV disease does not seem to be an unsolvable problem (see Sect. 2.14).

## References


Collin HB, Abelson MB (1976) Herpes simplex virus in human cornea, retrocorneal fibrous membrane and vitreous. Arch Ophthalmol 94: 1726–1729

Collum LMT, Grant DM (1987) A double-blind comparative trial of acyclovir and adenine arabinoside in combination with dilute betamethasone in the management of herpetic disciform keratitis. Curr Eye Res 6: 221–224

Hakin KN, Dart JK, Sherrard E (1989) Sporadic diffuse corneal endotheliitis. Am J Ophthalmol 108: 509–515

Holbach LM, Asano N, Naumann GOH (1998) Infection of the corneal endothelium in herpes simplex keratitis. Am J Ophthalmol 126: 592–594

Holbach LM, Font RL, Nauman GOH (1990) Herpes simplex stromal and endothelial keratitis. Granulomatous cell reactions at the level of Descemet´s membrane, the stroma, and Bowman´s layer. Ophthalmology 97: 722–728

Oh JO (1970) Endothelial lesions of rabbit cornea produced by herpes simplex virus. Invest Ophthalmol Vis Sci 9: 196–205

Ohashi Y, Kinoshita S, Mano T, Kiritoshi A, Ohji M (1985) Idiopathic corneal endotheliopathy. A report of two cases. Arch Ophthalmol 103: 1666–1668

Ohashi Y, Yamamoto S, Hishida K (1991) Demonstration of herpes simplex virus DNA in idiopathic corneal endotheliopathy. Am J Ophthalmol 112: 419–423

Olsen TW, Hardten DR, Meiusi RS, Holland EJ (1994) Linear endotheliitis. Am J Ophthalmol 117: 468–474

Porter SM, Patterson A, Kho P (1990) A comparison of local and systemic acyclovir in the management of herpetic disciform keratitis. Br J Ophthalmol 74: 283–285

Robin JB, Steigner JB, Kaufman HE (1985) Progressive herpetic corneal endotheliitis. Am J Ophthalmol 100: 336–337

Sundmacher R (1981) A clinico-virologic classification of herpetic anterior segment diseases with special reference to intraocular herpes. In: R Sundmacher (ed) Herpetic eye disease. Bergmann, Munich, pp 203–208

Sundmacher R (1983) Orale Acyclovir-Therapie virologisch nachgewiesener intraokularer Herpes simplex Virus-Infektionen. Klin Monatsbl Augenheilk 183: 246–250

Sundmacher R (1984) Endotheliitis corneae. Begriffsbestimmung and klinische Abgrenzung. Klin Monatsbl Augenheilk 184: 163–167

Sundmacher R (1997) Diagnose und Differentialdiagnose der Endotheliitis und Trabekulitis. In: A Kampik, F Grehn (Hrsg): Entzündungen des Augeninnern. Bücherei des Augenarztes. Enke, Stuttgart, 138: 96–102

Sundmacher R, Neumann-Haefelin D (1979) Herpes simplex virus-positive and –negative keratouveitis. In: A Silverstein, R O´Connor (eds): Immunology and immunopathology of the eye. Masson, New York / Paris, pp 225–229

Sundmacher R, Neumann-Haefelin D (1979) Herpes-simplex-Virus-Isolierung aus dem Kammerwasser bei fokaler Iritis, Endotheliitis und langdauernder Keratitis disciformis mit Sekundärglaukom. Klin Monatsbl Augenheilk 175: 488–501

Sutcliffe E, Baum J (1984) Acute idiopathic corneal endotheliitis. Ophthalmology 91: 1161–1165

Vannas A, Ahonen R (1981) Herpetic endothelial keratitis. Acta Ophthalmol 59: 296

Vannas A, Ahonen R, Mäkitie J (1983) Corneal endothelium in herpetic keratouveitis. Arch Ophthalmol 101: 913–915

Witschel H, Sundmacher R (1980) Virusendotheliitis als Ursache konnataler Hornhauttrübungen. Ber Dtsch Ophthalmol Ges 77: 503–507

Zheng X, Yamaguchi M, Goto T, Okamoto S, Ohashi Y (2000) Experimental corneal endotheliitis in rabbit. Invest Ophthalmol Vis Sci 41: 377–385

# HSV Trabeculitis and Acute Secondary Glaucoma

Section 2.8

## Core Messages

- In HSV trabeculitis, severe acute secondary glaucoma is caused by infection of the trabecular endothelial cells, which swell and lyse, and thus obstruct the outflow channels.
- Acute pressure rise in HSV trabeculitis, and also in HSV corneal endotheliitis (Sect. 2.7) and HSV iritis (Sect. 2.9), is correlated with presence of culturable HSV in the aqueous humor.
- Acute pressure rise in herpes eyes calls primarily for therapy with systemic antiviral agents plus steroids. Additionally, general glaucoma therapy is necessary, but only in the second line.
- If an acute pathologic pressure rise is found in an eye with an otherwise unclear inflammation of the cornea or the iris, herpetic etiology ranges first in the differential diagnosis.

HSV trabeculitis is still a partly speculative term, because we are unable to directly visualize the trabecular meshwork in vivo, and cannot be sure what is actually going on in its cells and its lumen. But we have a hypothesis, of course, which says that herpes simplex viruses do not only infect corneal endothelial cells (see Sect. 2.7) but also the related endothelial cells of the trabecular meshwork. These trabecular meshwork cells may swell and lyse as a result of the HSV infection itself, but far more swelling and lysis is brought about by the secondary immune attacks on them. Cell swelling and lysis with cell debris and inflammatory cells in the lumen can increase the outflow resistance of the trabecular meshwork so much, that the resultant acute glaucoma may mimic acute angle closure glaucoma with pressures as high as 60–70 mm Hg.

The following observations and considerations may serve as accumulated circumstantial evidence that the pathophysiological hypothesis of viral trabeculitis is basically correct:

1. HSV can infect corneal endothelium (see Sect. 2.7). It can most probably also infect its neighbor, the trabecular endothelium, which is developmentally closely related.
2. It has been shown, that herpes eyes enucleated for absolute glaucoma show a massive intratrabecular inflammation.
3. In HSV trabeculitis, high pressures develop with so little associated anterior chamber inflammation that a massive inflow of inflammatory material is not a valid explanation. The most likely explanation, however, is an acute obstruction by swelling (and lysis) of sufficiently many trabecular endothelial cells.
4. It is also hypothesized that such acute obstruction is to occur in the Posner–Schlossman syndrome (acute glaucomatocyclitic crisis), which shows an even more disproportionate pressure rise with minimal inflammatory signs in the aqueous humor. Interestingly, some Posner–Schlossman cases were recently correlated with the presence of CMV (see Chap. 4).
5. Acute pathologic pressure rise in HSV trabeculitis, and also in HSV corneal endotheliitis (Sect. 2.7) and HSV iritis (Sect. 2.9), is correlated with presence of culturable HSV in the aqueous humor.
6. Last but not least, therapeutic experiences speak in favor of direct endothelial infection in HSV trabeculitis: The higher the pressure, the less it is possible to reduce it by acetazolamide or other glaucoma therapy alone. Only together with a basic therapy of high-dosed systemic antiviral agents plus steroids, does the pressure reliably decrease within reasonable time.

The correlation between intraocular HSV replication and acute intraocular pressure rise needs some more consideration. The pathologic pressure rise must not necessarily be high. It suffices to suspect HSV etiology of an inflammation in the anterior segment of the eye if the pressure in the diseased eye is clearly elevated above the level in the partner eye, e.g., 20 versus 14 mm Hg. In such situations, HSV could regularly be cultured from aqueous taps. While HSV endotheliitis and HSV iritis only lead to slight increase in introcular pressure, the increase resulting from severe trabeculitis is the most dramatic. This does not mean that the basic pathophysiology must be different. On the contrary, it is well conceivable that every pressure rise in case of intraocular HSV replication is caused by HSV trabeculitis, and that only the amount of infected and thus affected endothelial trabecular cells makes a difference in pressure response. While such considerations are certainly partly "academic", the following are important practical conclusions:

- Acute elevated intraocular pressure in herpes eyes with intraocular inflammation must be taken as a sign of intraocular HSV replication, even if the pressure rise is relatively low.

- Intraocular HSV replication always calls for a basic therapy with high dose *systemic* antiviral agents plus moderately dosed steroids (e.g., 800 mg ACV 5 qd plus 20 mg fluocortolone).
- If an acute pressure rise is found in an eye with an otherwise unclear inflammation of the cornea or the iris, a herpetic etiology ranges first in the differential diagnosis.

## Detailed analysis of Fig 2.78

***Clinic:*** From gross clinical appearance, the patient in Fig. 2.78 was primarily also suspected to suffer from acute angle closure glaucoma with moderate pain, ptosis, deeply red and hard eye (on palpation), dilated and distorted pupil, and moderately edematous cornea with reduced vision (a). As this was a known herpes eye with deep anterior chamber, an acute herpetic secondary glaucoma was the correct diagnosis. After forced pupillary dilation (Fig. 2.78b), the anterior segment was investigated through a moderately edematous cornea, which contained some herpes scars and possibly also some newer interstitial infiltrations. Multiple precipitates were visible on the endothelium. As the whole cornea was edematous from the high pressure, a correlation between precipitates and corneal edema – as necessary for the diagnosis of endotheliitis – was impossible at this stage of disease. The aqueous was not clearly visible, Tyndall not recognizable. However, significant amounts of inflammatory cells were certainly not present. Anterior chamber depth was normal. Iris pigment epithelium sheets adhered to the anterior lens capsule.

***Diagnosis:*** Severe acute HSV trabeculitis. Minor endotheliitis, and/or iritis, and/or interstitial keratitis are possibly associated.

***Differential diagnosis:*** The herpetic etiology of the trabeculitis is undisputable. The presence and acuity of accompanying other deep herpetic diseases cannot unequivocally be confirmed at this stage of disease:

- Interstitial cell infiltrates of HSV interstitial keratitis can be suspected, but there is too much diffuse corneal edema to be sure.
- HSV endotheliitis can also be suspected. Mostly, it goes together with trabeculitis. For a positive diagnosis, a close topographic correlation with circumscribed corneal edema would be necessary. This is impossible as long as the cornea is totally swollen. The total corneal edema is pressure-induced.
- Form and distribution of the visible precipitates fits well with an accompanying HSV iritis (many large precipitates on the basal endothelium with triangular distribution). The other typical signs of HSV iritis (focal dilator muscle dysfunction plus focal pigment epithelium defects, see Sect. 2.9) are not (yet) visible. They will come out clearly in the course of the disease, if HSV iritis coexists. The pigment epithelium sheets on the anterior lens capsule are no sign of HSV iritis. More probably, they are simply the result of iris damage in the course of excessive pressure rise with subsequent exudation of fibrin and gluing of the pigment epithelium to the lens capsule.

***Therapy:*** As long as the massive trabeculitis threatens survival of the eye by the dangerous pressure of 60–70 mm Hg, the hypothetical presence of other deep HSV diseases plays no role in therapeutic decisions. They will be cotreated with trabeculitis therapy, anyway: Basic therapy consists of 800 mg ACV orally 5 qd (or equivalent intravenous infusions) plus 20–30 mg of oral fluocortolone (or other equivalent steroid). Maximal mydriasis must be contained. Symptomatic systemic glaucoma therapy (e.g., with azetazolamide) is also necessary, but comes only third in the therapeutic rank of order. Given alone, glaucoma therapy will have no effect. Other measures may also be helpful but are certainly only fourth rank (topical antiviral-steroid combination, topical glaucoma therapy).

Without this therapy, the pressure may stay invariably high for weeks and may cause severe optic nerve and corneal endothelial damage. Also with maximal therapy, no rapid response can be expected. After 3–5 days, however, pressure should slowly come down, and with clearing cornea more details will become visible around the anterior chamber. That will then make controlled adjustments of therapy possible.

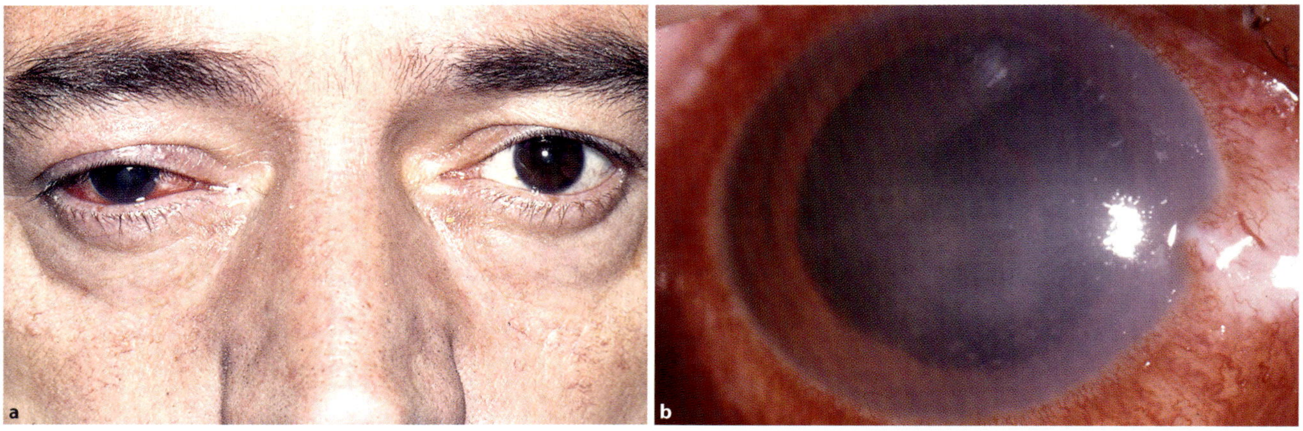


Fig. 2.78a,b Severe acute HSV trabeculitis with a deeply red eye and high intraocular pressure (see text)

## Analysis of Fig 2.79

Figure 2.79 is shown as a reminder of the old technique of estimating the intraocular pressure by comparative bilateral digital palpation. In these high-tech times, such a technique may seem obsolete to many. This is not the case. Every ophthalmologist should as often as possible practice in order to acquire sufficient experience in the detection of even minor pressure differences between a diseased eye, which cannot be evaluated by applanation tonometry, and its healthy partner eye, in which the reference pressure is measured by applanation. This is the only way to relatively reliably detect pathologic intraocular pressures in eyes with severe corneal disease or after keratoplasty or in patients who cannot open the diseased eye wide enough. Pressure differences of 4–5 mm Hg are certainly recognizable by experienced persons, and this is sufficiently precise for emergency decisions relating to secondary glaucoma problems.

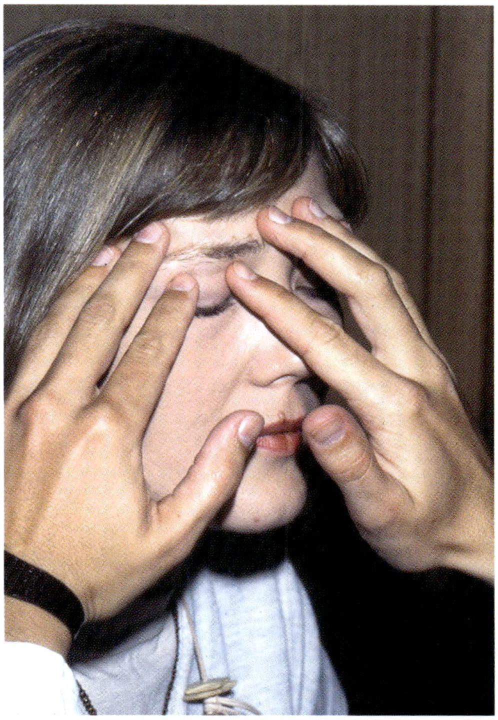

Fig. 2.79 Estimate of the intraocular pressure by comparative bilateral digital palpation

## Analysis of Fig 2.80

The case in Fig. 2.80 is a rarity. Buphthalmus is nearly always a disease which develops intrauterine. In that stage of development, the sheaths of the eye are easily expanded beyond normal limits by high intraocular pressure. Already very soon in life, this "plasticity" is lost. After the age of about 2, high intraocular pressure can no longer dilate a normal eye. The *postpartal* development of buphthalmus requires, therefore, that persistently high intraocular pressure develops very early in life. The boy in Fig. 2.80 was reportedly born with two normally sized and normally appearing eyes. He started to develop severe recurrent eye infections in his right eye a couple of months *after birth*, and only at the age of three, his mother noticed a difference in size between both eyes. This difference had since then remained stable. When we saw the boy at the age of 12 (Fig. 2.80a), the buphthalmic cornea with Haab lines was severely scarred and vascularized with normal pressure. Vision was limited to perception of hand movements only, and the required perforating keratoplasty was, of course, not performed, because the optic nerve was atrophic, and deep amblyopia would additionally make all function-restoring attempts useless. Epicritically, the boy suffered from recurrent corneal and intraocular HSV diseases with severe secondary glaucoma, above all, from recurrent HSV trabeculitis with persistently high pressure. It must have started in the first year of life, but was not diagnosed and not treated correctly. Consequently, the boy functionally lost this eye. A spontaneous reduction of the high intraocular pressure must have occurred after trabeculitis attacks had ceased. The general message from such experience is that recurrent eye inflammations in early childhood – especially unilateral eye

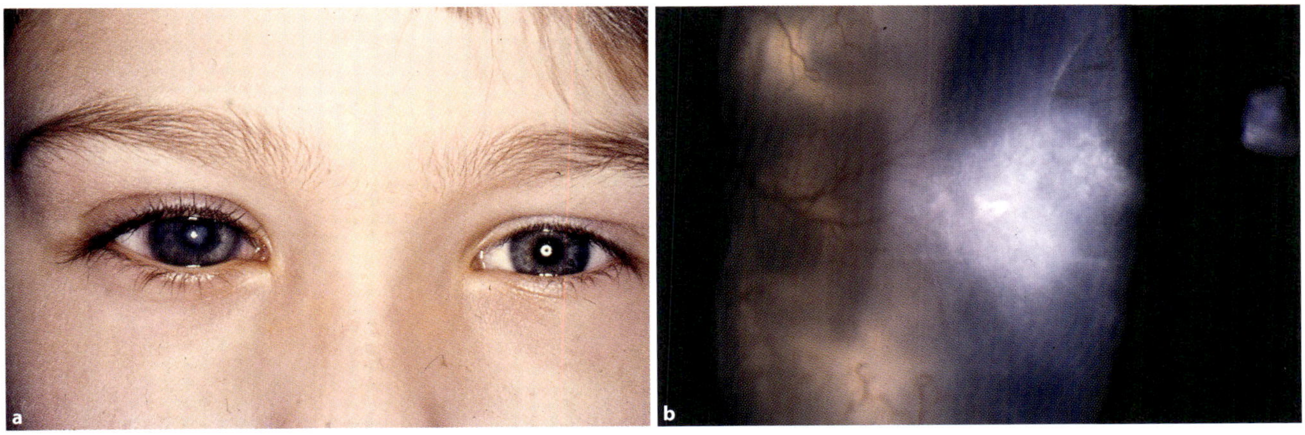

Fig. 2.80 Unilateral *postpartal* secondary buphthalmus (**a**) in a boy with early postpartal recurrent intraocular HSV disease with scarring and Haab lines (**b**)

inflammations – must be suspected as herpetic until proven otherwise. For detailed investigation and diagnosis, general anesthesia is necessary. Unilateral secondary glaucoma, however, could already have been suspected easily without anaesthesia, i.e., by digital palpation (Fig. 2.79).

## Analysis of Fig 2.81

Posner–Schlossman syndrome (PS) presents clinically different from HSV trabeculitis:

- In PS, no or only minimal conjunctival injection exists (Fig. 2.81a), while in HSV trabeculitis we may have a deeply red eye (Fig. 2.78a).
- In PS, only single endothelial precipitates attract diagnostic attention as pathologic signs (Fig. 2.81), with the cornea staying mostly clear, while in HSV trabeculitis, we normally have lots of associated pathologic signs in all parts of the anterior segment (Fig. 2.78b), in addition to endothelial precipitates.

But Posner–Schlossman syndrome presents also with striking pathophysiological similarities to HSV trabeculitis:

- Both are recurrent diseases with disease attacks leading to acute secondary glaucoma with significant rises in pressure.
- In both, acute massive swelling of trabecular endothelial cells is thought to initiate the acute pressure rise.
- In both, endotheliitic precipitates are present, which by themselves play no glaucomatogenic role. They are a diagnostic sign, however, of what is presumably simultaneously going on in the trabecular meshwork. The corneal endotheliitis is invariably correlated with trabeculitis.
- In both cases, the pressure rise is disproportionately high when compared with the endotheliitic signs.

Therefore, it comes as no surprise that Posner–Schlossman syndrome – or some of its variants – has long been suspected to be caused by viruses of the herpes group. While HSV and VZV have lost much of its previously favored status as candidate viruses, CMV is currently the most probable herpes virus that causes Posner–Schlossman-like diseases (see Chap. 4).

## Analysis of Fig 2.82

Figure 2.82 demonstrates that, with the Posner–Schlossman syndrome, we observe only a mild endotheliitis with minor endothelial cell edema at the corneal endothelial level (a), which by itself does not lead to corneal edema. Only if the acute pressure rise is

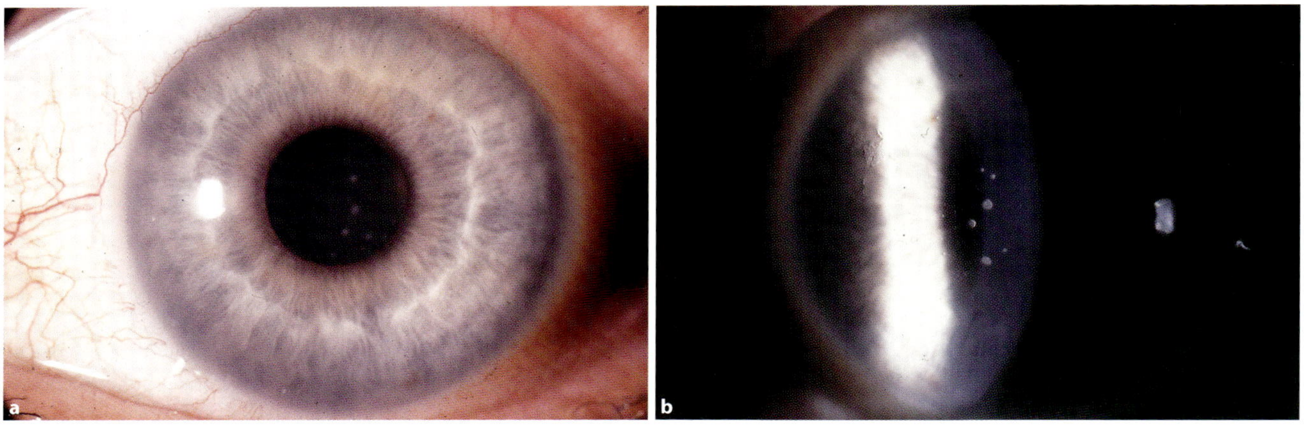

Fig. 2.81a,b Pathophysiologically related disease: Posner–Schlossman syndrome with diagnostically important endotheliitic precipitates

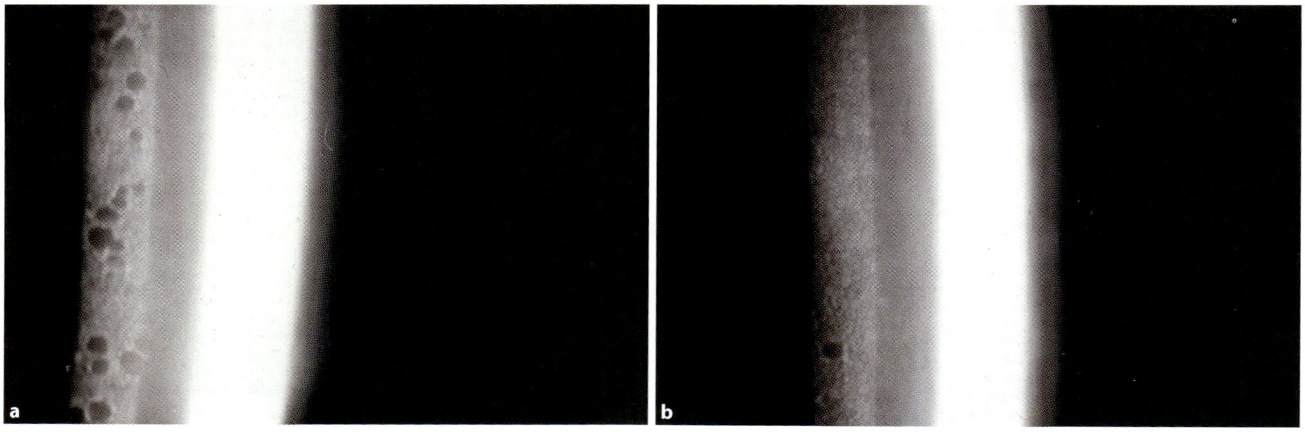

Fig. 2.82 Central corneal endothelium at the beginning of Posner–Schlossman syndrome (**a**), and 2 weeks thereafter (**b**)

high enough, whole corneal areas may intermittently swell for a short time period. As soon as the pressure is reduced, the corneal edema disappears again without sequelae. With specular microscopic investigation, we may follow the course and the gradual disappearance (b) of the corneal endothelial cell edema, which probably reflects what is simultaneously going on in the endothelial cells of the trabecular meshwork.

## References


Alvarado JA, Underwood JL, Green WR, Wu S, Murphy CG, Hwang DG, Moore TE, O´Day D (1994) Detection of herpes simplex viral DNA in the iridocorneal endothelial syndrome. Arch Ophthalmol 112: 1601–1609

Amano S, Oshika T, Kaji Y, Numaga J, Matsubara M, Araie M (1999) Herpes simplex virus in the trabeculum of an eye with corneal endotheliitis. Am J Ophthalmol 127: 721–722

Dawson CR, Togni B, Moore TE (1968) Structural changes in chronic herpetic keratitis. Arch Ophthalmol 79: 740–747

Falcon MG, Williams HP (1978) Herpes simplex kerato-uveitis and glaucoma. Trans Ophthalmol Soc UK 98: 101–104

Grehn F, Sundmacher R (1982) Zur Pathogenese und Therapie des Posner-Schlossman-Syndroms. In: G Krieglstein, W Leydhecker (eds): Medikamentöse Glaukomtherapie. Bergmann, Munich, pp 95–99

Groh MI, Seitz B, Schumacher S, Naumann GOH (1999) Detection of herpes simplex virus in aqueous humor in iridocorneal endothelial (ICE) syndrome. Cornea 18: 359–360

Madjlessi F, Marx W, Reinhard T, Althaus C, Sundmacher R (2000) Impressions-Tonometrie und Applanations-Tonometrie bei pathologischen Hornhäuten im Vergleich mit der intraokularen Nadel-Druckmessung. Ophthalmologe 97: 478–481

Marx W, Madjlessi F, Reinhard T, Althaus C, Sundmacher R (1999) Mehr als vier Jahre Erfahrung mit der elektronischen intraokularen Nadel-Druckmessung bei irregulären Hornhäuten. Ein Erfahrungsbericht. Ophthalmologe 96: 498–502

Mitchell SM, Phylactou L, Fox JD, Kilpatrick MW, Murray PI (1996) The detection of herpesviral DNA in aqueous fluid samples from patients with Fuchs´ heterochromic cyclitis. Ocular Immunol Inflamm 4: 33–38

Sundmacher R (1981) A clinico-virologic classification of herpetic anterior segment diseases with special reference to intraocular herpes. In: R Sundmacher (ed) Herpetic eye disease. Bergmann, Munich, pp 203–208

Sundmacher R (1983) Orale Acyclovir-Therapie virologisch nachgewiesener intraokularer Herpes simplex Virus-Infektionen. Klin Monatsbl Augenheilk 183: 246–250

Sundmacher R (1997) Diagnose und Differentialdiagnose der Endotheliitis und Trabekulitis. In: A Kampik, F Grehn (eds): Entzündungen des Augeninnern. Bücherei des Augenarztes. Enke, Stuttgart, 138: 96–102

Sundmacher R, Neumann-Haefelin D (1979) Herpes simplex virus-positive and -negative keratouveitis. In: A Silverstein, R O´Connor (eds): Immunology and immunopathology of the eye. Masson, New York / Paris, pp 225–229

Sundmacher R, Neumann-Haefelin D (1979) Herpes-simplex-Virus-Isolierung aus dem Kammerwasser bei fokaler Iritis, Endotheliitis und langdauernder Keratitis disciformis mit Sekundärglaukom. Klin Monatsbl Augenheilk 175: 488–501

Teitelbaum CS, Streeten BW, Dawson CR (1987) Histopathology of herpes simplex virus keratouveitis. Curr Eye Res 6: 189–194

Townsend WM, Kaufman HE (1971) Pathogenesis of glaucoma and endothelial changes in herpetic keratouveitis in rabbits. Am J Ophthalmol 71: 904–910

Vannas A, Ahonen R, Mäkitie J (1983) Corneal endothelium in herpetic keratouveitis. Arch Ophthalmol 101: 913–915

Weber U, Sundmacher R (1988) Die systemische Acyclovirtherapie herpetischer Sekundärglaukome. Fortschr Ophthalmol 85: 85–87

Yamamoto S, Pavan-Langston D, Tada R, Yamamoto R, Kinoshita S, Nishida K, Shimomura Y, Tano Y (1995) Possible role of herpes simplex virus in the origin of Posner-Schlossman syndrome. Am J Ophthalmol 119: 796–798

# HSV Focal Serous Iritis

Section

2.9

## Core Messages

- HSV focal serous iritis exhibits typical biomicroscopic signs: circumscribed dysfunctions of the dilator muscle with subsequent focal iris pigment epithelium loss.
- HSV focal serous iritis may develop monosymptomatically without other associated herpetic eye disease.
- Only VZV iritis leads to similar pictures.

HSV iritis has already been briefly mentioned in the sections on HSV endotheliitis (Sect. 2.7) and HSV trabeculitis (Sect. 2.8). These three together make up the intraocular anterior segment HSV diseases. They lead to high (trabeculitis) or low (endotheliitis and iritis) intraocular pressure rises. Pressure rise in a herpes eye is always a strong indicator of intraocular HSV replication. Such disease should be treated with a systemic combination of antiviral agents plus steroids. In so far, the general therapeutic aspects of HSV iritis are the same as of its topographically related diseases.

Some developmental and pathophysiologic aspects of HSV focal serous iritis facilitate understanding of the clinical course:

1. HSV has a predilection for the iris muscle layer and the iris pigment epithelium layer. These develop from the anterior part of the embryonic optic cup and are equivalent to retina and retinal pigment epithelium in the posterior segment of the eye. These can also be infected by HSV (see Chap. 6). Different from iritis in ophthalmic zoster, the iris stroma and the endothelium of iris vessels, which are of different embryonic origin, are not easily infected by HSV.
2. According to this cellular predilection, HSV typically replicates in the double layer of *iris muscles and pigment epithelium* on the back of the iris. Mostly, the widely extended dilator muscle is topographically and functionally more involved than the sphincter muscle, which is concentrated around the pupil.
3. One or more circumscribed foci may be infected. Also the borders of the same focus can be infected in the course of subsequent recurrences, and an old focus can thus repeatedly enlarge. Diffuse infection of the iris has not been described.
4. First sign of focal serous HSV iritis is an irregular shape of the pupil with a deficit in dilator function in the area of the infectious focus. This becomes more evident as the pupil is medically more dilated. In this early stage of the disease, the iritic precipitates are still small and gray.
5. After several days and weeks, the precipitates grow larger and contain more and more pigment, which stems from lysed iris pigment epithelial cells.
6. Only with progressing pigment epithelial cell lysis, the area of focal disease becomes visible at the slit lamp as a sharply demarcated red "window" by retro-illumination.
7. The characteristic focal defects of the pigment epithelium persist indefinitely and allow a reliable retrospective diagnosis of previous herpes disease even in quiet eyes without a history of herpes.
8. HSV focal serous iritis is not only observed in herpes eyes with other associated HSV diseases, which then facilitate diagnosis. It may also present as a monosymptomatic recurrent iritis.
9. Up to 9% of non-traumatic iritis is estimated to be of HSV origin.

### Detailed analysis of Fig 2.83

***Clinic:*** The eye in Fig. 2.83 is moderately red with diffuse edema in the lower 2/3 of the cornea. The intraocular pressure is about 10 mm Hg higher than in the normal partner eye. Endothelial precipitates with triangular distribution are indistinctly visible through the hazy part of cornea. A focal dilator deficit is evident from 3–6 o'clock after medical pupillary dilatation. The iris color appears to be redder in that area and the structure somewhat thicker than in the rest of the circumference.

***Diagnosis:*** All criteria of HSV focal serous iritis are present. It is obvious, however, that there must also be additional associated intraocular disease. The extended corneal edema is *no* sign of focal iritis. Iritic precipitates never cause edema by themselves. An exclusively pressure-derived edema would affect the whole cornea and not only the lower part of it, as is the case here. The only explanation for the circumscribed edema of the cornea is

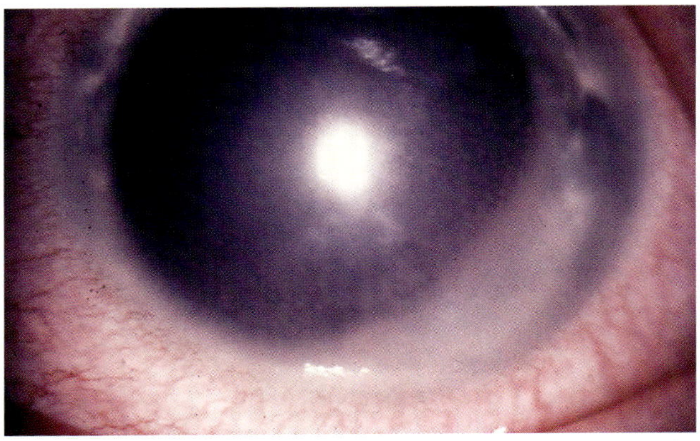

Fig. 2.83 HSV focal serous iritis with other associated intraocular HSV disease

*additional HSV endotheliitis* (see Sect. 2.7). The edema manifests itself quicker, the more the associated intraocular pressure rises. The pathologic pressure itself is mainly caused by an *associated slight HSV trabeculitis* (see Sect. 2.8)

***Differential diagnosis:*** The only possible differential diagnosis would be ophthalmic zoster, which is normally easy to exclude.

***Therapy:*** Basic therapy is with a full dose systemic combination of antiviral agents plus steroids, and medical mydriasis. Additional therapy should include symptomatic systemic glaucoma therapy and a topical combination therapy of antiviral agents plus steroids.

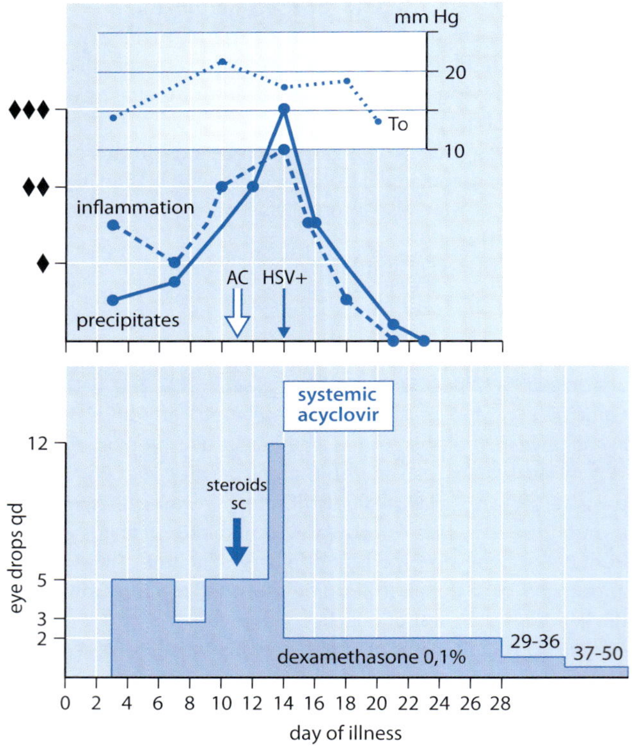


Fig. 2.84 Educative disease course of a monosymptomatic HSV focal serous iritis with different therapeutic strategies (see text) from: Sundmacher R (1983)

## Analysis of Fig 2.84

The treatment of a case of monosymptomatic focal iritis, as shown in Fig. 2.84, was started at a time when the pathognomonic signs for HSV etiology were *still unknown*. Therefore, initial treatment was only with topical steroids. Most strikingly, they did not reduce inflammation. On the contrary, with additional subconjunctival injection of crystalline steroids and hourly applications of steroid eye drops, the iritis deteriorated further with increasing amounts of cells in the aqueous humor and increasing amounts of precipitates, but without hypopyon. This being in strict contradiction to non-infectious iritis, a viral origin was suspected and an aqueous tap was performed. From this, HSV was cultured within 3 days, reflecting massive intraocular HSV replication. A systemic antiviral therapy with ACV was immediately started, and the steroids reduced to as little as three drops daily. This led to a stunningly quick disappearance of all iritic signs. Also the intraocular pressure fell quickly again to the patient's normal level.

## Analysis of Fig 2.85

Figure 2.85 shows a similar case as in Fig. 2.83 after some days of therapy, at a higher magnification. The cornea has cleared with some residual haze. One has a better look now at the area of focal disease between 5 and 7 o'clock with swollen iris, dilated iris vessels, and dilator deficit. The precipitates have mostly been dissolved by therapy. At this stage of disease, a red "window effect" would still not be clearly visible with retroillumination.

## Analysis of Fig 2.86

Figure 2.86 is an example of a monosymptomatic HSV focal serous iritis in its early stage. The cornea is clear. The iritic precipitates are arranged in triangular fashion with the largest ones near the chamber angle. Specular microscopy reveals no associated

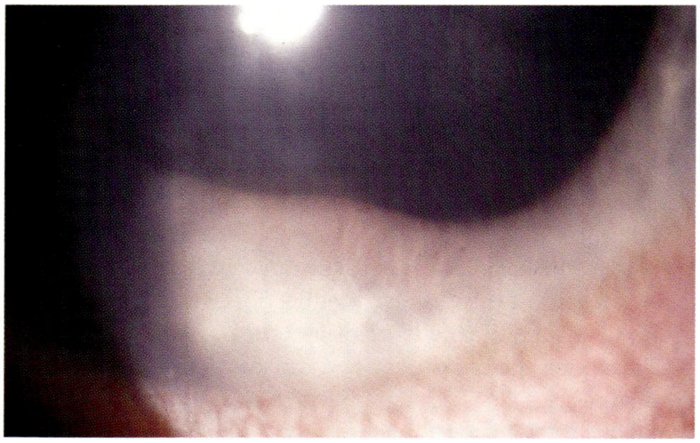

Fig. 2.85 Early stage of HSV focal serous iritis

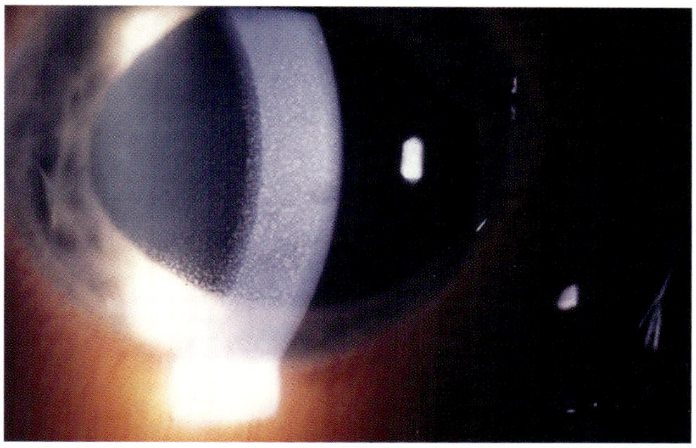

Fig. 2.86 Monosymptomatic HSV focal serous iritis

endothelial edema (i. e., no associated endotheliitis). The aqueous contains only moderate amounts of cells (1 ½ +) with a significant Tyndall phenomenon. The intraocular pressure is elevated only 4 mm Hg above the pressure in the partner eye. The dilator deficit associated with the focal infection is more discrete in this case, but is evident nonetheless: between 6 and 8 o'clock.

## Analysis of Fig 2.87

Figure 2.87a shows pigmented and unpigmented iritic precipitates of different sizes in the early phase of disease. They do not functionally affect the endothelium (no endothelial edema, clear cornea). At the right of Fig. 2.87a, the swollen area of focal disease is visible. With progressive lysis of iris pigment epithelium cells in the focal area, free pigment granules are incorporated into the iritic precipitates, which then turn brownish, while simultaneously shrinking under therapy (Fig. 2.87b). With complete healing of HSV focal serous iritis, precipitates disappear, occasionally leaving one or the other pigment granule on the endothelial layer. Black pigment granules may remain indefinitely on the iris stroma and the anterior lens capsule if iris destruction was severe enough (Fig. 2.87c).

## Analysis of Fig 2.88

In the early phase of this iritis case (Fig. 2.88a), the actual disease area may be suspected between 7 and 9 o'clock, as judged by the dilator dysfunction. In the same area, however, previous attacks of focal iritis have evidently already occurred also with involvement of the iris stroma. This gives a moth-eaten appearance (possibly sequelae from previous HSV iris vasculitis). A large area of total iris pigment epithelium loss already exists (Fig. 2.88b). This cannot stem from the early phase of the actual focal iritis. The presence of defects at this stage of actual disease proves, therefore,

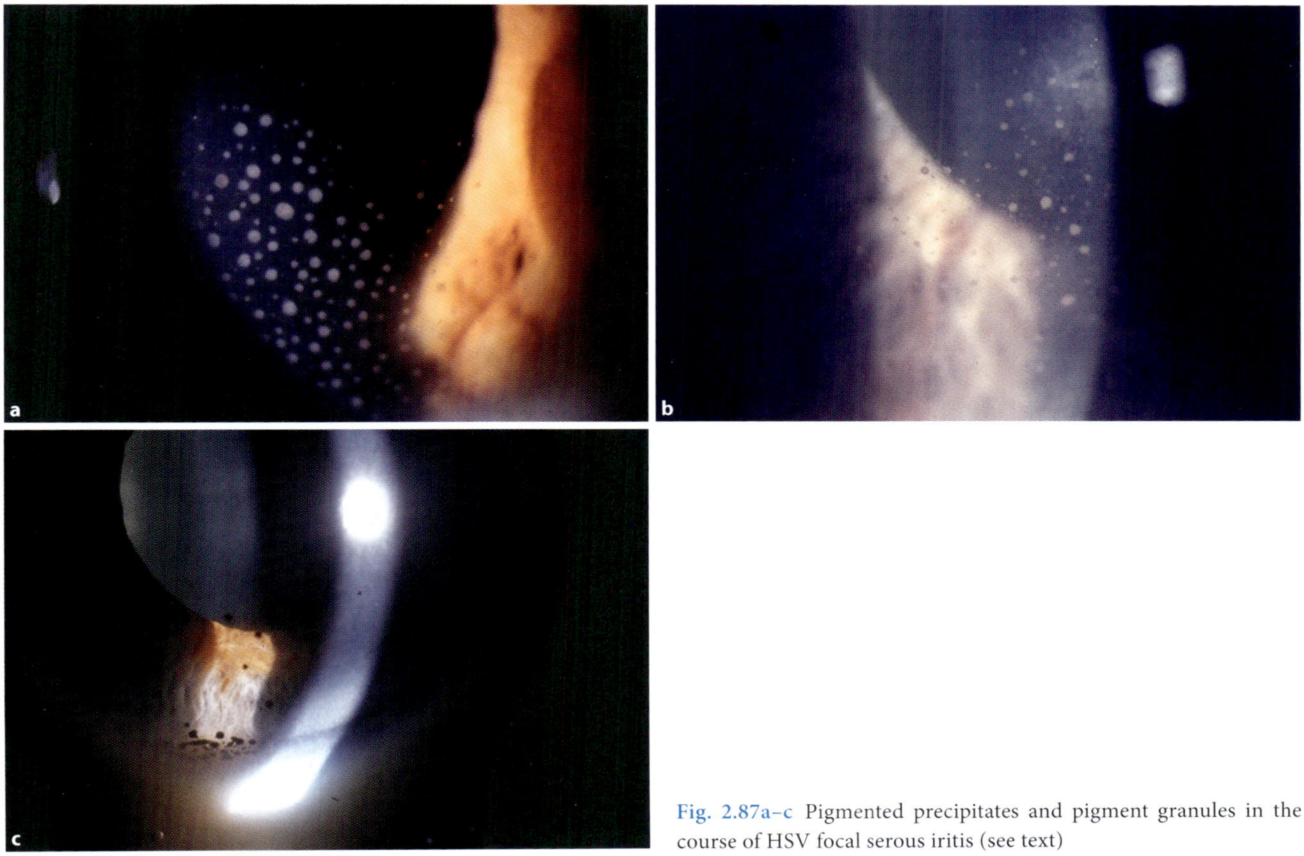

Fig. 2.87a–c Pigmented precipitates and pigment granules in the course of HSV focal serous iritis (see text)

that this area had already been diseased before in the course of a previous attack. After complete healing (Fig. 2.88c), it becomes evident that with the actual recurrence, focal disease has further expanded and enlarged in the 6 o'clock direction.

## Analysis of Fig 2.89

If we deal with more than one iritic foci, which are additionally tiny, the herpes diagnosis may be more difficult. In Fig. 2.89a, a major diseased area can be suspected between 9 and 11 o'clock by the dilator dysfunction. A second less evident area is between 4 and 5 o'clock, according to the discrete pupillary distortion. 3 weeks later (Fig. 2.89b), moth-eaten, small pigment epithelium defects appear in the suspected areas, but also at 12 o'clock, an area which initially looked normal. Such small, moth-eaten defects are not as typical for HSV etiology as the larger ones shown in the previous figures. Mostly, however, the history and the typical pupillary dysfunction are sufficiently significant to conclude herpes etiology.

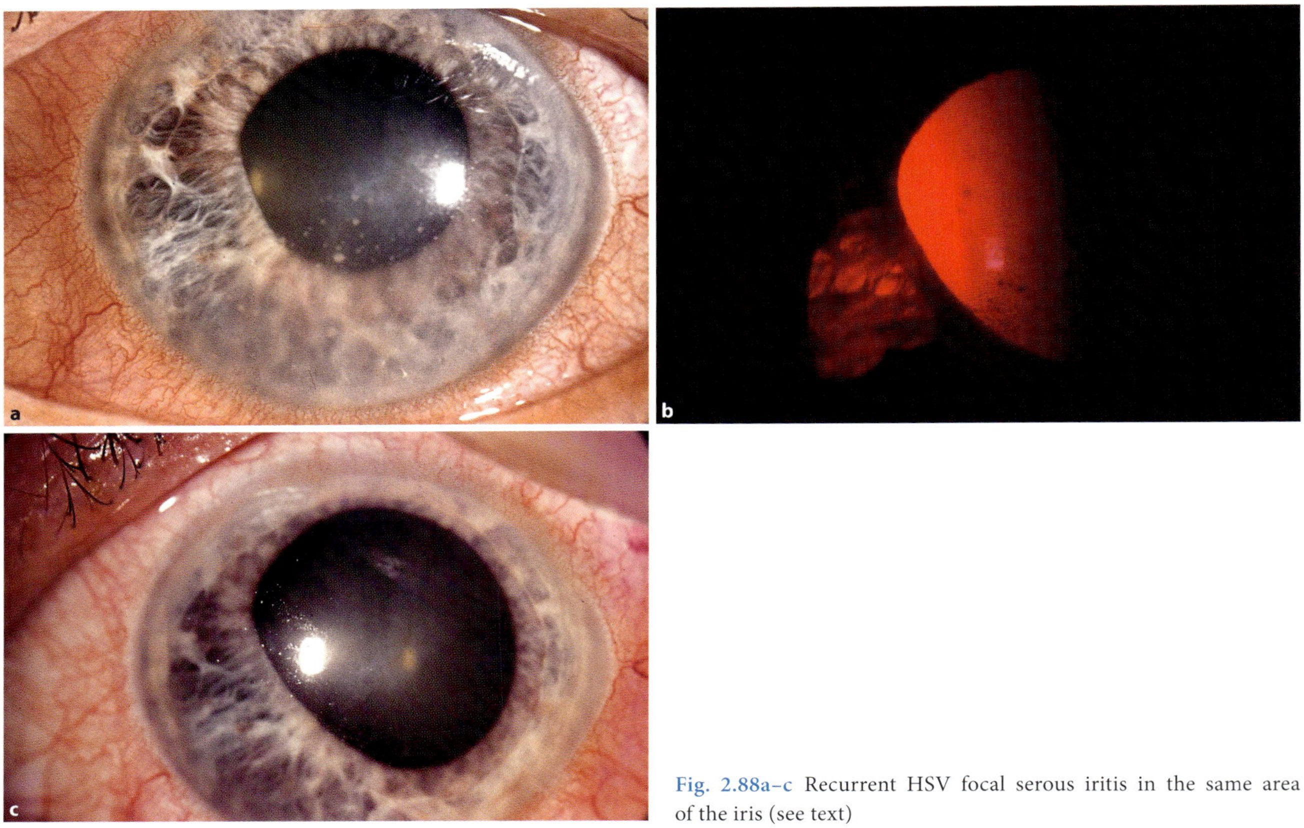

Fig. 2.88a–c Recurrent HSV focal serous iritis in the same area of the iris (see text)

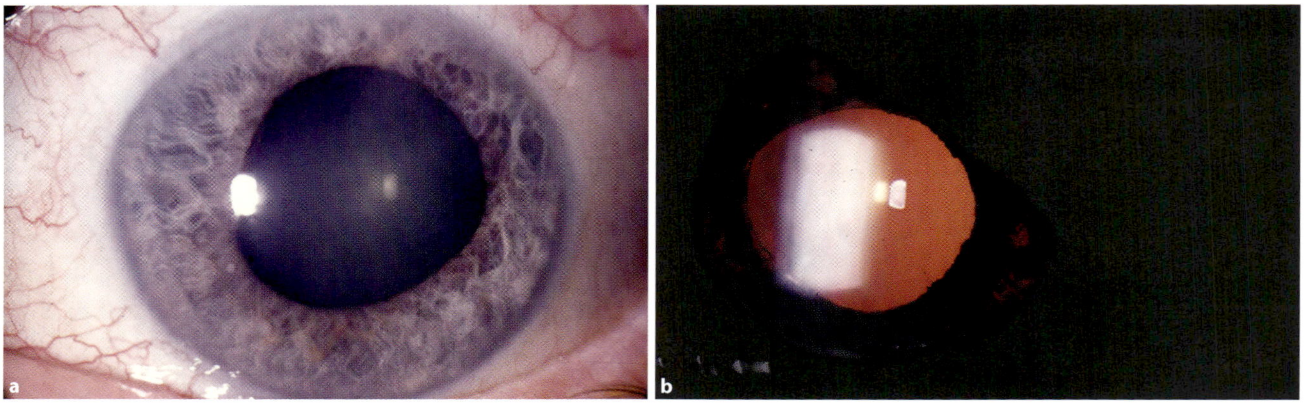

Fig. 2.89a,b Aspect of an iris with multiple tiny patches of HSV focal serous iritis (see text)

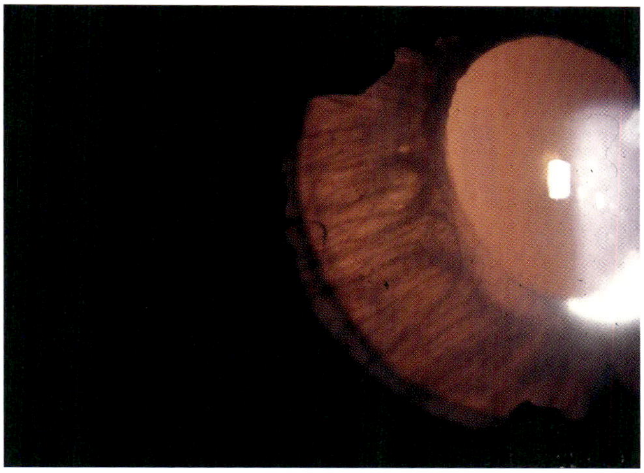

Fig. 2.90 HSV focal serous iritis comprising a large area of the pupillary margin

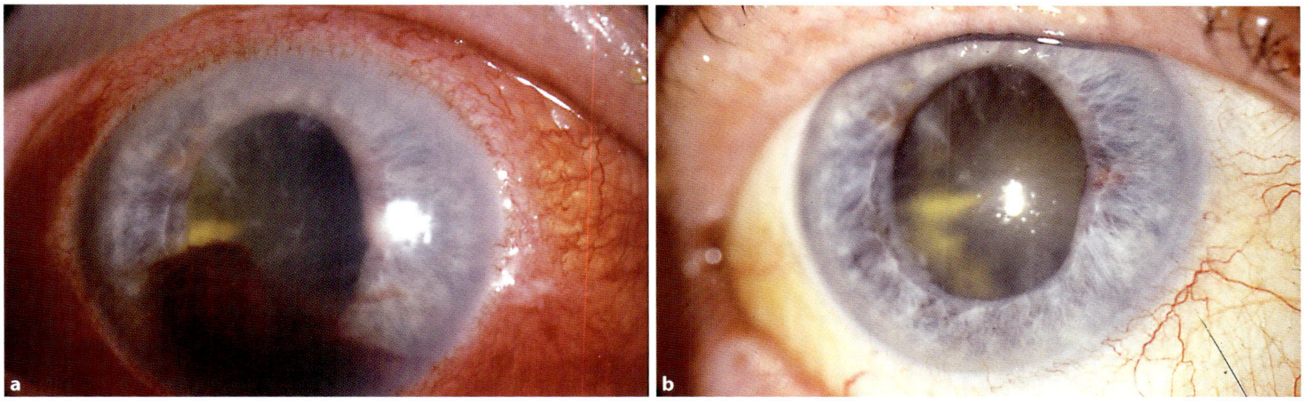

Fig. 2.91 Rare case with a large clotted hyphema in the early stage of HSV focal serous iritis (**a**). After healing, the area of focal disease can be identified more clearly by the pupil distortion and the blood remnants at the site of additional stromal vascular involvement (**b**)

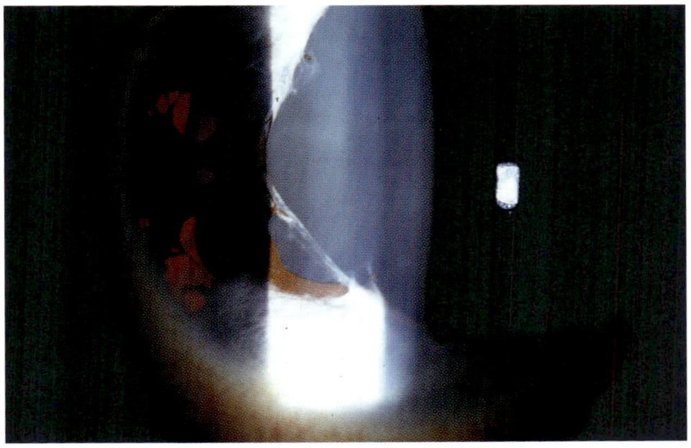

Fig. 2.92 *Differential diagnosis:* Full thickness focal iris destruction with massive vascular necrosis of the iris stroma. This case was elsewhere clinically classified as being of HSV origin. Because such severe iris destructions with massive vascular damage are much more typical for VZV focal iritis, however, the HSV etiology of such iris defects should be doubted until objectively proven

## Analysis of Fig 2.90

In the case presented in Fig. 2.90, retro-illumination shows a large patchy pigment epithelium defect comprising an extended area of the pupillary margin and thus of the iris sphincter muscle. One would expect focal sphincter weakness with such finding. This is not the case. Evidently, the sphincter is not so severely involved and not as severely damaged as the iris pigment epithelium in the same area. An analogous phenomenon can be found after cataract extraction through narrow pupils. There may be large patches of peripupillary loss of pigment epithelium, but the topographically associated sphincter still functions well.

If iris pathology is the only criteria available, differential diagnosis between HSV and VZV disease may be difficult. HSV and VZV focal iris defects are indistinguishable from biomicroscopic appearance alone (see Sect. 3.6). If iris vasculitis is associated, which can be diagnosed from iris bleeding and subsequent patches of destructive necrosis, then VZV etiology becomes the more probable the more destructive the disease course is (Fig. 2.92). For HSV disease, vasculitis and its sequelae are less common. However, occasionally they are also observed (Fig. 2.91).

## References


Herpetic Eye Disease Study Group (1996) A controlled study of oral acyclovir for iridocyclitis caused by herpes simplex virus. Arch Ophthalmol 114: 1065–1072

Kaufman HE, Kanai A, Ellison ED: Herpetic iritis (1971) demonstration of virus in the anterior chamber by fluorescent antibody technique and electron microscopy. Am J Ophthalmol 71: 465–469

Miserocchi E, Waheed NK, Dios E, Christen W, Merayo J, Roque M, Foster CS (2002) Visual outcome in herpes simplex virus and varicella zoster virus uveitis. Ophthalmology 109: 1532–1537

Schacher S, Garweg JG, Russ C, Böhnke M (1998) Diagnosis of herpetic uveitis and keratouveitis. Klin Monatsbl Augenheilkd 212: 359–362

Siverio CD, Imai Y, Cunningham ET (2002) Diagnosis and management of herpetic anterior uveitis. Int Ophthalmol Clin 42: 43–48

Sundmacher R (1981) A clinico-virologic classification of herpetic anterior segment diseases with special reference to intraocular herpes. In: R Sundmacher (ed) Herpetic eye disease. Bergmann, Munich, pp 203–208

Sundmacher R (1981) Die fokale Iritis durch Herpes simplex- und Varizellen-Zoster-Virus. Ber Dtsch Ophthalmol Ges 78: 73–76

Sundmacher R (1983) Orale Acyclovir-Therapie virologisch nachgewiesener intraokularer Herpes simplex Virus-Infektionen. Klin Monatsbl Augenheilk 183: 246–250

Sundmacher R, Neumann-Haefelin D (1979) Herpes simplex virus-positive and -negative keratouveitis. In: A Silverstein, R O´Connor (eds): Immunology and immunopathology of the eye. Masson, New York / Paris, pp 225–229.

Sundmacher R, Neumann-Haefelin D (1979) Herpes-simplex-Virus-Isolierung aus dem Kammerwasser bei fokaler Iritis, Endotheliitis und langdauernder Keratitis disciformis mit Sekundärglaukom. Klin Monatsbl Augenheilk 175: 488–501

Van der Lelij A, Ooijman FM, Kijlstra A, Rothova A (2000) Anterior uveitis with sectoral iris atrophy in the absence of keratitis. A distinct entity among herpetic eye diseases. Ophthalmology 107: 1164–1170

Witmer R, Iwamoto T (1968) Electron microscopic observation of herpes-like particles in the iris. Arch Ophthalmol 79: 331–337

Yamamoto S, Pavan-Langston D, Kinoshita S, Nishida K, Shimomura Y, Tano Y (1996) Detecting herpes simplex virus DNA in uveitis using the polymerase chain reaction. Br J Ophthalmol 80: 465–468

# HSV Scleritis

Section

2.10

## Core Messages

- HSV scleritis is rarely observed in herpes eyes. It is mostly not a therapeutic problem.

The vast majority of all scleritis cases is associated with vasculitis, either infectious, or autoimmunological, or both of them in sequence. Contrary to VZV, as HSV has no specific predilection for vascular endothelium, HSV vasculitis and HSV scleritis are rare.

If scleritis flares up in a herpes eye, the pathophysiologic background (infectious versus immunogenic) will generally remain unsettled. It is certainly not a mistake to treat it for at least 3 weeks with a systemic combination of high dosed antiherpetic agents plus moderately dosed systemic steroids, which covers both pathogenic possibilities, before eventually carrying on with a monotherapy of steroids under close control.

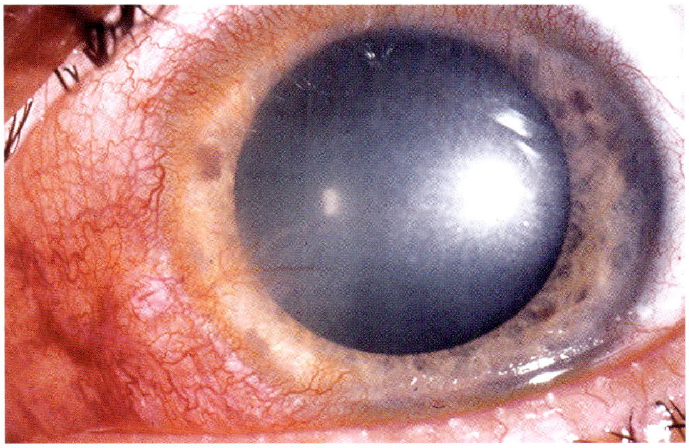

Fig. 2.93 HSV scleritis in an eye with vascularized corneal scars

## Detailed analysis of Fig 2.93

***Clinic:*** An area of circumscribed diffuse scleritis extends from the limbus between 7 and 9 o'clock (Fig. 2.93). Peripherally, a small nodule is visible in front of the swollen plica region. The cornea exhibits scars with some subtle infiltrations from a recent recurrence of HSV interstitial keratitis. When the scleritis was first noticed, the patient was on a topical combination therapy, which was already tapered out to ACV ointment 5 qd and steroid eye drops 2 qd at the time.

***Diagnosis:*** Diffuse and nodular HSV scleritis in a herpes eye with a recent attack of HSV interstitial keratitis.

***Differential diagnosis:*** None.

***Therapy:*** Systemic combination therapy of 800 mg ACV 5 qd plus 20–30 mg of fluocortolone qd for at least 3 weeks, tapering out thereafter.

## References


Green LK, Pavan-Langston D (2006) Herpes simplex ocular inflammatory disease. Int Ophthalmol Clin 46: 27–37

Sainz de la Maza M, Hemady RK, Foster CS (1993) Infectious scleritis: report of four cases. Documenta Ophthalmol 83: 33–41

# Metaherpetic Corneal Disease

Section

2.11

## Core Messages

- Metaherpetic corneal healing disorders (epithelial and deep metaherpetic corneal ulcers) develop *after* preceding viral HSV keratitis.
- To promote healing of metaherpetic ulcers, adequate resurfacing measures are mostly sufficient.
- Ongoing antiviral therapy may critically impede healing and is therefore mostly disadvantageous.

The term "metaherpetic" describes diseases that develop *after* preceding *viral HSV* disease. In the strict sense, it refers to superficial and deep healing disorders of the cornea (*metaherpetic epithelial and deep corneal ulcers*). Only these metaherpetic "core" diseases will be presented and discussed in this section.

Other non-viral diseases after HSV disease, which may also be called metaherpetic in the *broad sense*, are presented in other sections, above all in Sect. 2.14 on intraocular surgery and keratoplasty in HSV eyes: corneal scars and vascularization, bullous keratopathies, and chronic metaherpetic glaucoma.

The pathophysiologic reasons, which cause metaherpetic corneal healing disorders, are difficult to analyze in individual patients. A varying combination of the following is generally suspected to be operative:

- Neurotrophic disturbances after neuronal damage
- Postinfectious dry eye conditions following neuronal damage and infectious destruction of production sites of tear film components
- Toxic effects of topical antiviral therapy on the regenerating corneal cells
- Partial inhibition of limbus stem cell function
- Ongoing invasion into a corneal defect of inflammatory cells with liberation of lytic enzymes
- Blink reflex anomalies, due to reduced corneal sensitivity with enhanced instability of the tear film on an irregular corneal surface, and with lagophthalmus sequelae

The common sign of metaherpetic healing disorders is that a front of regenerating epithelium is halted and piled up at the borders of a lesion. The epithelium looks compromised and ill. It does not easily succeed in sliding on the defect in front of it. This is strikingly different from the easiness with which microbial ulcers resurface after termination of infection, irrespective of how destroyed is the ulcer base.

As metaherpetic corneal disease comes immediately after preceding viral HSV disease, it is conceivable that some overlap exists between viral and metaherpetic disease states, and that in the beginning of metaherpetic healing disorders, minor amounts of HSV may still be present in the cornea for some time. This is impossible to investigate and to prove in the individual patient. Such principal uncertainty does not affect, however, the general therapeutic policy for metaherpetic eye diseases. From clinical experience, it is agreed that they heal with adequate resurfacing measures only. Ongoing therapy with antiviral agents is not needed for such healing. On the contrary, antiviral therapy is dangerous because of its potential cytotoxic side effects. If it is exceptionally felt that antiviral therapy should be given in a borderline case with suspected viral as well as metaherpetic pathophysiology for a few more days, then an antiviral regime with minimal negative impact on epithelial regeneration should be chosen. Currently, that would be systemically by ACV.

### Detailed analysis of Fig 2.94

***Clinic:*** In Fig. 2.94, in the lower pupillary area, a small epithelial ulcer persists with little if any healing progress (a). The rounded margins of the ulcer contain a small zone of grey opaque cells shoved together and piled up. The ulcer base is relatively clear. Fluorescein staining shows that the epithelial cells in the grey borderline have not yet made tight junctions (b). The epithelial ulcer lies within a much larger zone of troubled epithelium with hazy epithelial structures and punctate keratopathy.
***Diagnosis:*** An immediately preceding HSV dendritic keratitis and the typical signs of severely disturbed epithelial regeneration make the diagnosis of metaherpetic epithelial ulcer easy.
***Differential diagnosis:*** There are no signs of residual HSV replication in the ulcer margins (no microdestruction pattern, see Fig. 2.19). On the contrary, the thickened borders of grey, piled-up epithelium are the consequence of severely disturbed epithelial regeneration and migration. From its outline, the ulcer could be mistaken for a steroid-induced geographic ulcer, especially if immediately stained with fluorescein (b) and not thoroughly investigated before *without stain* (a). Unstained, the thickened grey

border zone makes a differential diagnosis easy: geographic ulcers do not contain such thickened epithelial zones.

***Therapy:*** If the patient is still under antiviral therapy, the most important measure is to immediately end such treatment (one could also often say "over-treatment"). Thereafter, resurfacing measures must be taken as possible in the individual patient. The minimum would be a conventional dry eye therapy with ointments and artificial tears *without preservatives.* Mostly, a short term course with a soft therapeutic contact lens plus artificial tears without preservatives every two hours is more effective. However, such a therapy requires that the patient is compliant and that adequate controls are possible, at least in the beginning. The contact lens can mostly already be removed after about 10 days. Thereafter, conventional dry eye therapy should go on as required by the corneal epithelium.

It is to be noted that with much prolonged contact lens therapy, the risk of new HSV recurrences rises. Epithelial HSV recurrences in contact lens wearers take a very untypical course. A dendritic figure and the pathognomonic microdestruction pattern are mostly missing. Therefore, if an ulcer recurs or enlarges under a contact lens in a herpes eye, contact lens therapy must immediately be finished and the newly formed ulcer must be suspected to be of HSV origin and treated as such until proven otherwise.

## Analysis of Fig 2.95

The grey border zone of the metaherpetic epithelial ulcer in Fig. 2.95 is even broader than in Fig. 2.94. This does not mean that healing would be more efficient. With such a constellation, it can often be observed that during 1 day the central defect is nearly closed, but during the subsequent day, the loosened epithelium has broken out again with the defect being larger than before. It is remarkable that the neovascularization reaches the area of metaherpetic ulcer but does not invade it. The impression exists that neovascularizations of this kind are not always helpful in terms of accelerating healing by quicker resorption of infiltrates. On the contrary, they seem to increase the epithelial instability. It can be suspected that this comes by extravasation of leukocytes from the vessels. The leukocytes invade the ulcer margins, liberating lytic enzymes there, and thus further destabilize the epithelial regenerative process. Especially for such recalcitrant cases, short-term soft contact lens therapy is a good choice.

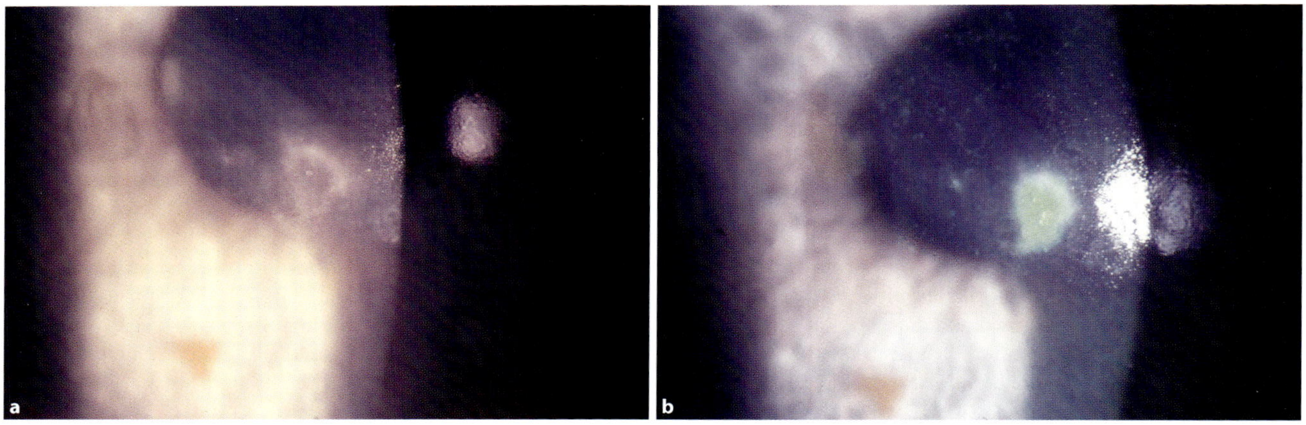


Fig. 2.94a,b Metaherpetic epithelial ulcer. **a** Unstained. **b** Fluorescein

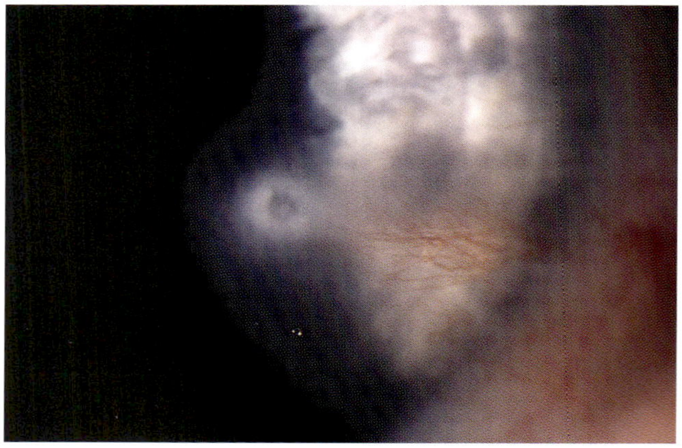

Fig. 2.95 Persistent metaherpetic epithelial ulcer in front of a band of corneal vessels

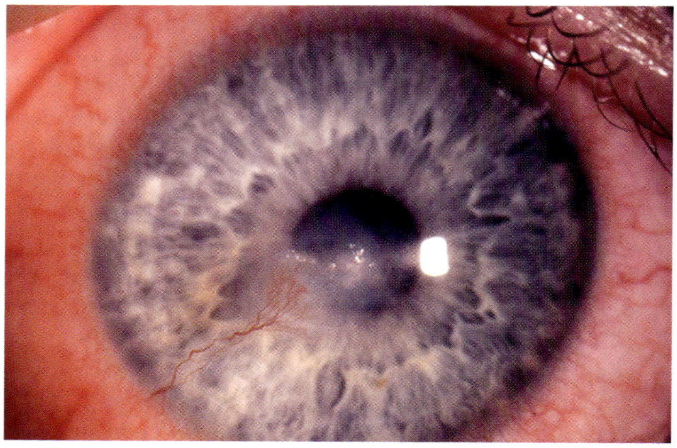

Fig. 2.96 Frequently recurring metaherpetic epithelial erosion in the corneal center

## Analysis of Fig 2.96

Figure 2.96 shows a frequently recurring epithelial erosion after deep ulcerative HSV keratitis in the corneal center. Laterally, where the approaching corneal vessels have already invaded the disease area, the overlying epithelium is nearly stable. In the center, however, no comparable epithelial consolidation takes place. The vessels make no quick attempt to invade into this area. In such a case, a soft contact lens plus artificial tears without preservatives are also the most efficient way to promote healing.

## Analysis of Fig 2.97

Only by knowing the history of a preceding HSV dendritic keratitis, the circumscribed bullous epithelium in Fig. 2.97 which extends far over the pupillary margin to the left, can be classified as metaherpetic erosion. The second clue for the herpetic origin is easy to evaluate: the patient is not in pain. From biomicroscopy alone, however, the disease cannot be differentiated from idiopathic recurrent erosion or from a recurrent erosion with map-dot-fingerprint dystrophy. The pathophysiology of all these erosive diseases is similar. We deal with genetic or acquired anomalies of corneal basal membrane production. The classification as metaherpetic is important for therapy as well as for prognosis. While one would consider to treat frequently recurring idiopathic or dystrophic erosions more actively, e. g., by a dense anterior stromal puncture, this is unnecessary with recurrent metaherpetic erosions. Once they have healed under a soft contact lens and have further been treated for a while with a dry eye regime, subsequent recurrent erosions are barely to be expected. On the contrary, with idiopathic and dystrophic erosions, the prognosis is much worse in this respect, even after anterior stromal puncture.

## Detailed analysis of Fig 2.98

***Clinic:*** The eye in Fig. 2.98 is only moderately red, the aqueous barely shows inflammation. The cornea exhibits diffusely distributed faint scars from previous attacks of HSV interstitial keratitis. Recently, another recurrence of HSV ulcerating interstitial keratitis has taken place (similar to Fig. 2.57). The infiltrates have mostly resolved under combination therapy. The ulcer itself, however, has become deeper and deeper. The regenerating epithelium did not succeed in surpassing the steep ulcer borders. Centrally, only a thin stromal layer still covers Descemet's membrane. Development of a descemetocele cannot be excluded.

***Diagnosis:*** Metaherpetic deep corneal ulcer.

***Differential diagnosis:*** None.

***Therapy:*** Conservative resurfacing therapy with ointments, which has already been tested (see ointment pearls at the upper limbus), may still be successful in the long run. However, that would take many weeks or even months. If surgery is no option and a quicker healing than with ointments only is desired, then a soft contact lens with frequent controls may be tried, but only in patients with excellent compliance. However, as the stromal defect is so deep, a surgical amnion cover would be the most helpful therapy. Such an amnion cover immediately reduces the risk of a descemetocele and considerably furthers healing (see Sect. 2.14).

## Analysis of Fig 2.99

Compared with Fig. 2.98, the ulcer in Fig. 2.99 shows more residual infiltrates in the ulcer base and around its borders (a). The stromal defect is deepest in the upper half (b) and more shallow in the lower half, where more infiltrates still persist. Once these have disappeared, a uniformly deep ulcer is to be expected. The relative amount of infiltrates in and around a herpetic ulcer is the only sign which gives us a clue as to its actual viral or metaherpetic pathophysiology. In Fig. 2.99, there are less infiltrates than in typical viral ulcers (e. g., Fig. 2.56). On the other hand, there are more infiltrates than in clearly metaherpetic stages (e. g., Fig. 2.98). One may classify such a case as a transitional stage between viral and metaherpetic pathophysiology. Therapeutically, the important basic therapy is the same as for every clear metaherpetic ulcer. The residual viral component will mostly fade away spontaneously without ongoing antiviral therapy. However, it is certainly not wrong, if such transition cases are also given an antiviral systemic cover with moderate doses of ACV (400 mg 3–5 qd) for one or two more weeks – just as a precaution.

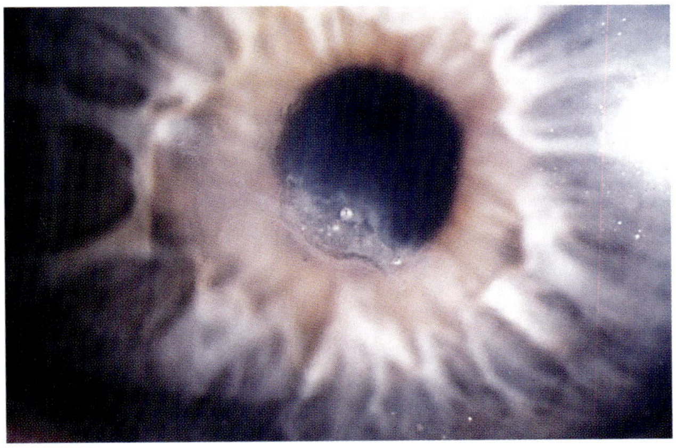

Fig. 2.97 Metaherpetic recurrent erosion

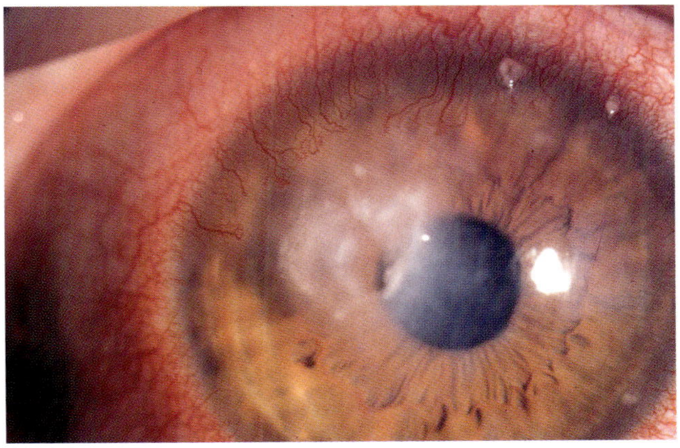

Fig. 2.98 Metaherpetic deep corneal ulcer

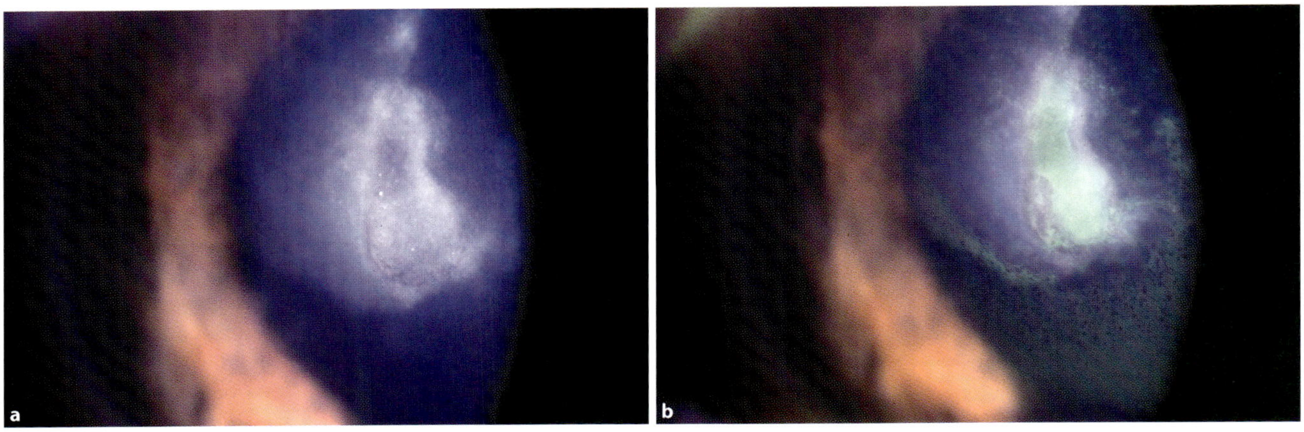


Fig. 2.99a,b Deep herpetic ulcer with mostly metaherpetic characteristics. **a** Unstained. **b** Fluorescein

## Detailed analysis of Fig 2.100

***Clinic:*** The giant ulcer in Fig. 2.100 developed from a HSV ulcerating interstitial keratitis, which was treated with too many topical steroids in addition to ACV ointment. Ointment remnants cover the ulcer base and make a judgement of residual infiltrations difficult. But there do not seem to be many. From 4 to 6 o'clock, an especially deep large oval defect presents near the limbus. Here, perforation of the cornea is an impending complication. Collarettes of pathologic regenerating epithelium are visible at the left border of the ulcer.

***Diagnosis:*** Deep metaherpetic ulcer with impending perforation near the limbus

***Differential diagnosis:*** Some residual viral activity cannot be excluded and must be considered therapeutically.

***Therapy:*** The deep oval defect near the limbus is the greatest threat. If the cornea perforates in that site, a perforating high risk keratoplasty has to be made. This can be avoided by immediate rescue surgery (amnion cover after cleaning of the ulcer base, see Sect. 2.14). Any potentially persisting viral activity should concomitantly be systemically treated (e.g., 400 mg ACV 5 qd plus fluocortolone 20 qd or equivalent steroid). Thus, a very dangerous situation can be cleared with minimal risk, and it may even be hoped that the remaining clear upper half of the cornea might later allow sufficient vision without perforating keratoplasty.

## Analysis of Fig 2.101

The longstanding deep central metaherpetic ulcer in Fig. 2.101 offers no realistic chance for sufficient vision after conservative healing, which will take many more months. An amnion cover can be performed for quicker consolidation. For noteworthy visual rehabilitation, however, a perforating keratoplasty will be the best solution. The only remaining choice to make is between immediate keratoplasty à chaud and a keratoplasty postponed to a later, more "quiet" stage after a preceding amnion cover. Which way is best for a patient is dependent on personal and logistic circumstances, e.g., the availability of a transplant and the decision whether or not an optimally HLA-matched graft is desired. In the latter case, one has to calculate additional waiting times, and then an intermittent amnion cover is certainly the optimal immediate measure. Generally, however, the prognosis for

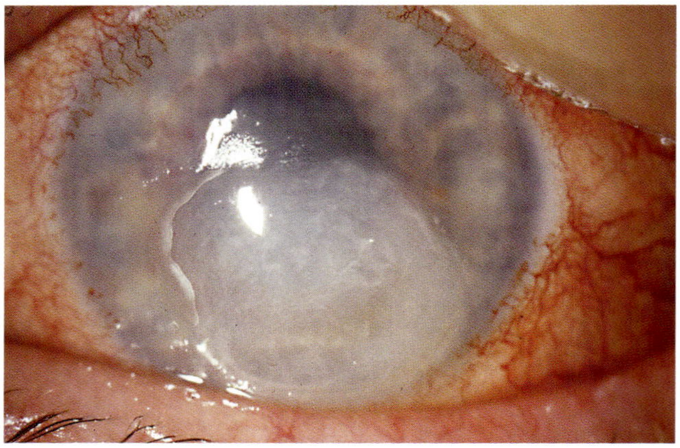

Fig. 2.100 Giant deep metaherpetic ulcer

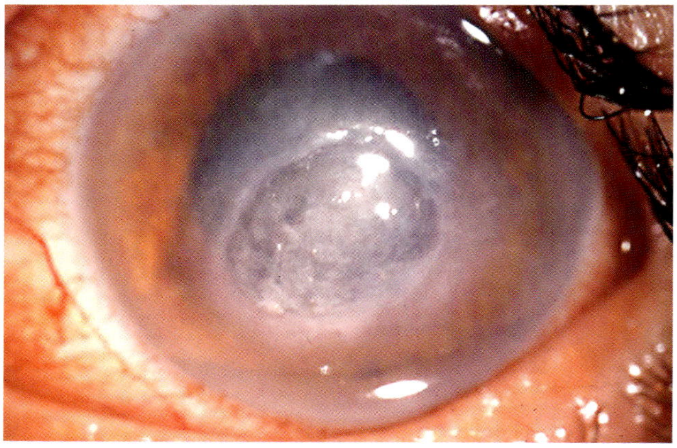

Fig. 2.101 Large deep central metaherpetic ulcer

keratoplasty à chaud with random transplants in herpes eyes is so excellent with adequate post-surgical care that the wide-spread fear of keratoplasties *à chaud* is unjustified. The advantage of immediate surgery is that overall drug therapy and its potential side effects are less. The same is true for the overall costs.

## Analysis of Fig 2.102

Figure 2.102 is a historic document from the early times of antiviral therapy, when only IDU was available with its now well-known cytotoxic side effects. HSV replication has after all been stopped and all infiltrating cells removed. However, every epithelial regeneration has also been stopped. The viral disease has been "overtreated". One could also call it "overkill". This example illustrates the principal danger of inadequately ongoing antiviral therapy for the development of metaherpetic ulcers. IDU is no longer used. However, the currently used antiviral agents also have at least some cytotoxic side effects which cannot be ignored when dealing with metaherpetic complications.

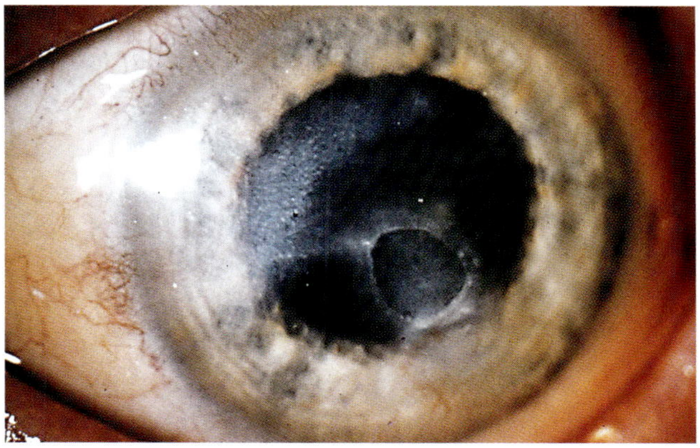

Fig. 2.102 Sharply demarcated deep metaherpetic ulcer with no infiltration and no effective epithelial regeneration after too intensive topical IDU treatment

## References


Algan B (1978) Considérations sur la kératite métaherpétique. Klin Monatsbl Augenheilkd 172 : 609–616

De Haas EBH (1962) Desiccation of cornea and conjunctiva after sensory denervation. Significance of desiccation for pathogenesis of neuroparalytic keratitis. Arch Ophthalmol 67: 79–92

Kaufman HE (1964) Epithelial erosion syndrome: metaherpetic keratitis. Am J Ophthalmol 57: 983–987

Kaufman HE (1967) Disease of the corneal stroma after herpes simplex infection. Am J Ophthalmol 63: 878–882

Kaufman HE, Brown DC, Ellison EM (1968) Herpes virus in the lacrimal gland, conjunctiva and cornea of man. Am J Ophthalmol 65: 32–35

Kok van Alphen CC, Völker-Dieben HJM (1981) Impairment of tear-production in corneal herpetic disease. In: R Sundmacher (ed) Herpetic Eye Diseases. Bergmann, Munich, pp 215–219

Mackie IA (1978) Role of corneal nerves in destructive disease of the cornea. Trans Ophth Soc UK 98: 343–347

Metcalf JF (1982) Corneal sensitivity and neurohistochemical studies of experimental herpetic keratitis in the rabbit. Exp Eye Res 35: 231–237

Singh D, Singh M, Singh R, Amritsar (1981) Herpetic keratitis causing lacrimal hyposecretion and xerosis. In: R Sundmacher (ed) Herpetic Eye Diseases. Bergmann, Munich, pp 211–214,

Sundmacher R, Neumann-Haefelin D (1976) Keratitis metaherpetica. Klinische und virologische Befunde. Klin Monatsbl Augenheilk 169: 728–737

Van Bijsterveld OP, de Koning EWJ (1984) Trophic herpetic corneal ulcers. In: FC Blodi (ed) Herpes Simplex Infections of the Eye. Contemporary Issues in Ophthalmology vol 1. Churchill Livingstone, NY, pp 29–45

# Clinically Manifest Primary HSV Infections

Section

**2.12**

## Core Messages

- An estimated 98% of primary ocular HSV infections are not identified because they either remain subclinical or pass as quickly transient slight conjunctivitis without raising attention.
- If primary HSV infection is severe enough to cause disease, the clinical signs are typically different from those of recurrent HSV disease.
- Clinically manifest primary HSV infections should be treated systemically with antiviral agents.

An estimated 98% of primary ocular HSV infections are never identified because they either remain subclinical or pass unrecognized as quickly transient slight conjunctivitis, without raising attention. Consequently, nearly all HSV ocular disease, which is diagnosed for the first time, is already secondary, endogenously recurrent disease from the pathophysiologic point of view (see Sect. 2.1). Only in an estimated 2%, primary infection manifests itself clinically as disease. These diseases are easily recognizable as herpetic, and, in addition, they exhibit unique clinical signs which make them identifiable as primary infections. An IgM analysis is mostly unnecessary for confirmation. Primary HSV diseases should be treated systemically with antiviral agents in order to limit primary HSV spread in the eye and in the associated ganglionic tissue as much as possible.

The difference between primary and secondary recurrent disease is, of course, the absence or presence of immune reactions at the beginning of the episode. Primary infection starts without impeding or modifying immune reactions. These increase only gradually thereafter until they have become efficient enough to terminate viral replication.

In the recurrent disease situation, immune reactions modify disease from the beginning. Either disease is primarily inhibited and peripheral viral shedding remains without pathologic sequelae, or disease develops in the presence of a local antiviral defence which is too weak. An important aspect is that immune reactions not only limit disease activity, but that they often also increase or sustain it. The latter may at least partly be a reason why secondary HSV disease manifests itself so much more frequently than primary disease.

Primary HSV infections are no longer only observed in childhood, as was still the case half a century ago. Nowadays, more and more primary HSV infections do not occur before adolescence or early adulthood, depending on the general hygienic conditions and the social milieu. This time, the shift in primary infections goes along with an increased risk of acquiring HSV-2 instead of HSV-1 through sexual activities. HSV-2 has been suspected to cause more severe human disease than HSV-1. Even if the difference should not be dramatic, HSV-2 has a different sensitivity towards antiviral agents than HSV-1. HSV-2 is totally resistant, e.g., against BVDU. The general time shift and the infection routes of primary infection may thus have influence on the severity and treatment of subsequent eye disease in herpes patients.

While the diagnosis of clinically manifest primary HSV disease and its treatment are mostly easy, some questions remain, which relate to the pathophysiologic differences between primary and secondary disease:

- Why do primary HSV infections remain mostly subclinical?
- What predisposes a primary infected human being to develop severe primary disease?
- Is this predisposition the same in all human beings, or does a variable combination of different causes (infectious dose of HSV, pathogenicity of the HSV strain involved, entry site, genetically different susceptibility of the host tissues towards HSV, and other reasons) explain the differences?
- What makes secondary recurrent infections so often clinically manifest?
- Patients with clinically severe primary infection do not have to expect a more severe course of *recurrent* HSV disease than patients in whom primary infection passed unrecognized. What is the reason for this?

To date, scientifically proven answers are unobtainable.

### Detailed analysis of Fig 2.103

***Clinic:*** The girl gives an impression of general infection with malaise, left-sided inflammatory ptosis, red tearing left eye with crusted exudate on the lower lid margin, and cutaneous herpes efflorescences below the left nostril with swollen lips (Fig. 2.103).

The preauricular lymph nodes on the left are palpable and tender. Body temperature is slightly above normal. The mother shows a healing herpes blister on the lower lip.

***Diagnosis:*** Clinically manifest primary HSV infection at three mucosal sites (ocular, nasal, and oral), transferred from the mother. The primary infection typically concerns one eye only with serous conjunctivitis and no other involvement of cornea or lid margins. The right eye has remained totally normal, and it will stay normal and unaffected by recurrences, if forced superinfection by scratching or rubbing is avoided. Future endogenous recurrences can manifest themselves either as monosymptomatic oral or ocular disease – always at the sites of primary infection – or also as combined oral-ocular disease.

***Differential diagnosis:*** None. IgM analysis was performed for documentation only, and it proved the diagnosis. If the causal infection of the mother would have been unknown, and if the girl´s herpes blisters under the left nostril would not have existed, at least a suspicion of HSV primary infection would have arisen nonetheless because of the *heavily exudating* conjunctivitis. Such a conjunctivitis is a feature of *exogenous* microbial or viral infections, but never a feature of endogenously recurring HSV disease. Therefore, the differential diagnosis would have been made between some microbial infection and primary viral infection, above all of HSV or ADV origin. A laboratory check-up would have given the correct diagnosis.

***Therapy:*** 7–10 days of systemic ACV therapy are recommended in order to limit primary HSV spread in the eye and in the associated ganglionic tissue as much as possible.

***Prophylaxis:*** Clinically manifest primary infections offer the chance to prepare for recurrence triggers. In children and adolescents, above all general infections and fever are operative. Thorough education about the risks and signs of local recurrences is important, as is the advice to immediately see an ophthalmologist once the left eye again starts to become symptomatic. For security, one should also organize to start self-prophylaxis with 400 mg ACV 3 qd (or 200 mg ACV 5 qd) every time, the development of an ocular recurrence is suspected. This is especially important if consulting an ophthalmologist is not always possible in time. Of course, such self-prophylaxis must not be perpetuated without seeking ophthalmological help as quickly as possible.

## Analysis of Fig 2.104

The gross impression of the right eye region of the young man in Fig. 2.104a is similar to that in Fig. 2.103a: Moderate inflammatory ptosis and a red tearing eye. Different to Fig. 2.103a, we are dealing not only with acute exudating conjunctivitis but also with a blistering blepharitis involving the lid margins along the lashes. The blisters are large, and, in this form and extension (Fig. 2.104b), they are never seen in ordinary recurrent blepharitis. Giant blisters are pathognomonic for clinically manifest primary HSV disease. The likely pathophysiologic explanation for this phenomenon is that immune reactions, which would limit the spread of herpes blisters, are absent in the beginning of primary infection. This leads to much larger diseased areas than in recurrent situations.

## Detailed analysis of Fig 2.105

***Clinic:*** The patient in Fig. 2.105 suffers from an exsudating conjunctivitis, which in itself gives no direct diagnostic clue. The lower lid margin, however, exhibitis pathognomonic HSV signs: The intermarginal epithelium has nearly totally been lost, and the intermarginal area is covered by a slimy layer. The subtotal loss of the intermarginal epithelium can easily be overlooked. It is more clearly visible, when the lid margin is cautiously wiped with a cot-

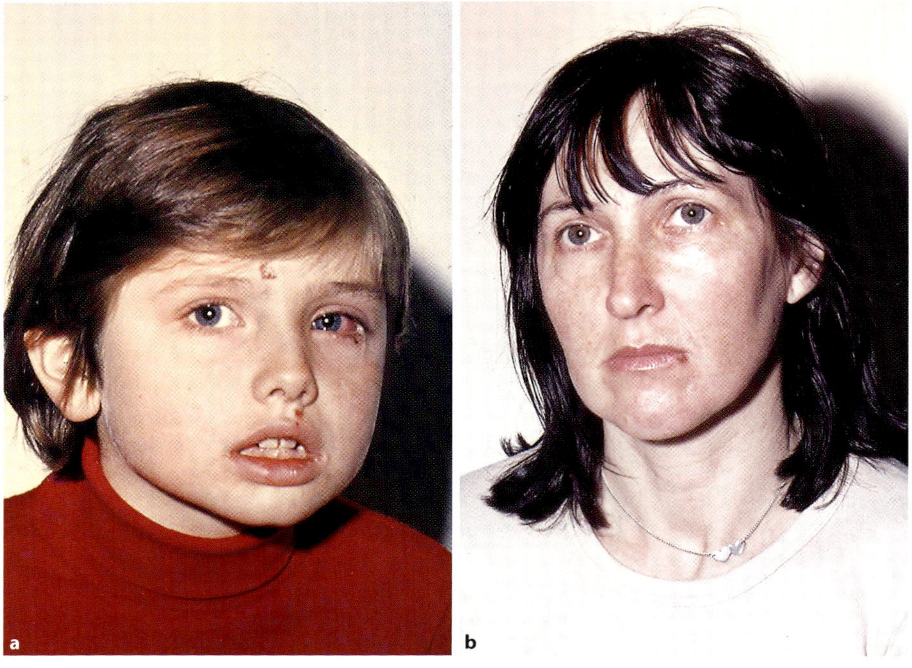

Fig. 2.103 Clinically manifest primary HSV disease in a girl (**a**) infected via her mothers recurrent labial herpes (**b**)

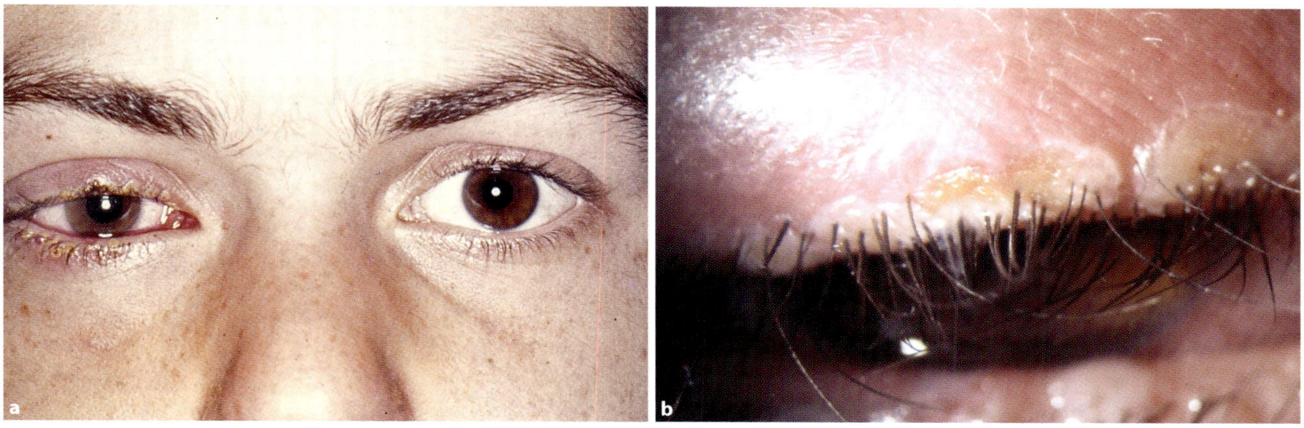

Fig. 2.104a,b Typical "giant blisters" in the early stage of clinically manifest primary HSV blepharitis (see text)

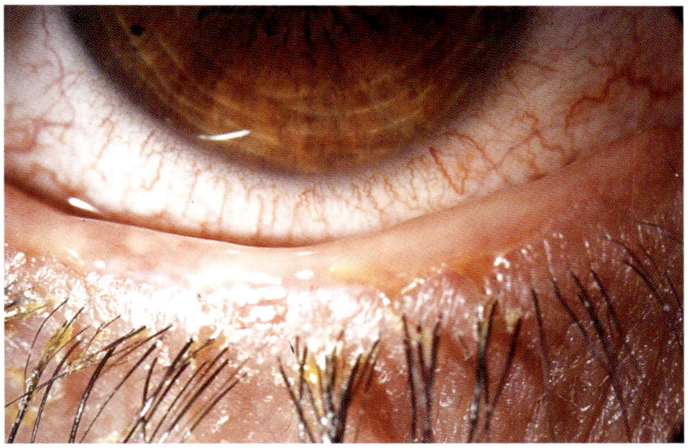

Fig. 2.105 Intermarginal blepharitis comprising the entire lower margin in clinically manifest primary HSV infection

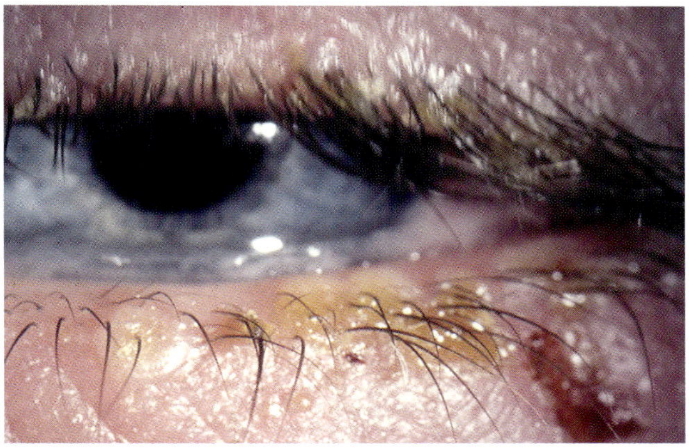

Fig. 2.106 Clinically manifest primary intermarginal HSV blepharitis

ton tip, and the surface thereafter stained with fluorescein and/or Bengal rose.

***Diagnosis:*** Intermarginal blepharitis in clinically manifest primary HSV infection.

***Differential diagnosis:*** None. The general pathognomic importance of intermarginal blepharitis for HSV etiology has already been pointed out in Sect. 2.3. Here, it remains shown that extended intermarginal lesions, like in Fig. 2.105, are never encountered in normal recurrent disease (compare Fig. 2.12). Such extended forms of intermarginal blepharitis are a reliable sign of primary infection.

***Therapy and prophylaxis:*** See Fig. 2.103.

## Analysis of Fig 2.106

Figure 2.106 shows another case of clinically manifest primary HSV blepharitis. There is not yet an extended intermarginal erosion, but two large vesicles comparable to those in Fig. 2.104 are discernible in the middle of the picture. They will quickly lose their epithelial roof and then coalesce to form a large intermarginal ulcer. The excessive exudate stems partly from the blepharitis and partly from the accompanying conjunctivitis.

## Analysis of Fig 2.107

Figure 2.107 is chosen to show that extended and so much coalescing and exudating lid lesions with typical herpes vesicles in the adjacent dermis are practically pathognomonic for clinically manifest primary HSV disease. Comparing this to Fig. 2.14, a differential diagnosis of eczema herpeticum in a patient with endogenous eczema would be a differential diagnostic possibility. This can be excluded, however, by Fig. 2.107a, which shows that the facial dermis outside the diseased right lid area is totally normal with no signs of endogenous eczema whatsoever.

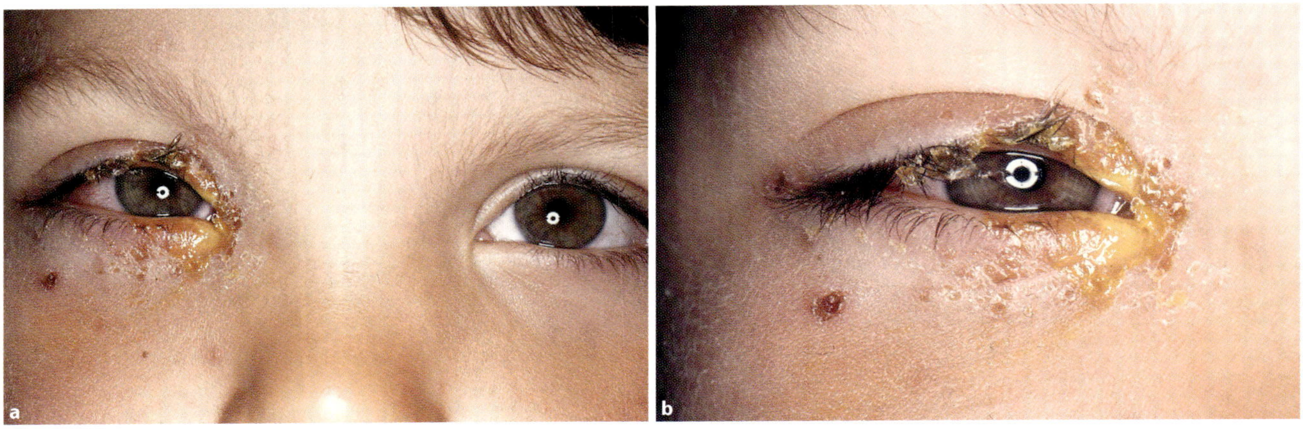

Fig. 2.107a,b Clinically manifest primary HSV blepharitis and intermarginal blepharitis

## Analysis of Fig 2.108

Figure 2.108a shows a case with severely exudating muco-serous conjunctivitis, Fig. 2.108b a muco-serous conjunctivitis with small areas of membranous conjunctivitis and epithelial cell loss in the lower cul-de-sac, Fig. 2.108c a severe necrotizing conjunctivitis. Each of these types of acute exudating conjunctivitis is *not typical by itself* for herpes infection or primary HSV infection. The possible etiologies range from a large variety of non-viral causes over microbial infections to other viruses, especially adenoviruses, and also to non-infectious immunologic causes. The HSV etiology must be proven in the laboratory in every single case. If a herpes etiology has thus been proven, however, it is also undisputable that it can only be clinically *manifest primary* HSV conjunctivitis. A *recurrent* HSV conjunctivitis *never* takes such a severe exudating or necrotizing course.

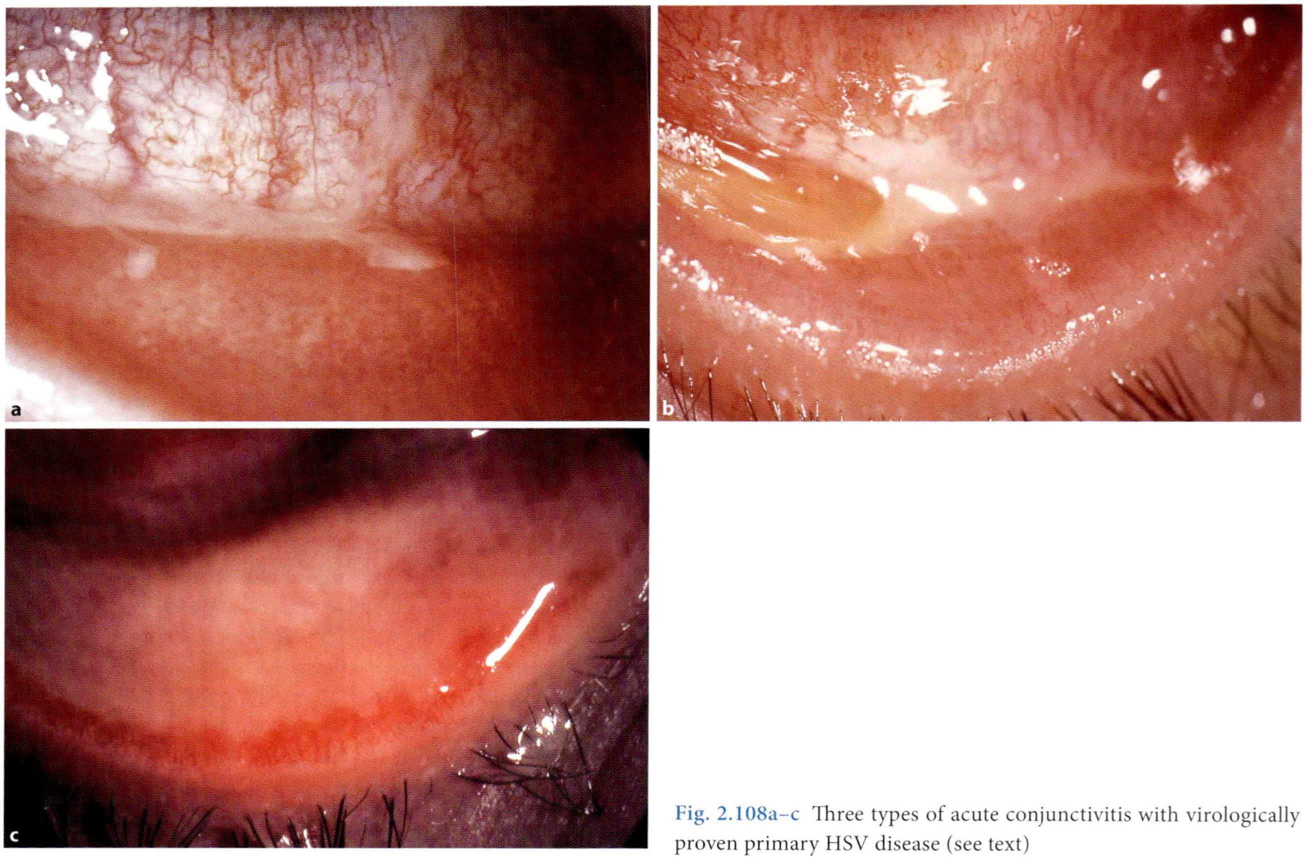

Fig. 2.108a–c Three types of acute conjunctivitis with virologically proven primary HSV disease (see text)

## Analysis of Fig 2.109

Taking into account the moderate amount and type of inflammation which is usually associated with recurrent herpes disease, it becomes clear from Fig. 2.109, that the grade of residual inflammation after 2 weeks of illness is much greater than it should be with any type of recurrent disease. The lid edema is still large as is the periorbital edema (Fig. 2.109a). The two cutaneous herpes efflorescences are deeply umbilicated with central defects, which still await filling-up by cellular regrowth. The conjunctiva is still edematous (Fig. 2.109b). This is never seen to such an extent in recurrent disease. In addition, an unusually massive follicular conjunctival reaction has developed. This indicates that significant HSV replication is still going on in the conjunctiva, and that the risk of viral persistence developing in the conjunctiva with a rather prolonged course of follicular conjunctivitis exists. All these signs together allow a reliable clinical diagnosis of manifest primary HSV infection.

## Analysis of Fig 2.110

The limbal efflorescence shown in Fig. 2.110 is *pathognomonic* for HSV etiology. It is *observed only in primary HSV infection*. The Bengal rose stain makes the sharp outlines and the reticulate structure of the efflorescence especially well visible. It remains unclear why HSV has a predelection for this transition zone between conjunctival and corneal epithelium only in primary HSV infections.

## Analysis of Fig 2.111

Figure 2.111 shows a HSV limbitis, which comprises nearly the whole limbal circumference in primary infection. Unlike Bengal rose, which stains directly the diseased or dead epithelium (Fig. 2.110), fluorescein can only make visible the gross topography of the efflorescences by leaking through broken tight junctions into the subepithelial space. Without staining, HSV limbitis cannot be directly visualized. It can only be suspected by a swol-

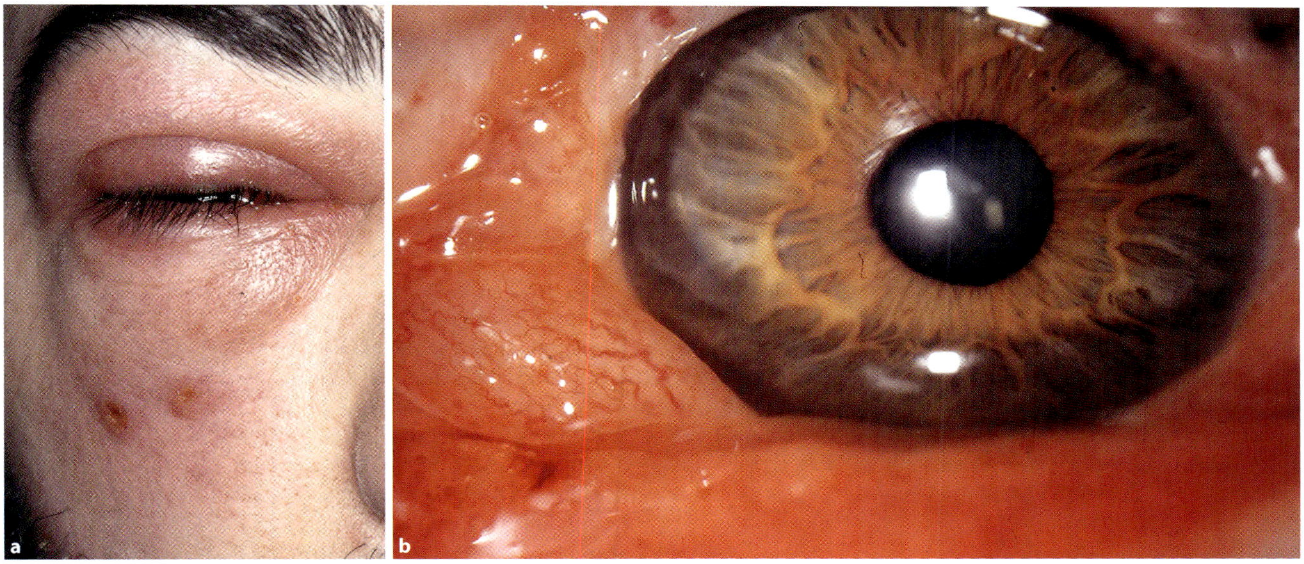


**Fig. 2.109a,b** Clinically manifest primary HSV infection in a young man, 2 weeks after onset (see text)

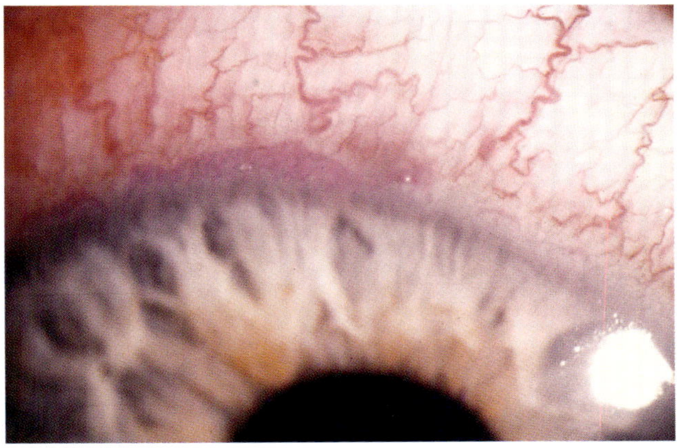

**Fig. 2.110** *Pathognomonic HSV limbitis* in clinically manifest primary HSV infection (Bengal rose)

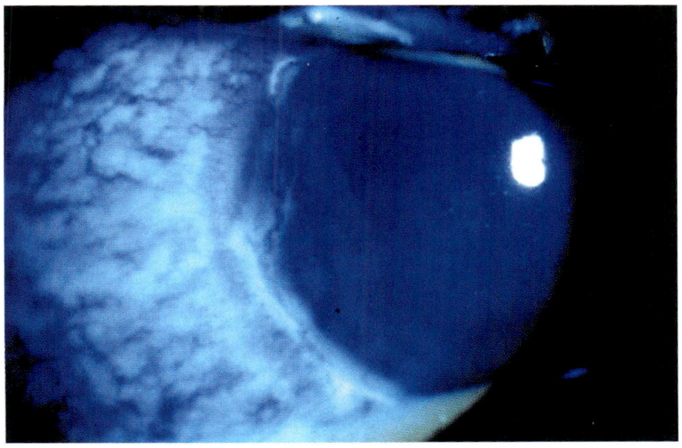

**Fig. 2.111** *Pathognomonic limbitis* in primary HSV infection (fluorescein)

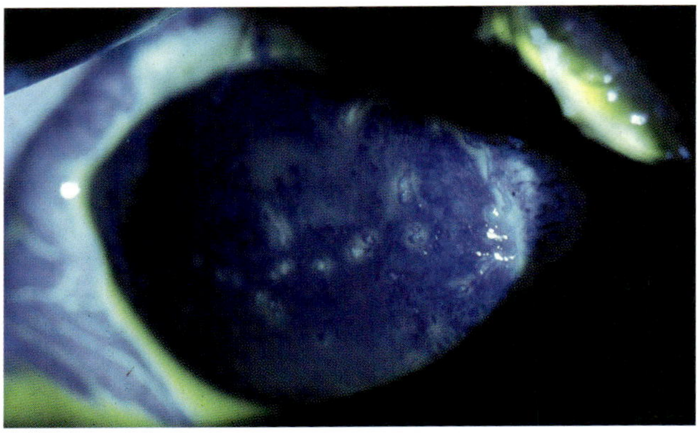

Fig. 2.112 Disseminated punctate, stellate, and dendritic HSV efflorescences in primary HSV infection, plus *pathognomonic* limbitis (fluorescein)

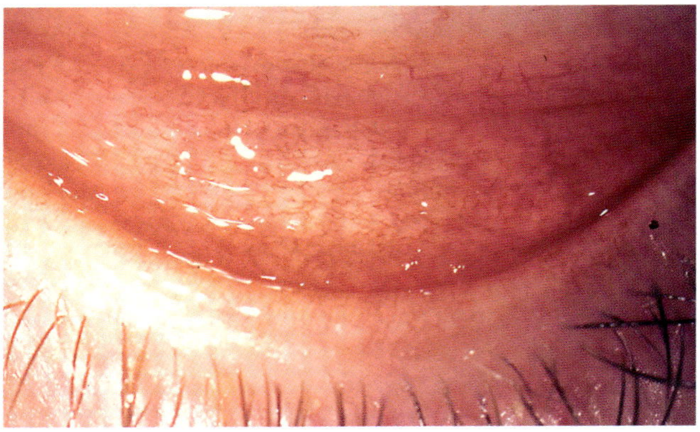

Fig. 2.113 Differential diagnosis: Chronic follicular conjunctivitis of unknown etiology

len appearance of the limbal area and is therefore often overlooked. For safe diagnosis, either Bengal rose or fluorescein staining is necessary.

## Analysis of Fig 2.112

The disseminated punctate, stellate, and dendritic HSV efflorescences are by themselves pathognomonic for HSV etiology, but *not* for primary infection. The biomicroscopic fine structure of these lesions is identical in primary and recurrent disease! Moreover, the distribution on the cornea of the efflorescences is no differentiating criteria for primary versus recurrent disease. There are just two signs in Fig. 2.112 that are typical for clinically manifest primary HSV disease. First, the exudative conjunctivitis, which can be seen on the left-hand side, would be atypical for recurrent disease and, second, there is above all a limbitis visible on the right side of the limbus, which is pathognomonic for primary disease (compare Figs. 2.110 and 2.111).

## Analysis of Fig 2.113

Aside from macrofollicles in chlamydial and molluscum contagiosum conjunctivitis, conjunctival follicles can have so many different etiologies that their mere presence gives no hint as to their etiology, and not even a hint to general viral etiology (Fig. 2.113). They may occasionally grow immediately after primary HSV infection if HSV persists for some time in the conjunctival tissues (see Fig. 2.109). But once the virus has been successfully eliminated from the conjunctiva, such follicles disappear. Accordingly, they are even rarer observed with established antiviral immunity, i. e., in the recurrent situation. Then they are probably associated with either peripheral HSV persistence or with extraordinarily frequent HSV shedding from the neurons into the conjunctiva (Fig. 2.17). Without longstanding presence of HSV antigens in the conjunctiva – which practically always also indicates presence of the virus itself – chronic follicular HSV conjunctivitis is difficult to imagine.

## References


Ameye C, Maudgal PC, Missotten L (1985) Primary ocular HSV infections in adults. In: PC Maudgal, L Missotten (eds) Herpetic Eye Diseases. Doc Ophthalmol Proc ser 44, pp 133–140

Beigi B, Algawi K, Foleye-Nolan A, O′Keefe M (1994) Herpes simplex keratitis in children. Br J Ophthalmol 78: 458–460

Colin J, Le Grignou A, BAikoff G, Chastel C (1980) Three cases of dendritic herpetic ulcerations of the conjunctiva. Am J Ophthalmol 4: 608

Darougar S, Wishart MS, Vishwalingham ND (1985): Epidemiological and clinical features of primary herpes simplex virus ocular infection. Br J Ophthalmol 69: 2–6

Ostler HB (1976) Herpes simplex: the primary infection. Surv Ophthalmol 21: 91–99

Poirier RH (1980) Herpetic ocular infections of childhood. Arch Ophthalmol 98: 704–706

Sundmacher R (1981) A clinico-virologic classification of herpetic anterior segment diseases with special reference to intraocular herpes. In: R Sundmacher (ed) Herpetic eye diseases. Bergmann, Munich, pp 203–208

Wald A, Benedetti, Davis G, Remington M, Winter C, Corey L (1994) A randomized, double-blind, comparative trial comparing high- and standard-dose oral acyclovir for first-episode genital herpes infections. Antimicrob Agents Chemother 38: 174–176

Posavad CM, Koelle DM, Corey L (1998) Tipping the scales of herpes simplex virus reactivation: the important responses are local. Nat Med 4: 381–382

Sundmacher R (1984) Trauma und Herpes. Fortschr Ophthalmol 81: 409–415

Sundmacher R (1986) Keratitis dendritica nach Hornhautfremdkörper. Klin Monatsbl Augenheilk 188: 307–309

Wald A, Zeh J, Selke S, Warren T, Ryncarz AJ, Ashley R, Krieger JN, Corey L (2000) Reactivation of genital herpes simplex virus type 2 infection in asymptomatic seropositive persons. N Engl J Med 342: 844–850

Zheng X, Loutsch JM, Shimomura Y, Gebhardt BM, Hill JM, Kaufman HE (1999) Reactivation of herpes virus after lamellar keratoplasty. Jpn J Ophthalmol 43: 257–261

# Intraocular Surgery and Keratoplasty in HSV Eyes

Section

2.14

This section gives an overview of the most frequently used methods to restore vision in herpes eyes. Emphasis is laid on the indications for each method and on the potential complications and their handling. Differential diagnosis of postkeratoplasty complications is amply presented with clinical examples. For detailed technical aspects and problems, the reader is referred to specialized surgical publications. The different topics are structured as follows:



## 2.14.A General Rules for Surgery in Herpes Eyes

There are no principal limitations for surgery in herpes eyes. All types of surgery which are judged to be necessary or useful can principally be performed, nearly any time, even in severely inflamed eyes. This is made possible by the availability of systemically applicable potent antiviral agents, especially of ACV.

### 2.14.A.1 Systemic ACV Prophylaxis and Therapy of Herpes Complications

Three levels of systemic ACV application can be defined. The ACV dose doubles with each higher level:

1. Systemic *ACV prophylaxis* with 200 mg ACV 5 qd (or 400 mg ACV 3 qd). This dose effectively protects "quiet" herpes eyes from endogenously recurrent HSV disease as long as it is given. It is regularly recommended as a safety shield inhibiting herpes complications in conjunction with surgery in "quiet" herpes eyes.
2. Systemic *ACV therapy* with 400 mg ACV 5 qd. This is the normal dose for treatment of clinically symptomatic HSV disease. It is applied in all surgical situations where active HSV disease is still present or has only recently become subclinical.
3. *Maximal* systemic ACV *therapy* with 800 mg ACV 5 qd. It is recommended only for those cases where surgery has to be done in an emergency situation with much infiltration of the cornea or with severe disease of more than one part of the anterior segment of the eye.

It must be admitted that the real risk of triggering endogenous herpes recurrences by corneoconjunctival or intraocular surgery is unknown. It may well be that it is far lower than commonly assumed (see Sect. 2.13). The rare documentation of traumatically induced HSV disease (see Sect. 2.13) and the reportedly small risk of triggering a recurrence in herpes corneas by excimer laser treatment support such a view. As no reliable figures are available from the literature, and as systemic ACV prophylaxis of HSV recurrences is so easy and safe, not having applied ACV prophylaxis in a surgical herpes patient might be difficult to justify if herpetic disease flares up a couple of days after surgery.

### 2.14.A.2 Cataract and Glaucoma Surgery

With a prophylactic systemic ACV cover, *cataract surgery and intraocular lens implantation* in herpes eyes as well as any kind of *glaucoma surgery* for chronic secondary glaucoma have the same chance-risk profile as in normal eyes. We recommend

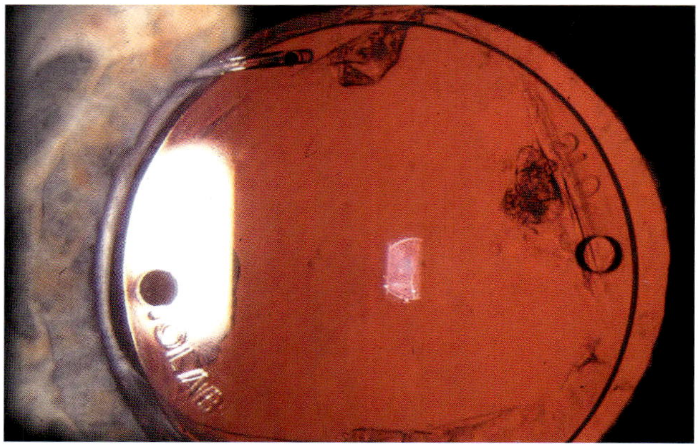

Fig. 2.115 Intraocular lens implantation under ACV cover in a herpes eye

maintaining full antiviral protection as long as the eye has not returned to its normal uninflamed state. Thereafter, HSV recurrences could potentially manifest themselves more frequently than before. The experience has been, however, that the incidence of recurrences is certainly not greater in the time period after surgery than in the time period before. The contrary may even be true in some patients after surgical "normalization". The herpes eye in Fig. 2.115 remained quiet after IOL implantation with no intraocular or corneal HSV recurrences for more than 20 years. I followed several patients suffering from frequent intraocular HSV recurrences with severe secondary glaucoma. When this became chronic and could no longer be treated medically, goniotrephination under ACV cover became necessary. Contrary to what was to be expected, the fistulae worked perfectly in these eyes in spite of the long inflammatory history of the conjunctiva. Glaucoma did not recur for decades, and no further intraocular HSV recurrences were observed. Such is only anecdotal experience, and goniotrephination is certainly not recommended as a surgical means against intraocular HSV recurrences. However, this anecdotal experience is nonetheless reassuring and may help to reduce the still widespread unjustified reservation against surgery in herpes eyes.

## 2.14.B Emergency Surgery with Different Tissue Covers

This type of surgery was developed in the old days, when effective antiviral drug therapy was unavailable, and when there was no other way to save severely infiltrated, melting, or already perforated herpes eyes than by covering them firmly with conjunctiva or cornea – i.e., with a biological wound dressing. It was hoped, that the eye would finally heal under the biocover, and so it regularly did.

Surgeons who have never experienced the need to resort to conjunctival flaps or to full thickness sclerocorneal buttons in severe herpes disease may look at these methods as being archaic and superfluous. But they are still needed in special situations. Therefore, these experiences are included in this atlas.

It is true that the indication for conjunctival flaps and corneal buttons as biodressing has largely decreased in the last decades. This loss of importance of the old methods has been accelerated by the success of a new cover method, which has started booming only in the last decade, i.e., the amnion membrane cover.

### 2.14.B.1 Conjunctiva

The oldest emergency surgery is covering a non-healing ulcerating herpes cornea with a conjunctival flap. Most frequently Gundersen´s technique is used.

While reconstructive perforating keratoplasty à chaud is nowadays the quickest and the most efficient way for primary surgery in ulcerating eyes, there are still indications where postponement of primary keratoplasty and instead performance of a conjunctival flap is a wise decision, e.g.:

- Severe incurable general illness and limited life span
- Impossibility of the necessary postkeratoplasty therapy with immunosuppressive agents plus ACV systemically
- No possibility to seek regularly ophthalmologic help and advice after keratoplasty
- Severe non-compliance of patients with drug or alcohol addiction
- Impossibility of any controlled treatment in mentally retarded patients
- Patient´s own decision not to undergo another keratoplasty after previous failures, but rather to content himself with a "quiet" covered eye

For the proper technique – which is not always easy – surgical textbooks must be consulted. The flap should not be too thin and not too thick, and it should be large enough. Before covering, the corneal surface must be cleaned from all epithelium and inflammatory debris. For this procedure, a thermomechanical debridement method with a heated metallic tip is ideal, because one can simultaneously destroy the thermolabile herpes viruses by heat.

If desired, a cosmetically irritating aspect of a "white eye" (Fig. 2.116c) can be fairly normalized by fitting a thin cosmetic eye prosthesis or a cosmetic soft contact lens on top. Under the conjunctival flap, HSV replication invariably stops. The inflammation subsides and the underlying cornea heals. If necessary, it is possible to remove the flap later on and perform a perforating keratoplasty, if the conditions and prospects for keratoplasty have meanwhile been sufficiently improved.

### 2.14.B.2 Cornea

Another surgical technique, which was first performed in Moscow some 50 years ago, is by suturing a full thickness sclerocorneal button on the heavily diseased herpes cornea. This method is especially recommendable if the conjunctiva is too

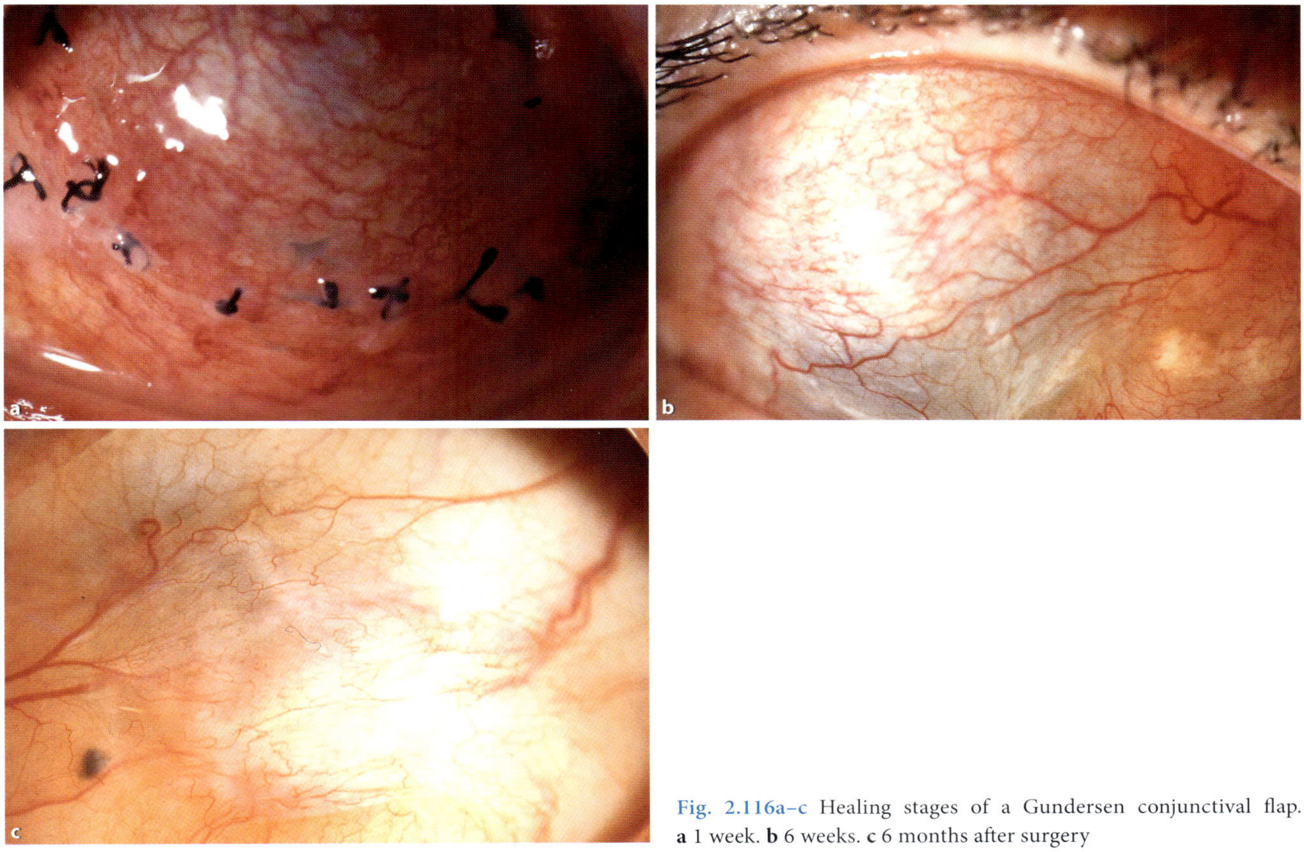

Fig. 2.116a–c Healing stages of a Gundersen conjunctival flap. **a** 1 week. **b** 6 weeks. **c** 6 months after surgery

weak or too short for Gundersen´s technique, or if a biocover is needed only temporarily until keratoplasty becomes possible within weeks or months.

## Analysis of Fig 2.117

This method is illustrated by the follow-up pictures of a patient, in whom no medical therapy would stop his ulcerating HSV keratitis from progressing to perforation (Fig. 2.117). An immediate keratoplasty à chaud was not advisable because the herpetic infiltrations reached the limbus already and could not sufficiently be removed by trephination (Fig. 2.117a, b). The diseased cornea and limbus were covered by a large full-thickness sclerocorneal graft fixed to the perilimbal sclera by nylon sutures (Fig. 2.117c). The donor cornea was left for nearly five months untouched in situ. Only loosened sutures were removed. In this time period, the donor cornea was progressively infiltrated by leukocytes and partially invaded by vessels (Fig. 2.117c, d) resulting in a sometimes irritating purulent aspect. It could be seen, however, that the underlying eye itself became more and more quiet. After 3–4 months, the donor cornea began to gradually dissolve. The remnants were surgically removed after five months (Fig. 2.117e). Already one month later, the patient's cornea had recovered to its best achievable state with areas of bullous keratopathy, some vascularization, and limbal thinning (Fig. 2.117f). Perforating keratoplasty restored vision successfully and permanently one year later (Fig. 2.117g).

### 2.14.B.3 Amnion

Currently, the most frequently used surgical healing aid for deep herpetic ulcers is by an amnion membrane sutured directly on the corneal defect. The advantages of this procedure are:

- Amnion contains molecules that transmit helpful anti-inflammatory signals into the underlying infiltrated cornea.
- Unlike with conjunctival flaps and sclerocorneal buttons, the whole anterior segment of the eye remains easily controllable. No pharmacokinetic barriers are built up against topical therapy.
- The amnion mostly dissolves spontaneously after having served its purpose, and only the corneal sutures must be removed when they loosen spontaneously.

There are also disadvantages and limitations of this method:

- Surgery with the delicate amnion material requires some skills.
- Accordingly, amnion sheets often loosen too early, which makes re-operations necessary.
- Unlike with conjunctival or full thickness corneal covers, which can also be used in far advanced cases (i. e., descemetoceles or even pin point perforations), amnion membranes are safe only for cases with still sufficient stromal layers left on Descemet´s.

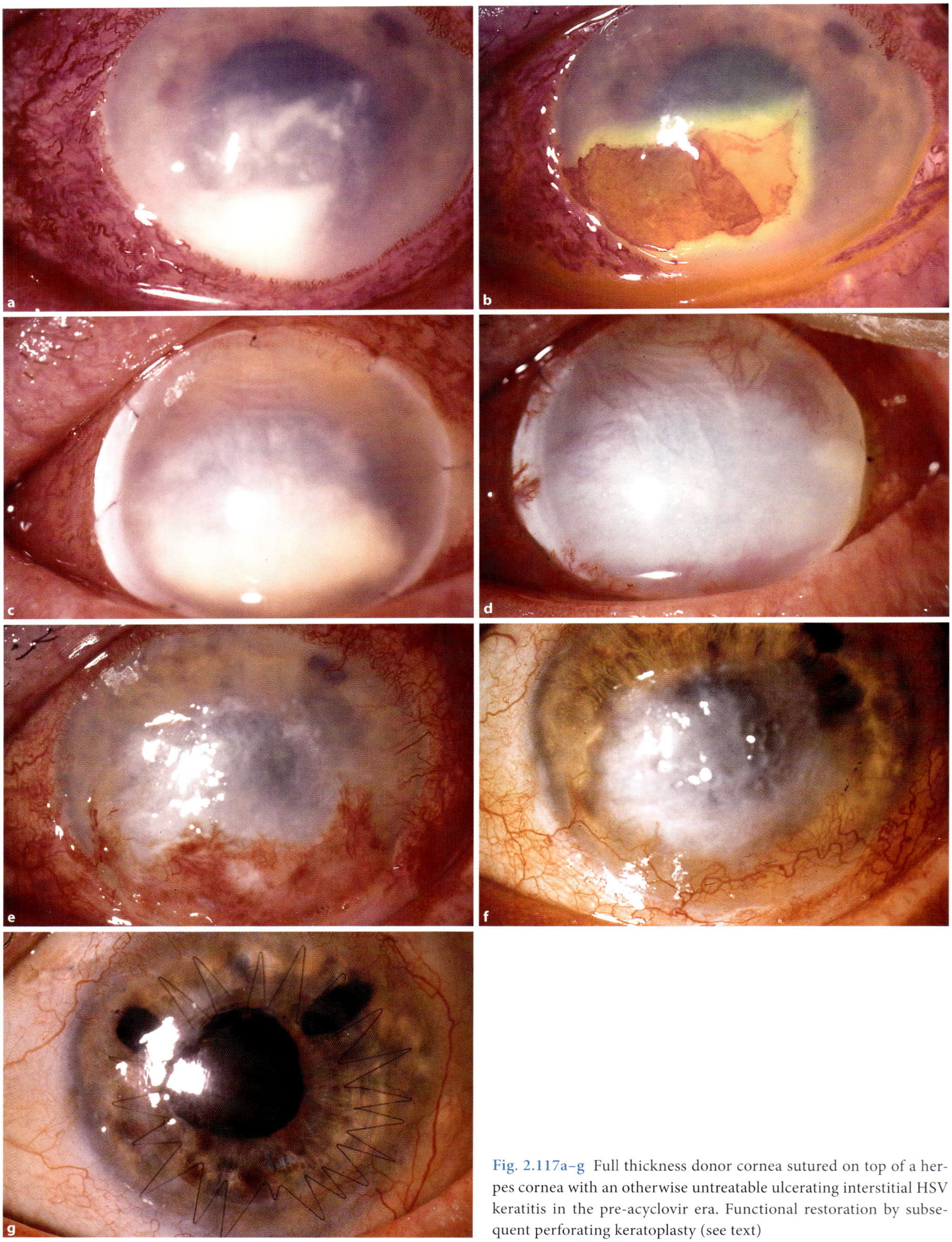

Fig. 2.117a–g Full thickness donor cornea sutured on top of a herpes cornea with an otherwise untreatable ulcerating interstitial HSV keratitis in the pre-acyclovir era. Functional restoration by subsequent perforating keratoplasty (see text)

As with every type of biodressing, the ulcer must first be cleaned (e.g., by thermomechanical debridement) before the amnion can be sutured on. If no *systemic* antiviral combination therapy is available, an amnion cover is too subtle, too insecure, and too dangerous to rely on. In such situations, a conjunctival or corneal cover is still to be preferred. Some surgeons apply soft therapeutic contact lenses for a while as a second mechanical shield on top of the amnion. I have not found this really necessary and have rather preferred to additionally secure the surface with a proper combination of ointments comprising also ACV.

### Analysis of Fig 2.118

The patient with the deep herpetic ulcer in Fig. 2.118a was not yet prepared to undergo perforating keratoplasty, which retrospectively would have offered him the quickest rehabilitation with the least overall drug investment and the least costs. Instead, a solution which accelerates healing and leaves a chance for regaining satisfying vision *without* perforating keratoplasty was preferred. This was a surgical cover by an amnion membrane (Fig. 2.117b, 1 week after surgery). The healing was achieved as predicted (Fig. 2.118c, four months after surgery, without amnion membrane). The function, however, did not match the patient's expectations. So the patient had to decide again, whether or not he should dare to undergo perforating keratoplasty as a second procedure, or content himself with a reduced function and the perspective of a further increasing recurrence rate, as is frequently the case with such eyes.

## 2.14.C Optical Improvement of an Irregular Corneal Surface

Sometimes, functional impairment of herpes eyes results more from an irregular corneal surface than from dense corneal scars. Therefore, it is worthwhile to test the functional effect of hard contact lenses on vision before making a decision for perforating keratoplasty. In this context, excimer laser therapeutic ablation may also be worth considering as a method to escape the need for homokeratoplasty in selected cases.

### 2.14.C.1 Contact Lenses

In Sect. 2.11 on metaherpetic diseases the usefulness of *therapeutic soft contact lenses* for accelerating healing of superficial metaherpetic ulcers has already been addressed. It has also been addressed that contact lenses unfortunately change the aspect and the fine structure of epithelial efflorescences so

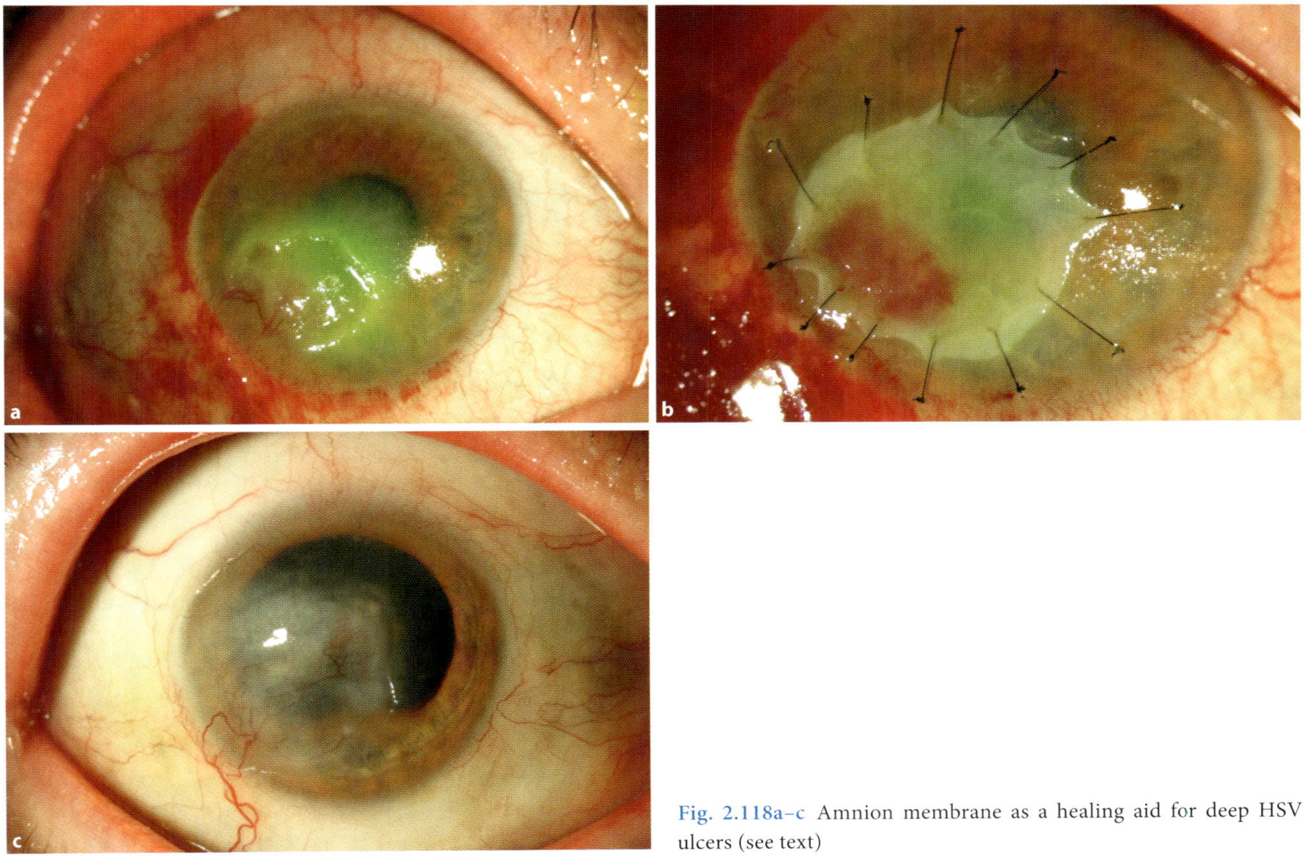

Fig. 2.118a–c Amnion membrane as a healing aid for deep HSV ulcers (see text)

much (especially the pathognomonic microscopic features of HSV dendrites) that intercurrent HSV epithelial recurrences may develop unnoticed, which is a potential danger. Also, it must be held probable, at least theoretically, that a constantly varying irritation by contact lenses, especially by "hard" contact lenses, may trigger herpes recurrences, as small as this danger may clinically be (see Sect. 2.13).

Apart from these reservations, fitting of a *diagnostic "hard"* contact lens is often indispensable, when the indication for perforating keratoplasty has to be weighed against alternative options.

A *flexible "hard"* contact lens *made of highly oxygen permeable materials* is provisionally fitted, and best corrected contact lens vision is evaluated. The results of contact lens vision as compared with corrected vision without contact lenses give valuable information about the relative impact of an irregular corneal surface, of corneal scars, lens opacities, and of macular function. All these influences should be known when estimating the functional prognosis for a perforating keratoplasty.

If the results of a diagnostic contact lens test are such that fitting for permanent optical correction appears promising, then this option should be consequently tried.

Often, a stabile fit with "hard" contact lenses will be impossible because of too much surface irregularity. Then, this option has to be given up. Large soft contact lenses, which center more easily, are not really recommendable as an alternative because their surface correcting potential is usually too low, and the impairment of corneal metabolism is generally higher with them than with movable flexible lenses.

The reduced corneal sensitivity of herpes eyes is a two-edged phenomenon. On one hand, it helps with a greater contact lens tolerance. On the other hand, it may be dangerous, because corneal damage by less than optimally fitted contact lenses is not always realized by the patient himself. Therefore, frequent routine controls of the fit of the contact lens and the corneal tolerance are important, at least in the beginning of "hard" contact lens wearing.

Comparing the chances and risks of "hard" contact lenses with those of perforating keratoplasty, one can state that contact lenses are tried far too seldom. Even if one succeeds "only" in restoring reading ability for a number of hours per day, this will sufficiently satisfy the personal requirements of many patients. If the contact lenses should become intolerable later on, or if they no longer provide sufficient vision, or if an intercurrent herpes recurrence deteriorates the corneal situation, then usually nothing has been missed or lost, and perforating keratoplasty can still be performed thereafter.

Quite a number of corneal surgeons seem to have a somewhat low opinion of contact lens specialists as far as the optical correction of significant corneal pathology is concerned. A frequently used justification for corneal surgery is that contact lenses were not tolerated by the patient. It has to be suspected that often enough they are not even tried, or the patients are not properly informed and not sufficiently motivated. Such a preoperative denigration of a contact lens option may have undesired drawbacks on the surgeon from unsatisfied, frustrated patients: An estimated 1/3 of all patients with perforating transplants can presently achieve best corrected vision *only with a "hard" contact lens.* Fitting such lenses on top of a corneal transplant is by no means easier or more successful than fitting it on a herpes cornea. In fact, the opposite is true.

### 2.14.C.2 Excimer Laser

Therapeutic laser ablation of superficial scars is a still debated procedure, because the results do not generally satisfy. Even if the surgeon restricts himself to minor corneal irregularities and very superficial scars and avoids deep ablations, the remaining irregular astigmatism of the newly created corneal surface may be still annoying, and best corrected vision may be achievable with additional "hard" contact lenses only. Therefore, laser surgeons are well advised not to promise satisfying vision without the help of additional contact lenses, and all that has been discussed on the interrelationship of contact lenses and perforating keratoplasty applies also to the interrelationship of contact lenses and therapeutic laser ablation. The latter offers not only the chance to improve vision by removing opacities and normalizing the corneal surface, additionally it offers the option to create a new corneal surface which allows a stable contact lens fit for the first time. This is nothing minor, but it is a potentially satisfying indication.

An often used argument against excimer laser surgery in herpes eyes is the potential triggering of herpes recurrences. This is not a valid argument. First, the overall risk of such a complication is low (see Sect. 2.13). Second, the risk of potentially triggered herpes recurrences can be reduced to about zero if the surgeon gives a prophylactic dose of systemic ACV at the time of surgery and for a number of days thereafter (see p. 88).

## 2.14.D Perforating Keratoplasty

Perforating homokeratoplasty remains the gold standard for rehabilitation of severely destructed herpes corneas. In spite of its many inherent problems – above all immune reactions, herpes recurrences, an often too high post-surgical astigmatism, and a limited lifespan of the donor cornea – perforating homokeratoplasty *on an average* offers the best chances for optimal functional rehabilitation. Contact lenses or laser ablations can mostly not offer this grade of improvement, and the various lamellar keratoplasty techniques – conventional ones as well as currently much promoted "deep anterior" or "posterior lamellar" ones – also offer no advantage over perforating techniques. Often, the opposite is true. One can content oneself, of course, with one or the other alternative method. By doing that, it must be accepted, however, that a reduction in risk invariably goes along with a reduction in chances for full visual rehabilitation. This applies also to a less risky variant of perforating keratoplasty, rotational *auto*keratoplasty. If this variant is chosen, the chances for full visual rehabilitation will also be lower than with perforating homokeratoplasty.

### 2.14.D.1 Rotational Autokeratoplasty

If a dense central scar leaves a sufficiently broad peripheral rim of clear cornea (Fig. 2.119a), a rotational autokeratoplasty can be offered to the patient as a less risky alternative to perforating homokeratoplasty. The principle is easy. A trephine is fitted decentralized in such a way that as much clear cornea as possible is excised at one side, and as much scar tissue as necessary to clear the pupillary area at the opposite side. The excised disc is then rotated 180 degrees and re-sutured (Fig. 2.119b). Thus, a sufficiently large part of clear cornea is moved from the periphery to the pupillary area.

The advantages of this procedure are:

- Immune reactions are impossible, because only the patient's own tissue is rotated. The greatest threat after perforating homokeratoplasty is thus avoided.
- Consequently, no potentially dangerous immunosuppressive therapy is necessary, except for low dosed steroids for just a couple of weeks.
- Another important, mostly overlooked advantage is the following: all sensory corneal nerves are cut by trephination with the effect that endogenously produced virus can no longer directly reach the corneal area within the trephination line. The clear cornea rotated to the center will thus be much safer from HSV recurrences after surgery than it had been before surgery. This advantage will last as long as no sensory nerve regrowth develops in the rotated corneal disc.

There are also disadvantages and limitations:

- This type of decentered keratoplasty creates a statistically higher postsurgical astigmatism. The differences in thickness of the cornea, which is about double as thick in the periphery than near the center, make an ideal wound adaptation impossible. On the other hand, the scarred parts of the disc lead to a different wound healing than the clear parts. Altogether, we deal with unpredictable effects on wound healing and corneal traction.
- The astigmatism is not only higher than after homokeratoplasty, it is also often more irregular, limiting the chances for optical correction with glasses only.
- A patient undergoing rotational autokeratoplasty must be warned, therefore, that the best achievable vision might be lower than after homokeratoplasty, and that the patient will probably additionally have to wear "hard" contact lenses in order to achieve optimal vision.

These pros and cons must be explained to the patient and properly weighed individually before making a decision regarding one or the other procedure.

However, it may be concluded that rotational autokeratoplasty merits more attention and consideration than is currently the case.

### 2.14.D.2 Homokeratoplasty

*Perforating homokeratoplasty* is the surgical gold standard for restoring vision in herpes eyes with severely damaged corneas. The results of keratoplasty for herpes are as good as those for keratoconus in the following cases:

- If proper prophylaxis with systemic immunosuppressive plus antiherpetic agents (ACV) is performed
- If all postsurgical complications are efficiently dealt with
- If the patient is compliant
- If the controlling ophthalmologist is experienced

This also applies to emergency procedures à chaud.

Patients must not wait for indicated surgery until his herpes eye has become "quiet".

The subsequent follow-up pictures of three patients may serve as examples for successful perforating homokeratoplasty, even in difficult herpes situations.

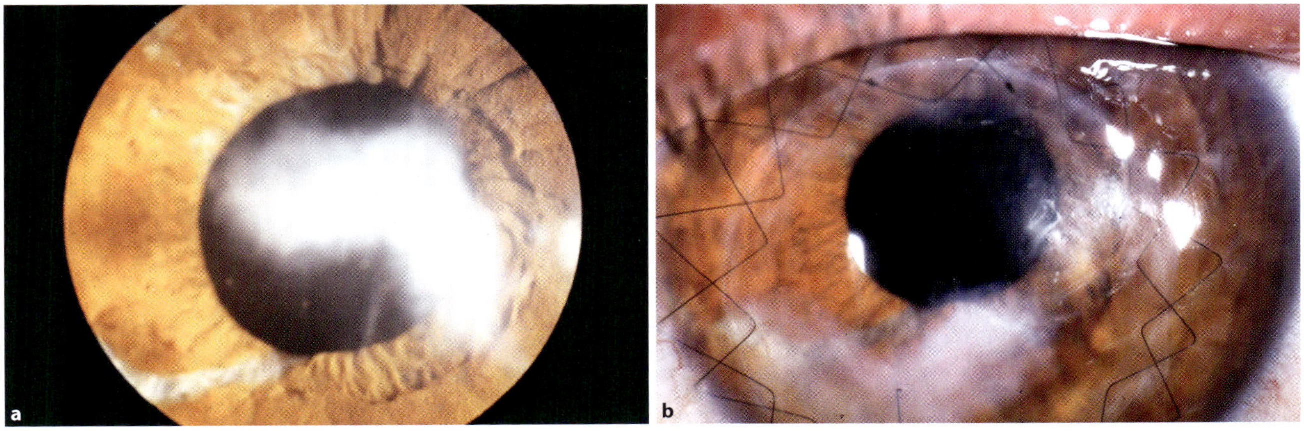

Fig. 2.119 *Rotational autokeratoplasty* in a herpes eye with dense central scar (**a**) rotated downwards to the limbus, moving clear cornea into the pupillary area (**b**)

## Analysis of Fig 2.120

The circular dense vascularization of the corneal stroma in Fig. 2.120a made this a high risk case. Additionally, the herpes scars contained residual infiltrates, and also there was certainly some replicating HSV in the cornea. Systemic combination therapy with ACV successfully suppressed HSV recurrences, and immunosuppressive therapy allowed for just one intercurrent endothelial immune reaction, which was immediately thereafter diagnosed and successfully treated with a crystal clear graft. As can be seen from Fig. 2.120b, the corneal vasculature mostly shrunk to ghost vessels. The graft stayed clear without further complications as long as the patient could be followed (five years).

## Analysis of Fig 2.121

The case in Fig. 2.121 was even more advanced than that in Fig. 2.120a. The central dense white infiltration area contained granulomatous reactions against Descemet´s. This, together with a frequently recurring central HSV ulcer, was the indication for keratoplasty in the active stage in order to remove all persistent HSV foci and all sites of granulomatous reactions, which were the cause for chronic non-healing disease. After surgery, the eye calmed down perfectly with no HSV recurrence and no immune reaction as long as the patient was kept under an efficient regime of systemic immunosuppressive agents plus systemic ACV (Fig. 2.121b). In the long run, such eyes may again experience HSV recurrences and immune reactions, but this must not invariably be so. Even if one or the other HSV recurrence complicates the late course after withdrawal of systemic ACV prophylaxis, the postoperative situation is by far better than the presurgical one: by perforating keratoplasty, the eye is turned from a blind, continuously inflamed, conservatively untreatable one into a seeing, quiet eye. By perforating keratoplasty, the many years of herpes illness are practically also "excised" and *the "disease timer" is turned back to the time before the first HSV disease* started. The chances for a vision-preserving therapy are good again.

## Analysis of Fig 2.122

The severe ulcerating interstitial HSV keratitis in Fig. 2.122a could presumably have been effectively treated by a systemic and topical combination therapy of ACV plus steroids. However, it would have taken months before the eye would have become "quiet".

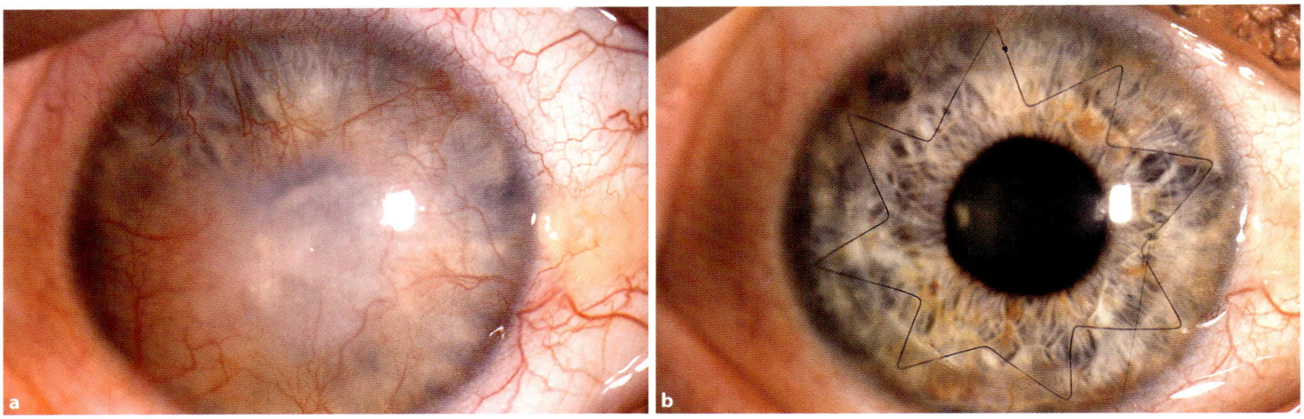


Fig. 2.120 Severely scarred and vascularized herpes cornea (**a**), clear graft 18 months after keratoplasty (**b**)

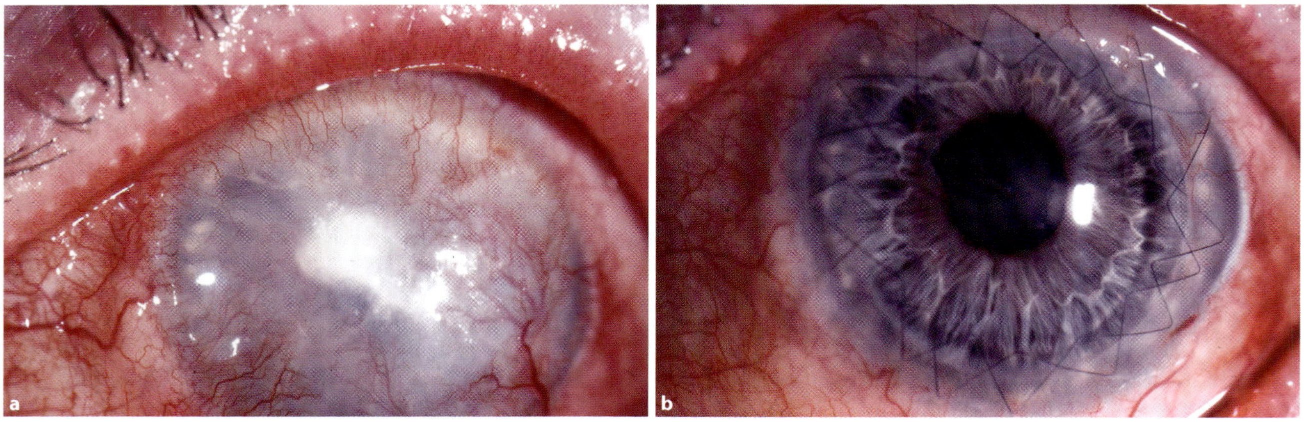


Fig. 2.121 Heavily scarred, vascularized, and infiltrated herpes cornea before (**a**) and 5 months after surgery (**b**)

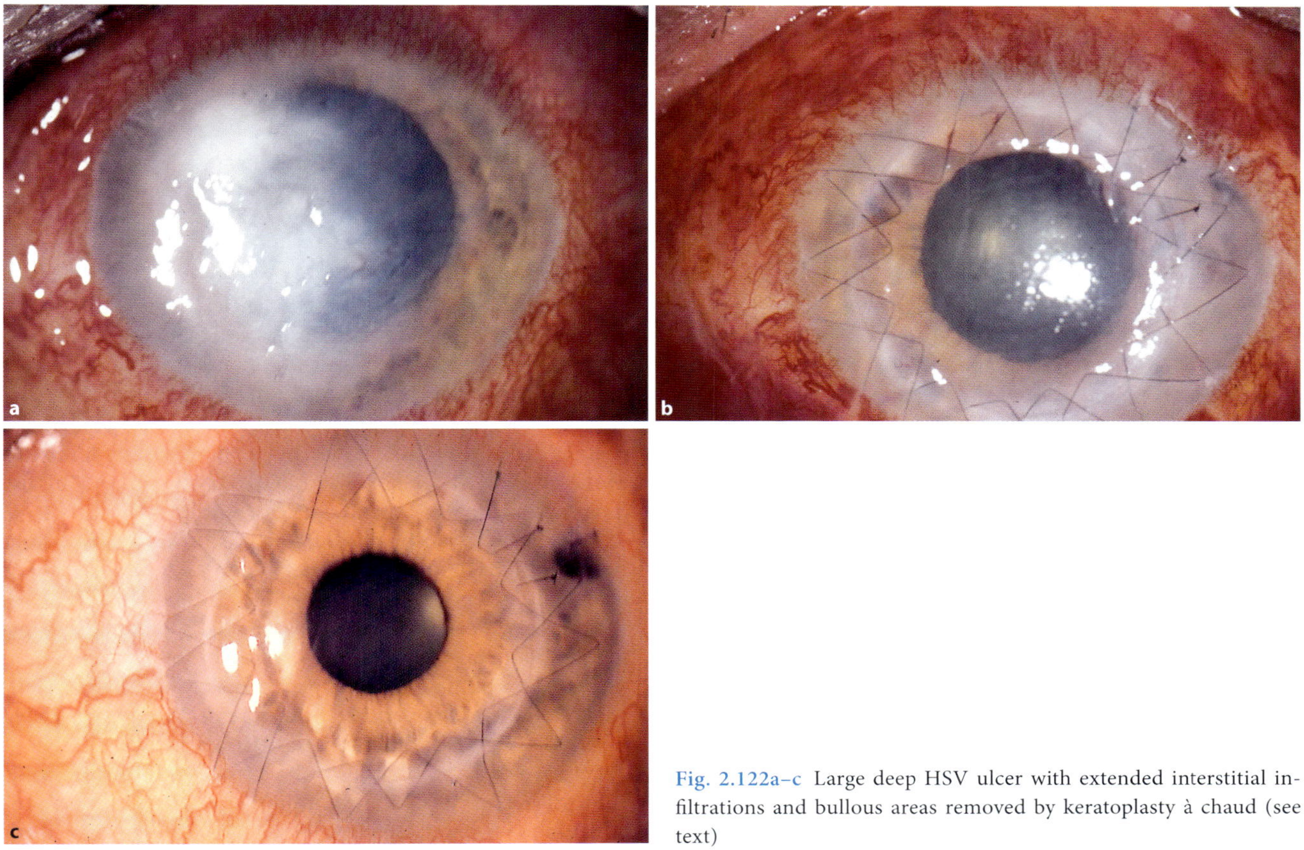

Fig. 2.122a–c Large deep HSV ulcer with extended interstitial infiltrations and bullous areas removed by keratoplasty à chaud (see text)

Thereafter, perforating keratoplasty probably would have had to follow in order to sufficiently restore function. Given the alternative choice to immediately undergo keratoplasty à chaud, the patient decided to go with keratoplasty in order to spare months of blindness, months of treatment, and overall expenses. That was the right decision for him: the eye had much improved already a couple of days after surgery (Fig. 2.122b). After four months (Fig. 2.122c), the "disease timer" in this eye was put back to the time before the first herpes disease now again with good chances to preserve good function of an eye which was previously blind and chronically inflamed.

The above shown three cases could be misunderstood as a general plea to perform more keratoplasty à chaud in severe HSV disease of the cornea. This is not what is intended. The intention is to show that those who possess sufficient diagnostic, therapeutic, and surgical abilities must not be anxious to perform keratoplasty à chaud. With proper skills, the results after keratoplasty à chaud are comparable to those of keratoplasty in "quiet" eyes.

Before deciding to go with a rapid emergency keratoplasty, however, the possibilities and chances for a *planned keratoplasty with a well-HLA-matched corneal graft* should also be considered and discussed. This is a still debated topic, although optimal HLA matching has definite advantages over random transplantation. The organization of efficient HLA matching is so time and money consuming, however, and the advantages are so rarely evident within the first years after surgery, that the excellent *long-term advantages* of matching have as of yet been mostly ignored. Corneal surgeons have still to be convinced, that optimal matching is codecisive for the *long-term survival* of corneal grafts, i.e., whether a graft survives only ten years, or 20 years and longer. The many complex aspects of matching cannot be discussed here. For introduction, the reader is referred to the small symposium booklet of Sundmacher (2003) or other recent summaries. If HLA matching can be organized, it is worthwhile to undertake this laborious, expensive, and longer way of rehabilitation. One should then refrain from keratoplasty à chaud with a random transplant, and should content oneself with "quietening" the inflamed eye as a presurgical measure, and postpone keratoplasty to the time when an excellently matched corneal graft would have become available. This is an especially important aspect for *all younger patients*.

While HLA matching improves long-term prognosis, the following five complications are decisive for short- and medium-term success of keratoplasty, i.e., the time range of 5–10 years after surgery.

#### 2.14.D.2.1 Dry Eye Complications

**Analysis of Fig 2.123**

Herpes eyes frequently suffer from tear film deficits. After keratoplasty, the surface problems usually become even more severe. Therefore, prophylactic dry eye therapy is mandatory as a basic measure after *every* keratoplasty in herpes eyes. It should be so efficient in protecting the epithelial surface that pseudodendrites as in Fig. 2.123 cannot develop. For differential diagnosis to HSV dendritic keratitis, refer to Sect. 2.5. If pseudodendrites arise, either dry eye prophylaxis was under-dosed, or the dry eye situation was so severe that conservative prophylaxis alone could not sufficiently protect the epithelium. Then, additional measures may become necessary, above all, occlusion of the lacrimal puncti or even intercurrent occlusion of the lids (see Fig. 2.124).
With pseudodendrites, the necessary postoperative steroid prophylaxis becomes impossible by the normal topical route. Then, steroids have to be given systemically or subconjunctivally (crystalline steroid depots) until the transplant epithelium has regenerated to such a degree as to again tolerate steroid ointments or eye drops. If the dry eye situation is so severe that no steroids at all can be given, this can usually be anticipated *before* surgery. In those rare cases and in severe diabetes, non-steroidal systemic immunosuppressive agents (mycophenolate mofetil, for example) are excellent alternatives to steroids.

**Analysis of Fig 2.124**

A *therapeutic soft contact lens* together with frequent applications of artificial tears (without preservatives) for treatment of pseudodendrites after keratoplasty is a two-edged measure, because it puts additional stress on the transplant. It is recommended for very experienced ophthalmologists only. Sometimes it is safer and easier to close the lids over the operated eye for a few weeks by simple *mattress sutures through the lid margins* leaving the inner lid fissure open for therapy and inspection (Fig. 2.124) until the epithelial surface of the transplant has become stable.

My personal experiences with botulinum injections into the upper lid in order to close the eye permanently but temporarily in severe dry eye conditions, are not really rewarding, and I do not recommend this method.

#### 2.14.D.2.2 Immune Reactions

Immune reactions and HSV recurrences are the major causes for irreversible transplant failure in herpes eyes. Immune reactions are more frequent than herpes recurrences (Fig. 2.125), and they lead much quicker to functional transplant failure. Therefore, they are acutely more dangerous than HSV recurrences, and if both develop together, which often is the case, therapy must primarily be directed towards stopping the immune reaction as quickly as possible. Only thereafter, one can focus on maximal treatment of HSV recurrences.

The risk of a transplant failure because of an immune reaction within the first 1–2 years after keratoplasty depends above all on the efficiency and duration of the postoperative immune-suppression. If prophylaxis is optimal, predisposing factors like grade of corneal vascularization, grade of inflammation, and limbal touch of the transplant play much less a role than commonly thought. Among the three aforementioned, the limbal position of a graft has the greatest negative impact.

While routine prophylaxis with systemic and topical steroids is mostly sufficient to control immune reactions after keratoplasty in herpes eyes, the often long duration of this steroid application is a rather two-edged measure, because it triggers the clinical manifestation of herpes recurrences at the same time. Therefore, these must always *also* be prophylactically inhibited by systemic ACV prophylaxis. As efficient as this ACV prophylaxis may be, it would certainly be preferable not to have to fight continuously against the virus-promoting steroid action. This can be achieved by performing the necessary immune prophylaxis with a non-steroidal systemic immune suppressive agent. Such an agent exists. It is *mycophenolate mofetil (MMF)*, which in combination with systemic ACV can be given for a year or

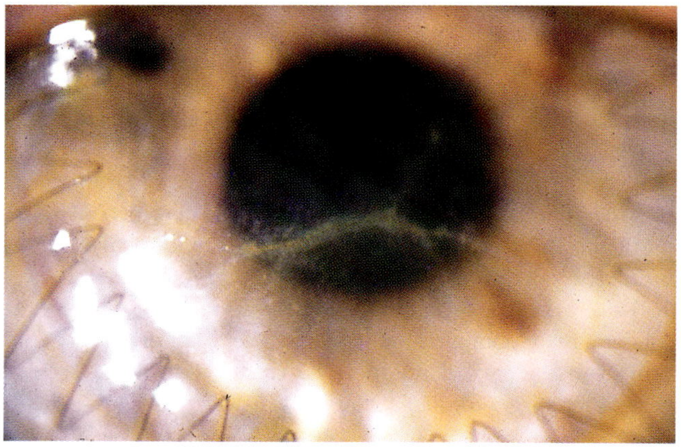

Fig. 2.123 Pseudodendrite on a corneal transplant in a herpes eye (fluorescein)

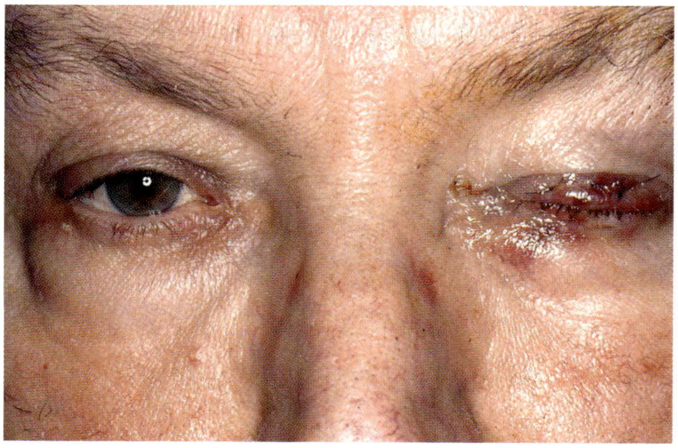

Fig. 2.124 Temporary surgical lid closure

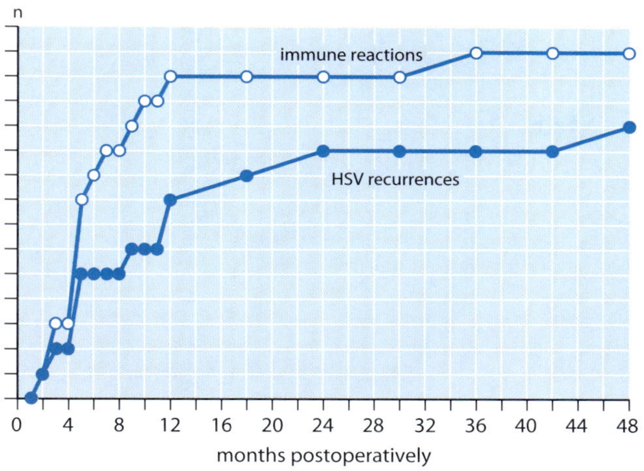


Fig. 2.125 Cumulative frequencies of immune reactions and HSV recurrences in 29 herpes patients after triple procedure (from: Sundmacher R., Wolf M., (1993)

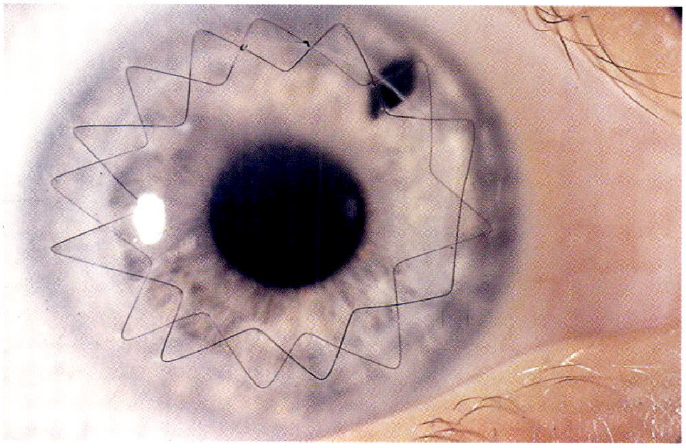

Fig. 2.126 Endothelial immune reaction with Khodadoust line

longer if necessary. MMF offers a reliable immune-suppressive protection (see Reis 2001).

The cumulative incidences of immune reactions and herpes recurrences after keratoplasty in Fig. 2.125 must not be misunderstood as reflecting average or optimal incidences. They just give a historic example with a historic immune-suppressive and antiviral prophylaxis, which can certainly be made more efficient by more effective drug combinations.

However, the curves in Fig. 2.125 contain messages which are generally helpful for the design of prophylaxis of complications and for long-term control of keratoplasty patients:

1. The greatest danger for immune reactions and herpes recurrences is within the first year after keratoplasty. A full-dose systemic protection (e.g., with MMF plus ACV) should therefore be given for the whole first postoperative year.
2. Thereafter, immune reactions become rare even without immune prophylaxis. Immune reactions may unexpectedly arise anew, however, even after many years.
3. New herpes recurrences are also rarely observed after one year even without antiviral prophylaxis. This complication is initially less frequent than immune reactions. However, as its potential threat seems to last indefinitely, over the years, one probably has to deal with more herpes recurrences than with immune reactions. The differential diagnosis between both of them is presented in detail in the picture part.

## Detailed analysis of Fig 2.126

***Clinic:*** Topical immune prophylaxis with steroid eye drops 3 qd had been tapered to 2 qd 3 weeks ago. The patient experienced some slight blurring of vision without other complaints and with the eye staying white. The upper half of the transplant exhibited a moderate edema with a sharp demarcation line of fine endothelial precipitates to the transparent corneal tissue. Only single cells were detected in the aqueous humor, and no Tyndall, and no elevated pressure.

***Diagnosis:*** Endothelial immune reaction with Khodadoust line creeping from the 12 o'clock position downward and now approaching the optic center of the pupil.

***Differential diagnosis:*** None. The relatively "quiet" eye without much inflammatory material in the anterior chamber and without redness is often seen with this type of acute immune reaction, especially if a basic steroid prophylaxis is still given. A Khodadoust line is one typical form of acute endothelial immune reaction after keratoplasty.

***Therapy:*** Steroid eye drops *hourly* for at least 12 hours during daytime and steroid ointment at night are the most effective measures. Additionally, subconjunctival injection of a crystalline steroid is advisable. Systemic steroids are not absolutely necessary if the patient is compliant with the topical therapy. It is necessary, however, to protect the eye with an efficient antiviral ACV regime against intercurrent herpes recurrences, which may be triggered by this high steroid therapy. Effective ACV prophylaxis is by 200 mg 5 qd (400 mg 3 qd) and should be given as long as the patient receives more than steroid eye drops 2 qd. Thereafter, the ACV prophylaxis can be stopped with the patient's disease still under control. An immunologically caused corneal edema, such as that in Fig. 2.126 often regresses completely leaving a clear transplant, if treated quickly and efficiently enough. The endothelial damage is demonstrable, however, by a reduced endothelial cell count of the transplant, which makes it more vulnerable for future immune attacks.

## Analysis of Fig 2.127

The case in Fig. 2.127 exhibits a more aggressive form of immune reaction with a Khodadoust line, which creeps up over the pupil area from the 6 o'clock position. The lower half of the transplant is already severely edematous with macroscopically visible corneal folds, and vision is correspondingly reduced. The aqueous humor contains more inflammatory material than in Fig. 2.126, and the conjunctiva is more inflamed. This is because the patient was already off of all immune-prophylaxis, when the endothelial immune reaction hit the transplant 11 months after surgery. With

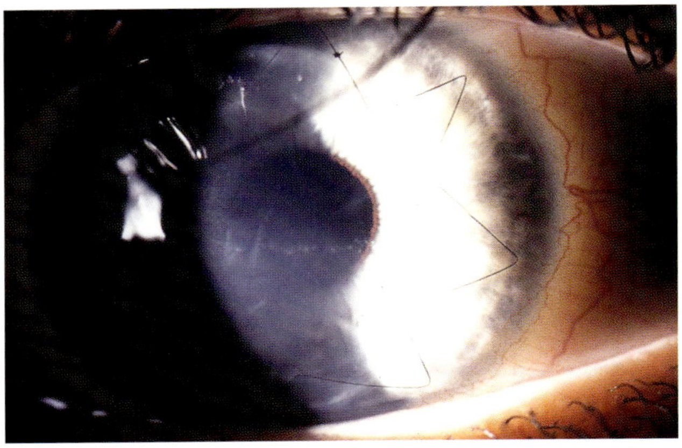

Fig. 2.127 A more aggressive endothelial immune reaction with Khodadoust line

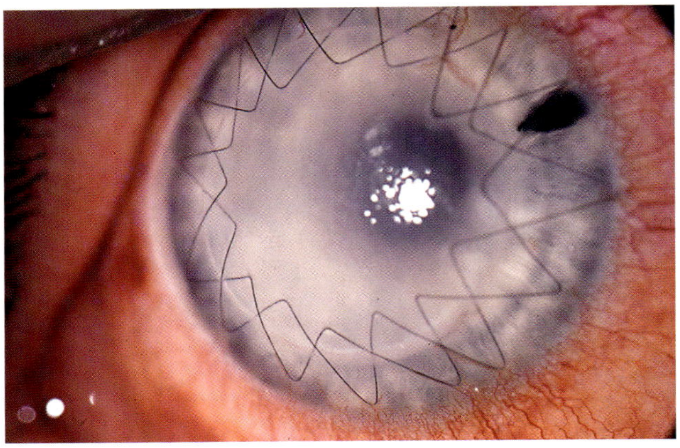

Fig. 2.128 Acute endothelial immune reaction, associated with a concomitant intraocular HSV recurrence

intensive therapy (see Fig. 2.126), this transplant also has a good chance to clear after a few weeks and to keep clear for many more years.

## Detailed analysis of Fig 2.128

***Clinic:*** Three months after surgery, topical steroid prophylaxis had been reduced from steroid eye drops 4 qd to 3 qd. No ACV prophylaxis was given. The patient experienced a rapid increase in eye redness together with a loss in vision within "a number of days". The conjunctiva was severely injected, and the transplant was completely edematous, however, with varying intensity. The intraocular pressure was elevated above that of the normal partner eye (about 35 mm Hg, as estimated by digital palpation). There were no details visible in the anterior chamber.

***Diagnosis:*** Peracute endothelial immune reaction, concomitant with intraocular HSV recurrence.

***Differential diagnosis:*** None. The increased intraocular pressure is a clear indicator for intraocular HSV replication and, thus, for an intraocular HSV recurrence. From what can be seen from the iris, a focal serous HSV iritis is not the problem. It seems that HSV trabeculitis is the main cause for the red eye as well as for the clearly elevated pressure. The pressure is not so high that it alone could be responsible for the massive total transplant edema. The donor corneal rim is clear. The transplant endothelium is, therefore, probably additionally damaged by an immune reaction attacking the complete endothelial backside of the transplant.

***Therapy:*** Considering both diseases involved, immune reaction is acutely the most dangerous one and must be treated topically, as outlined in Fig. 2.126. *Additionally*, a moderate dose of systemic steroids (30–40 mg of fluocortolone, or equivalents) is advisable. The normal antiviral prophylaxis, as outlined above, is insufficient here. We need effective systemic ACV *therapy*, at least 400 mg ACV 5 qd or, even better, the maximal ACV dose of 800 mg 5 qd, in order to stop the HSV trabeculitis. Without maximal ACV, the intraocular HSV disease would "explode" with so many steroids. As soon as the transplant starts to clear, tapering out of the systemic steroids can be started. The topical steroids and the systemic massive ACV therapy are still kept unchanged. Once the transplant has mostly cleared and most of the endothelial precipitates have gone, the topical steroid regime can also slowly be reduced. Concomitantly, the systemic maximal ACV therapy is reduced to normal therapeutic levels (400 mg 5 qd) and, a couple of weeks later, to prophylactic levels (200 mg 5 qd). Systemic ACV prophylaxis is kept on as long as the topical steroid regime is more than 2 qd.

## Analysis of Fig 2.129

Not rarely, the endothelial precipitates of a Khodadoust line become clearly visible only after a number of days (or even weeks) of intensive steroid therapy. Figure 2.129 is shown to remind that topical *steroid therapy must never be stopped before all precipitates have resolved.* Not even a single precipitate on the transplant must be left untreated. At the earliest 2–3 weeks after the last precipitate has gone, the last drop of steroids can also be withdrawn. Thus, the therapeutic sequence of the state in Fig. 2.129 could be:

- steroid eye drops 5–4 qd until only single separated precipitates remain on the endothelium,
- steroid eye drops 3 qd until the last precipitate has gone,
- thereafter, tapering from 2 qd to 1 qd to zero within 2–3 weeks,
- continued ophthalmological controls with 2, 4, 6, and 8 week intervals in order to detect an insidious recurrence of immune reaction, which the patient himself is unable to notice in time.

## Analysis of Fig 2.130

Acute immune reactions, as shown in the Figs. 2.126 to 2.129, may be therapeutically turned into chronic immune reactions. However, chronic immune reactions may also be a primary phenomenon (Fig. 2.130).

Typically, the endothelium of the graft is *sparsely* scattered with fine precipitates which cannot be found on the host endothelium. The endotheliitic nature of these precipitates is exhibited by their diffuse distribution (iritic precipitates would show a more triangular basal distribution), and also by some associated slight endothelial cell edema, best visible with an endothelial microscope.

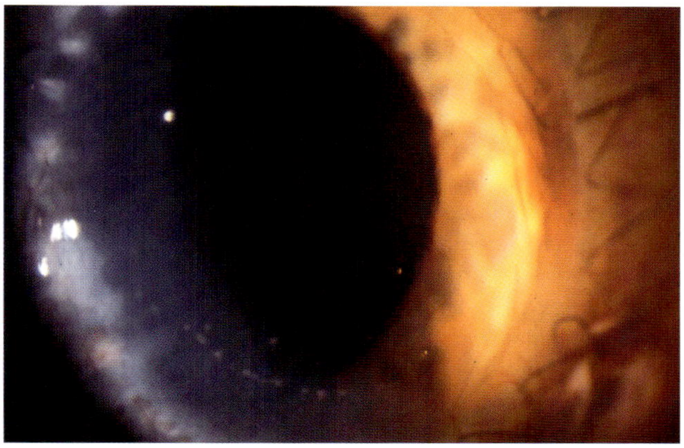

Fig. 2.129 Endothelial Khodadoust line in the course of treatment

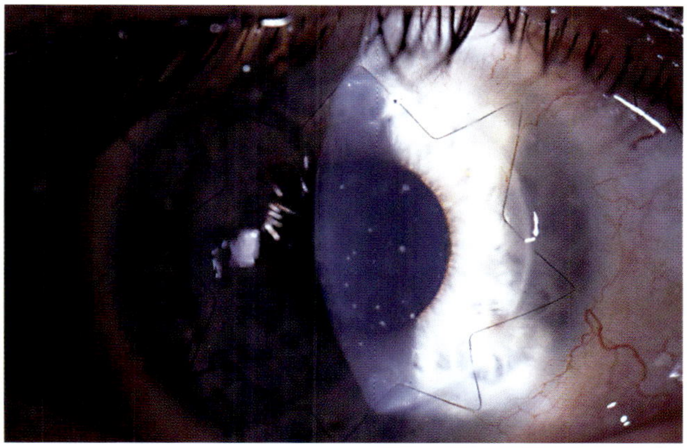

Fig. 2.130 Primary chronic endothelial immune reaction

The endothelial cell damage is so slow and focal in these cases, that the development of frank corneal edema takes months. Also, the eye may remain perfectly white and unsuspicious. The anterior chamber is free of inflammatory products, and the controlling ophthalmologist, who is unfamiliar with chronic immune reactions, regularly misunderstands the precipitates as inactive remnants of past intraocular inflammation, which need no further attention.

Chronic endothelial immune reactions do not call for hectic activity and not even for intensive therapy. It suffices to treat patiently with steroids eye drops 3 qd until the very last precipitate has gone and taper out thereafter, as described for Fig. 2.129. If handled this way, primary chronic endothelial immune reactions do not significantly limit function and life span of corneal transplants. No anti-herpetic cover is normally needed together with these limited daily doses of topical steroids, if more than one year has elapsed since surgery.

## Analysis of Fig 2.131

Much rarer than chronic endothelial is *chronic stromal immune reaction with nummuli* (Fig. 2.131). From their appearance, keratoplasty nummuli are indistinguishable from adenovirus nummuli. Both have the same pathophysiology, a cellular immune reaction against viral or HLA antigens in the cell membrane of the keratocytes. Taking all clinical signs and circumstances together, the differential diagnosis is mostly easy:

- Adenovirus nummuli do not develop without preceding inflammatory keratoconjunctivitis. They may also affect the host cornea of a keratoplasty eye.
- HLA-reactive nummuli arise insidiously only in the stroma of the donor cornea without preceding keratoconjunctivitis.
- Adenovirus nummuli often recur after topical steroid treatment, irrespective of how slowly the steroid was tapered out.
- HLA-reactive nummuli can also recur, even after months and years, if a change in the immune "surveillance" allows for a new immune attack. If treated long and sufficiently enough, however, they mostly disappear without recurrence.

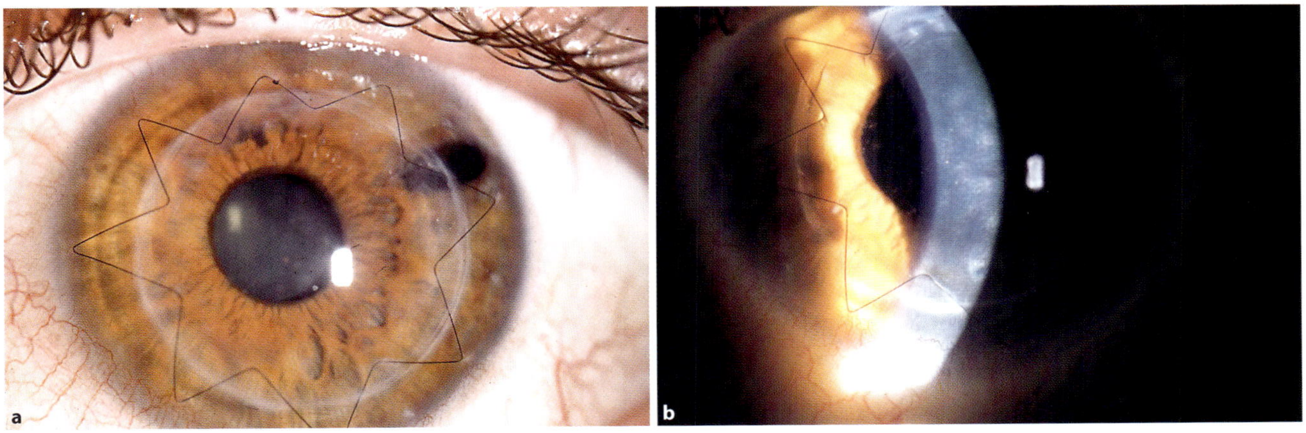

Fig. 2.131a,b Chronic stromal immune reaction with nummuli (see text)

- Although looking more impressive than chronic endothelial immune reactions, these chronic stromal reactions do not irreversibly damage the donor cornea within a number of weeks or months. The donor cornea can do well without some immunologically destroyed keratocytes. Above all, donor keratocytes can also partially be substituted by invading new host keratocytes.

Treatment is the same as with chronic endothelial immune reaction, starting with steroid eye drops 3 qd. An end point for therapy is much more difficult to define biomicroscopically because the disappearance of all infiltrating cells from the stroma is not easy to judge. It is recommended to treat additional 6–8 weeks beyond the point of presumed healing before tapering out. With such low doses of topical steroids, side effects are normally of limited importance. Also, no antiviral cover is needed together with low daily doses of steroid eye drops, if surgery took place more than one year before.

### 2.14.D.2.3 HSV Recurrences

After the dry eye complications and immune reactions, HSV recurrences are the third frequent complication after keratoplasty in herpes eyes, and they take the second most dangerous, after immune reactions.

Different to unoperated herpes eyes, where epithelial and stromal HSV disease is on an average the most frequent, HSV recurrences after keratoplasty in herpes eyes are most frequently observed *intraocularly*, with *HSV iritis* being the most frequent complication.

That has to do with the cutting of all corneal nerves in the course of surgical trephination. This blocks the free access of virus to the donor corneal stroma. A shedding of HSV from nasociliary nerve ramifications is possible only intraocularly or at the circumcision line in the cornea. Consequently, epithelial HSV recurrences can start only adjacent to the trephination line.

One would expect that dendritic recurrences along the trephination line and intraocular recurrences should have about the same incidence after keratoplasty. The fact that iritis is more frequently observed, must have an additional explanation, which I cannot give to date.

### Detailed analysis of Fig 2.132

***Clinic:*** 15 months after keratoplasty, the patient noticed an increasing redness of the eye with some slight visual irritation, but not much reduction. At this time he was already off all antiviral and immune suppressive prophylaxis. A suture correction had been necessary a week ago, and the patient claimed that discomfort and irritation had started "some days after". There had been no antiviral prophylaxis after suture removal. The pupil, which had been perfectly normal before, was now irregularly shaped without synechiae. The donor button was clear. Its endothelium was scattered with medium sized grey precipitates in a triangular distribution, some precipitates reaching more upwards on both sides of the button. The precipitates were also found on the basal host endothelium. The aqueous humor showed inflammatory cells 1 ½ + and some Tyndall. The intraocular pressure was slightly elevated above the level of the normal fellow eye (22 mm Hg versus 16 mm Hg).

***Diagnosis:*** Recurrent HSV iritis after keratoplasty in a herpes eye, presumably triggered by suture removal.

***Differential diagnosis:*** None. All typical signs of HSV iritis are present (see Sect. 2.9). Coexisting corneal endotheliitis should exhibit corneal or at least endothelial edema associated with the precipitates. This was not the case. A noteworthy HSV trabeculitis was also absent. With trabeculitis, the intraocular pressure rise should have been higher and the redness of the conjunctiva and episclera much more intensive. An endothelial immune reaction – which would have been the worst possible concomitant complication – could also be excluded, because of lack of any endothelial edema. It is possible that the intraocular recurrence was triggered by the corneal trauma of suture correction some days before. Such a complication would have been prevented by applying 400 mg ACV 3 qd for about a week after suture correction. In fact, as traumatic triggers of herpes recurrence seem to become operative rather rarely, systemic ACV prophylaxis after suture removal in herpes eyes is not a must, but it is recommended, especially if no routine control can be performed for about a week thereafter.

***Therapy:*** The same systemic and topical combination therapy with ACV plus steroids is applied as for HSV iritis in unoperated eyes (see Sect. 2.9). Care has to be taken not to overlook the potential development of an additionally evolving immune reaction triggered by the inflammatory irritations of HSV disease. If this occurs, the therapeutic dose of systemic ACV (400 mg 5 qd) must be at least maintained, and the topical steroid therapy immediately increased to hourly applications (see Fig. 2.126). Mostly, if treated quickly and consequently, such recurrent iritic complications leave no permanent functional damage.

### Analysis of Fig 2.133

Figure 2.133 illustrates that recurrent dendritic keratitis in the graft typically starts adjacent to the trephination line. This is explained by the cutting of all sensory nerves in this circumference. It is also conceivable that late recurrences are located more centrally in-

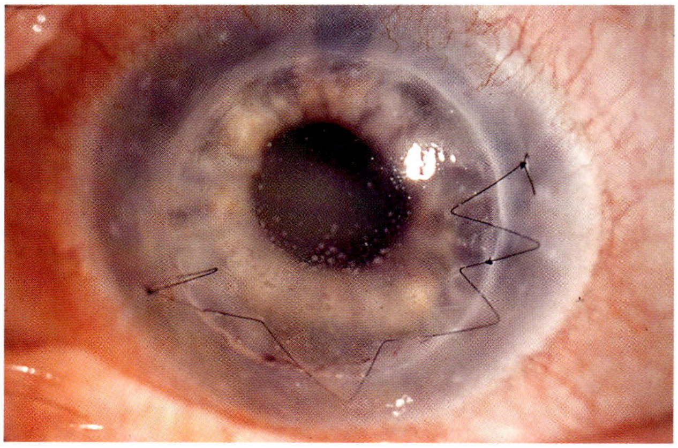

Fig. 2.132 HSV iritis after keratoplasty

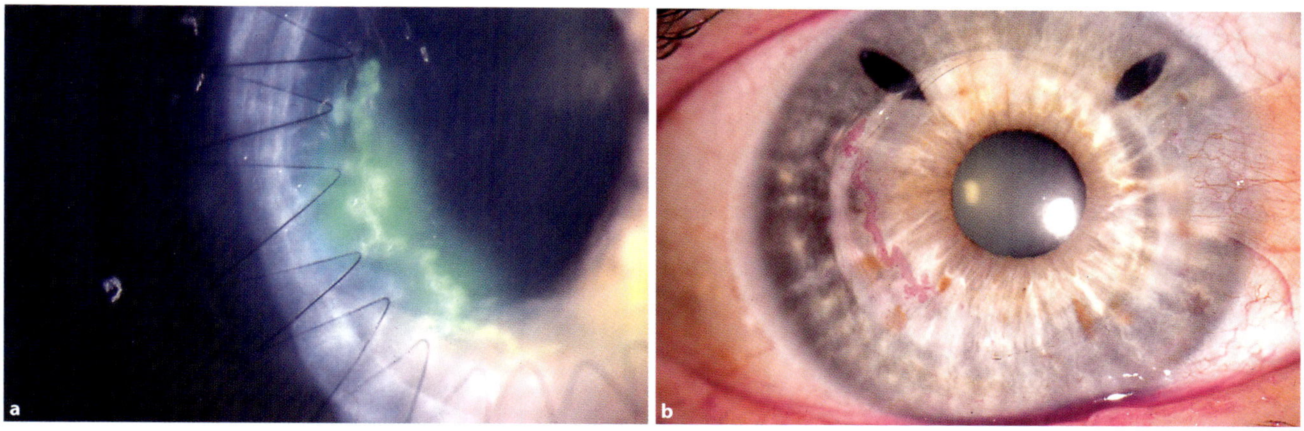

Fig. 2.133a,b Early and late recurrences of HSV dendritic keratitis in the graft. **a** Fluorescein. **b** Bengal-Rose

side the donor button, because there may be some nerve regeneration also in herpes eyes after keratoplasty – though much less than in keratoconus eyes. It is less easy to understand why the "normal" dendritic keratitis on a graft often develops centripetally and prefers to infect donor button epithelium.

*Treatment* is the same as for dendritic keratitis in unoperated eyes (see Sect. 2.5). If additional safety is desired against development of concomitant HSV recurrences at other sites of the eye, 200 mg ACV 5 qd (400 mg 2–3 qd) can be given prophylactically. A further increase in ACV dose to 400 mg 5 qd satisfies all prophylactic and therapeutic requirements one could imagine. Normally, such therapeutic and prophylactic intensity is not necessary, provided frequent ophthalmologic controls are feasible.

## Analysis of Fig 2.134

If recurrent dendritic keratitis develops unrecognized in a patient who is still under steroid prophylaxis, an expansion of the lesion to a superficial geographic ulcer may occur. This geographic lesion may then also involve the host cornea and the limbus area (Fig. 2.134, for geographic keratitis compare Figs. 2.29 to 2.31). Because of the severity of this complication, systemic ACV therapy (400 mg 5 qd) is advisable in addition to topical antiviral therapy. If the steroids cannot be reduced quickly (e.g., because of a yet insufficiently treated immune reaction), the systemic ACV must be maximally dosed (up to 800 mg 5 qd).

## Detailed analysis of Fig 2.135

***Clinic:*** This patient was still treated with steroid eye drops 4 qd for an endothelial immune reaction. No antiviral cover was given. When he noticed an increasing redness of the eye, he saw his ophthalmologist who found a shallow oval ulcer in the trephination line at 7 o'clock From there, epithelial defects suspicious of HSV etiology followed the trephination line to 6 and 8 o'clock, respectively.

***Diagnosis:*** Recurrence of a dendritic keratitis along the trephination line, partial expansion to geographic keratitis.

***Differential diagnosis:*** None. The pathognomonic epithelial microdestructions of HSV dendritic keratitis were clearly visible at

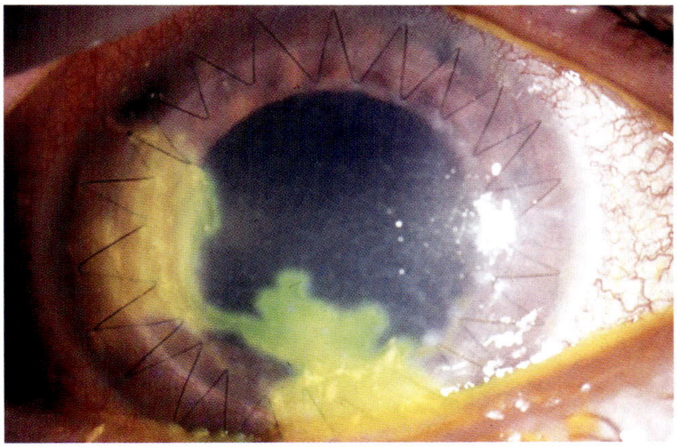

Fig. 2.134 Geographic expansion of an undetected dendritic HSV recurrence with ongoing topical steroid prophylaxis

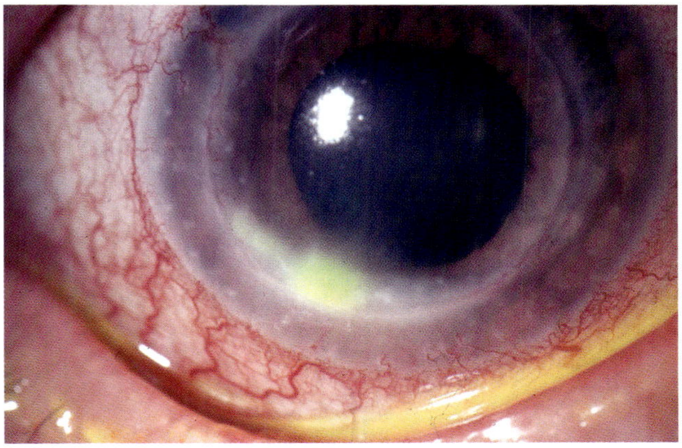

Fig. 2.135 Late epithelial HSV recurrence triggered by a still ongoing steroid therapy of an immune reaction

the endpoints of the efflorescence (see Sect. 2.5). The eye appeared relatively red for dendritic keratitis only and with concomitant steroid application. However, no other HSV recurrence was detected, especially no intraocular disease.

***Therapy:*** Large areas of the transplant were still hazy from immune reaction. Total withdrawal of the steroids would have meant a dangerous drawback for the recovery of the transplant. Therefore, it was decided to give the maximum systemic ACV dose (800 mg 5 qd), which would treat dendritic keratitis effectively and simultaneously inhibit additional HSV complications under a modified ongoing steroid therapy. The steroid eye drops were immediately stopped and substituted by 30 mg fluocortolone orally 1 qd plus a single subconjunctival injection of a crystalline steroid depot. Thus, direct application of the necessary steroids on the corneal epithelium was reduced. Additionally, ACV ointment was applied 5 qd. The dendritic keratitis healed promptly within a week, and the transplant did not deteriorate. Thereafter, systemic ACV was reduced to normal therapeutic levels (400 mg 5 qd), the systemic steroids were quickly tapered out, and steroid eye drops were re-instituted as needed. After two weeks, the systemic ACV was further reduced to prophylactic levels (200 mg 5 qd). These were given until the steroid eye drops could be reduced two 2 qd.

Such courses teach us that significant steroid therapy must always be accompanied by an antiviral cover in herpes eyes, and above all in herpes eyes after keratoplasty. If just 400 mg ACV 3 qd would have been given from the beginning of steroid treatment of the immune reaction, no such HSV complication would have occurred.

## Analysis of Fig 2.136

Figure 2.136 shows a historic case from the times when no effective antiviral therapy was available and a precise knowledge of the clinical appearance of HSV recurrences was also lacking. However, steroids were deliberately given in high doses to inhibit immune reactions. A small epithelial defect in the trephination line expanded quickly to geographic dimensions. From there, dense infiltrations expanded rapidly into the deep stroma of the donor button. The true nature of ulcer and infiltrations (i. e., dendritic recurrence in the trephination line with geographic ulceration and explosive interstitial HSV keratitis under steroid monotherapy) were not correctly identified. Instead, a severe immune reaction was thought to be the most probable diagnosis. When the steroids were finally withdrawn due to ulceration which was too severe, the donor button infiltrated even more rapidly. Finally, the only way to save the eye and avoid enucleation was to cover the ulcer by a conjunctival flap (see Fig. 2.116, same patient).

Such experiences make us appreciate how much progress we have made with the availability of systemically applicable ACV and with the principles of antiviral plus immune-suppressive combination therapy. Following these principles, downhill courses like that of Fig. 2.136 are no longer possible.

## Analysis of Fig 2.137

Sometimes, keratoplasty is performed for *corneal scars of unknown etiology*.

Neither patient, nor ophthalmologist, nor corneal surgeon had ever considered herpes in the case of Fig. 2.137, and if they had, they did not communicate. When this patient was sent for a second opinion, because of a non-healing epithelial ulcer at 6 o'clock in the trephination line, he stated on request to have never received the diagnosis of herpes. His doctor assumed that some chronic trophic problem was the cause for the ulceration, and he had given him systemic steroids instead of topical ones for immune prophylaxis. The ulcer´s borders did not reveal typical epithelial HSV microdestructions. There was no evident reason for a trophic complication. The position of the ulcer in the trephination line led to the suspicion of a HSV recurrence, which had taken a geographic appearance under steroid therapy. A combination therapy was immediately begun as described for Fig. 2.135. A PCR test confirmed the herpes etiology of the ulcer ten days later. At this time, the ulcer had already healed under systemic ACV plus some systemic steroids plus topical ACV ointment.

This case example is presented as a memento that *every corneal ulcer of unknown origin in a keratoplasty eye should be suspected*

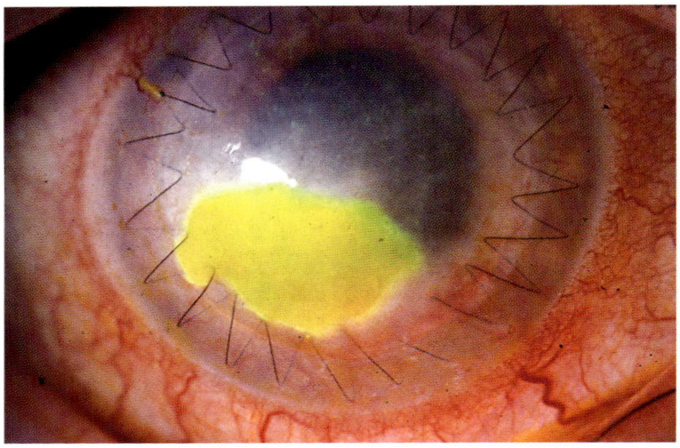

Fig. 2.136 HSV recurrence with large geographic keratitis and HSV interstitial keratitis

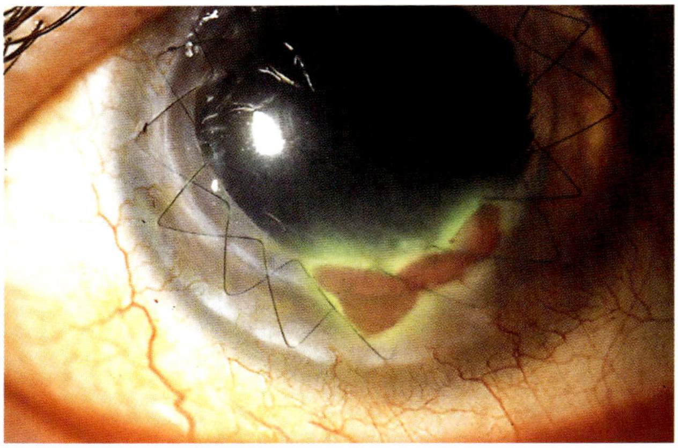

Fig. 2.137 HSV recurrence in a keratoplasty eye without herpes history (fluorescein, Bengal-Rose)

*as herpetic until proven otherwise. Currently,* PCR tests are the best way to prove or exclude herpes etiology. If the clinical suspicion of HSV etiology is strong – as in this case – antiherpetic combination therapy should immediately be instituted on suspicion only, and no time should be wasted by waiting for PCR results.

## Analysis of Fig 2.138

The course in Fig. 2.138 is extraordinary. Two keratoplasties had already failed in this herpes eye, each time with severe inflammations. The corneal transplant in Fig. 2.138a was the third one. *ACV prophylaxis was not yet routinely possible in those years,* but steroid prophylaxis was given (steroid eye drops 5 qd, systemic fluocortolone just tapered out). On a trip to South America, the patient was struck again by a severe inflammation in the keratoplasty eye and returned immediately for control and treatment. The transplant was edematous. Along the whole nasal circumference from 7 over 9 to 12 o'clock, host as well as donor cornea were massively infiltrated along the trephination line (Fig. 2.138b). There was a wound gap with fistulation of aqueous humor, and the intraocular pressure was zero. A diagnosis was made of a recurrence of *acute necrotizing HSV keratitis in the graft and the adjacent host cornea,* and maximally dosed combination therapy was instituted with systemic ACV, which had only recently become available, and with moderate doses of steroids. No antibiotics were added as there was no sign of microbial (super)infection. The anterior chamber exhibited only little inflammation. Immediate surgical closure of the opened keratoplasty wound was impossible because of the massive infiltrations, and an immediate re-keratoplasty was also impossible. Instead, high doses of azetazolamide were given in order to suppress aqueous humor production and thus facilitate spontaneous wound closure. This therapeutic policy saved the eye. The infiltrated areas scarred and the wound closed tightly. However, the function of the graft could not be sufficiently restored. Secondary calcifications were too massive (Fig. 2.138c). Therefore, the graft was exchanged half a year later, and with a combination prophylaxis of the duration of one year (ACV 200 mg 5 qd plus systemic and topical steroids), the fourth graft was finally a full success.

A morphologic *differential diagnosis* of the dense infiltrations on both sides of the trephination line (Fig. 2.138b) is impossible from the photograph only. The infiltrations closely resemble those of *recurrent amebic keratitis* (Fig. 2.145a). One has to have a good personal knowledge of the course and the pre-keratoplasty findings in such an eye to be sure that one deals with a recurrence of necrotizing HSV keratitis. Without such knowledge, a potential amebic etiology must be kept in mind, especially when the infiltrations do not respond as promptly to an intensive antiherpetic therapy as expected. For experiences with amebic infections, herpes, and keratoplasty see 2.14.E: Special Problem: Amebic Keratitis.

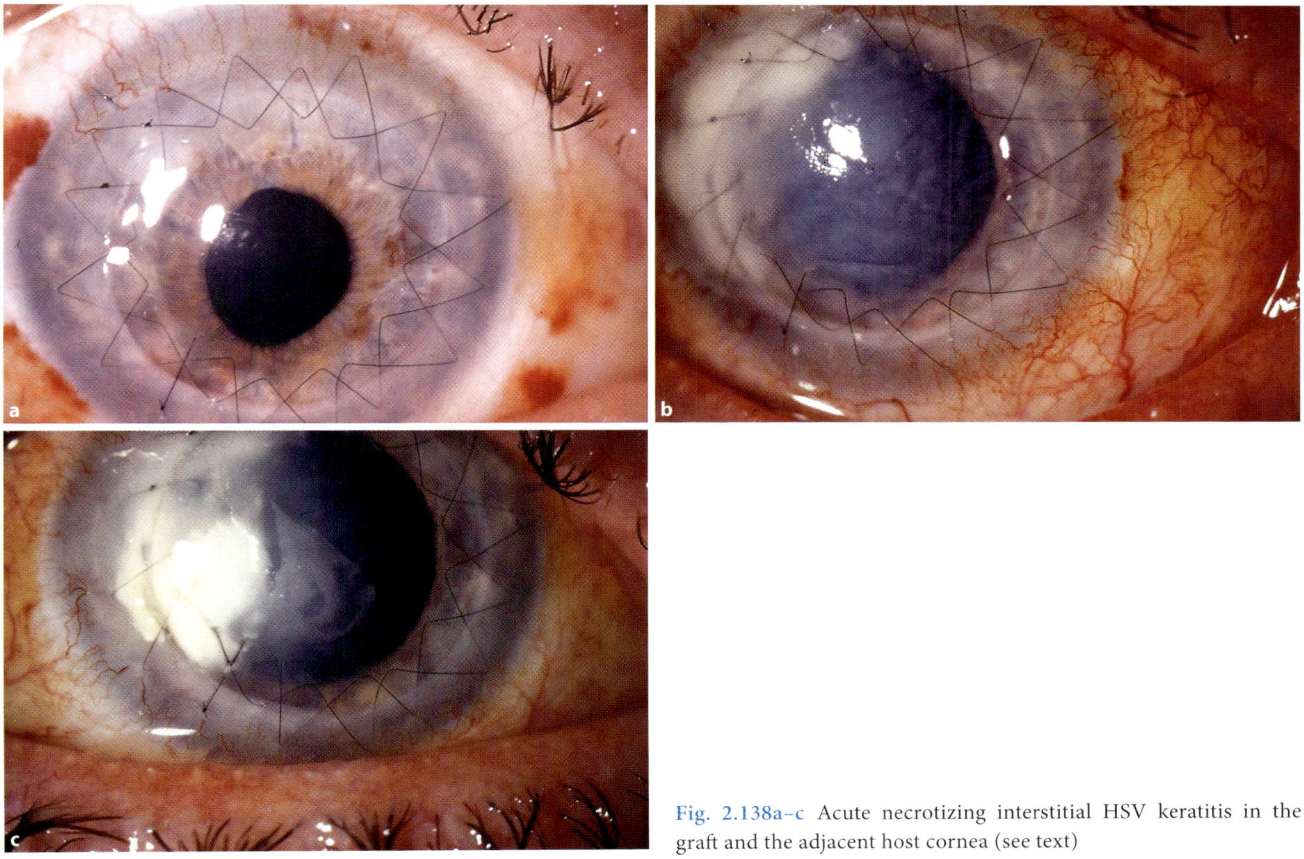

Fig. 2.138a–c Acute necrotizing interstitial HSV keratitis in the graft and the adjacent host cornea (see text)

### 2.14.D.2.4 Secondary Glaucoma

Glaucoma is an often overlooked severe problem which occurs following keratoplasty, and especially after keratoplasty in herpes eyes. It is the most frequent cause for "unexplained" graft failure within the first couple of years. Typically, neither immune reactions nor herpes recurrences are observed, and the graft becomes gradually edematous and grey without inflammation (see Fig. 2.139).

It comes as no surprise that secondary chronic glaucoma is disproportionately frequent in herpes eyes.

First, every intraocular HSV disease leads to acute pressure rise. The higher the pressure rise the more HSV trabeculitis is involved. This leads to increasing trabecular damage with every disease attack.

Second, the steroid responders among the keratoplasty patients further increase the risk of undiagnosed secondary glaucoma, leading not only to insidious transplant failure but, in the long run, also to papillary atrophy from glaucoma.

As every ophthalmologist is familiar with these risks, the question remains why is chronic glaucoma so often overlooked in keratoplasty eyes?

The problem is above all a basic diagnostic one: We are used to trusting the results of pressure measurements by applanation tonometry in normal eyes, and we assume that pressure measurements in abnormal eyes, i. e., eyes with corneal scars and distortions, and in keratoplasty eyes, will be as reliable. This is not the case. Aside from the difficulty that conventional pressure measurements are often impossible to perform in keratoplasty eyes, the resultant values are mostly wrong, and they are mostly too low. We know this from comparisons with the true intraocular pressure values as measured directly via cannula in the anterior chamber (see Figs. 2.140 to 2.142). Such direct measurements are no option for routine diagnosis. Currently, the only available alternative for routine use is to *estimate* the intraocular pressure by comparative digital palpation, as shown in Fig. 2.79. As old-fashioned as this may appear, it is the most important single measure in the hands of an experienced ophthalmologist for the detection of glaucoma in keratoplasty eyes.

The difficulties in evaluating the true intraocular pressure in keratoplasty eyes must have consequences for the therapeutic strategy. The general line should be not only to treat all cases with doubtlessly elevated intraocular pressure, but also all borderline cases: *in dubio pro therapia.*

A final remark to the problem of steroid responders in keratoplasty:

If they are high responders, there is no other way than to treat them from the beginning with non-steroidal immune suppressive agents, e. g., cyclosporine A or mycophenolate mofetil. If a high responder is detected only after having already developed severe glaucoma after keratoplasty, immune therapy must immediately be changed to non-steroidal agents, and the secondary glaucoma simultaneously be treated systemically and topically.

If we deal with low responders "only", it may suffice to get over some weeks or months of slightly elevated pressure by symptomatic therapy with azetazoleamide, until all steroids can finally be withdrawn.

#### Analysis of Fig 2.139

Figure 2.139a,b shows a typical frustrating course of a severely diseased herpes eye, in which immune reactions and herpes recurrences were successfully inhibited, but the chronic glaucoma was overlooked and led to insidious graft failure. The transplant very slowly became edematous and grey. The reason is progressive damage to the endothelial cells of the donor. While endothelial cells in normal eyes are quite resistant to damage by chronic glaucoma, donor endothelial cells are very easily damaged even by comparatively slight pressure rises. This is widely unknown. It is very important, therefore, to pay permanent attention to potential glaucoma damage in keratoplasty eyes.

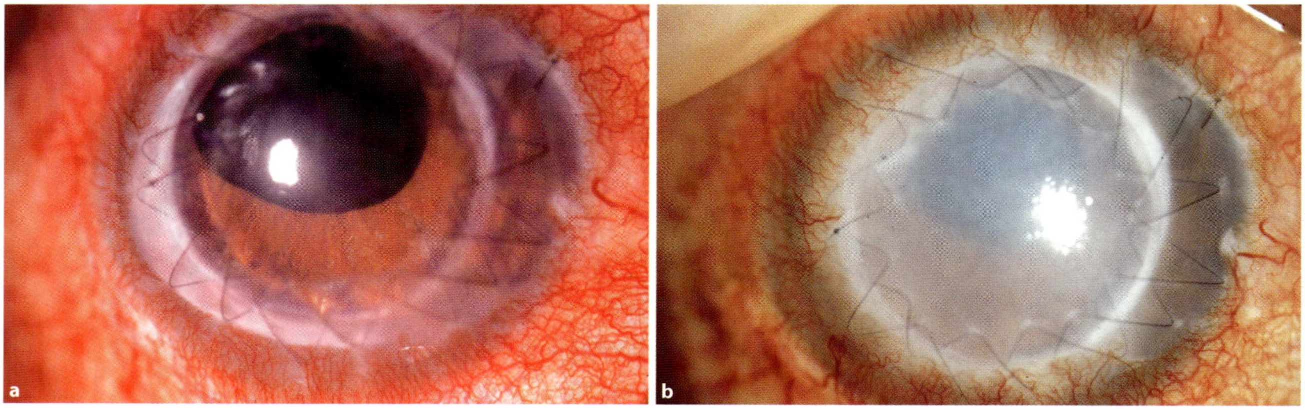


Fig. 2.139a,b Chronic failure (**b**) of an initially excellent transplant, (**a**) by undetected chronic secondary glaucoma

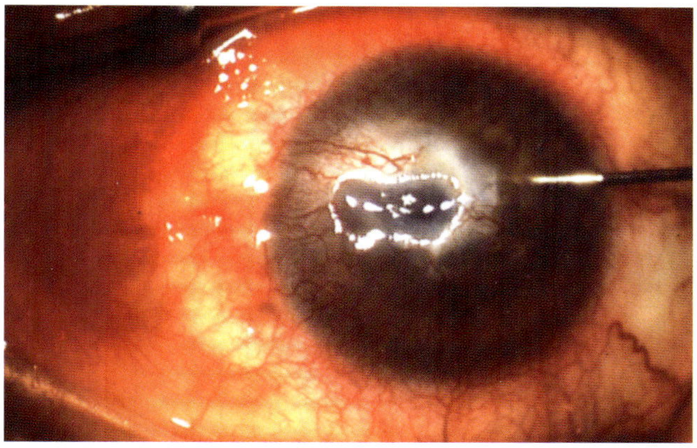

Fig. 2.140 Preoperative intracameral pressure measurement via cannula. Even if applanation tonometry is possible somewhere on such a pathologic cornea, the resulting values would not be reliable. The same holds true for applanation measurements on corneal grafts (see Fig. 2.142)

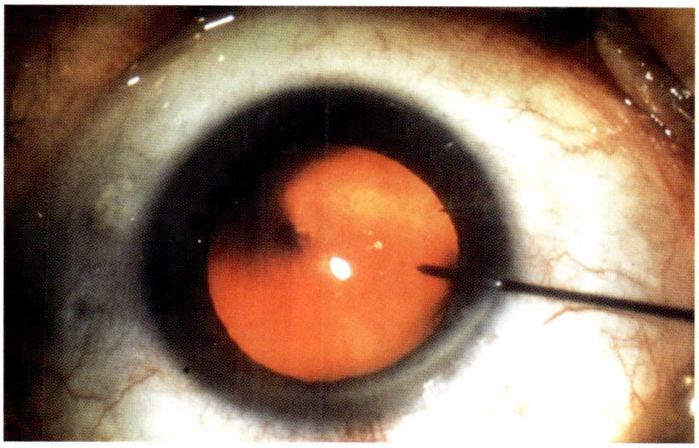

Fig. 2.141 Intracameral pressure measurement via cannula in an eye with irregular corneal surface for comparison with applanation values

### 2.14.D.2.5 Irritating Sutures

Loosening keratoplasty sutures are a general surgical problem and must not necessarily be discussed in this atlas. However, as suture loosening is frequent after keratoplasty in herpes eyes, this topic is also presented.

The most important predisposing factor for suture loosening is a pathologic destruction of Bowman's membrane in the host cornea, so that it cannot serve as a reliable anchor for the thin sutures. These tend to rapidly cut through, especially if suture tension was primarily too high. The second important factor is infiltrations that lyse parts of the corneal tissue. Both causes come together quite frequently in herpes eyes. The loosened suture loops irritate the corneal tissue, and this irritation can trigger immune reactions as well as herpes recurrences and can also promote microbiologic superinfections. The situation is quite dangerous, therefore, and calls for immediate surgical correction by (partial) suture removal and eventually new sutures. It should not happen that a controlling ophthalmologist, who himself is no corneal surgeon, tells a patient with suture loosening that he should see his surgeon "sometime". He must tell the patient that suture loosening is potentially dangerous and that the patient better sees his surgeon quickly.

A practical surgical advice may be added: The more destroyed the corneal host cell rim, the more important it is to use sutures with wide loop angles. The sutures which loosen quickest are single sutures. They have no loop angle, and full tension allows a rapid through cut. If surgeons use single sutures, especially in situations where the host cornea is "soft" and infiltrated, they will have to use lots of them, and many will have to be removed early as soon as they loosen, one after the other. Working with single sutures only is a continuous competition between rapidity of wound healing and rapidity of suture loosening and removal: which one is quicker and will wound healing prevail?

With a single running suture, the loops have small angles and some of them will also cut through and loosen focally. Correction of a single running suture under topical anaesthesia only is an exciting experience in some patients.

I have found that the best suture "in my hands" is a double running suture with eight loops each resulting in wide loop angles. If necessary, additional single sutures can be added for adaptation of gaping wound margins. These single sutures can be removed without disadvantage at any time. They become superfluous after a couple of weeks anyway. With such a suture strategy, suture loosening stops to be a significant problem in keratoplasty (Sundmacher R., 1995).

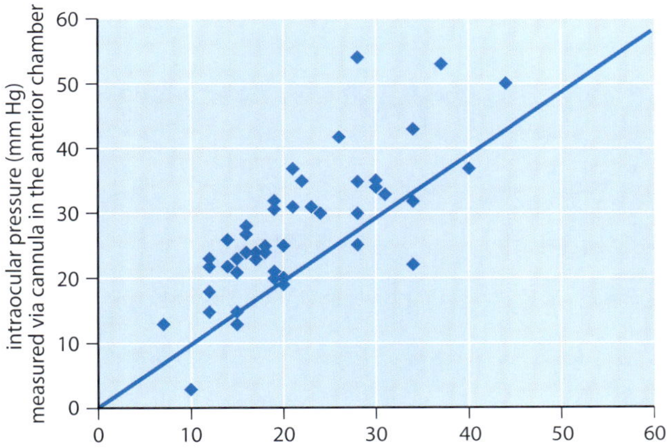


Fig. 2.142a,b Comparison of true intraocular pressure as measured via cannula with applanation tonometry in 49 keratoplasty eyes. Tonometry gives mostly too low values in this situation (from: Marx W. et al., 1999)

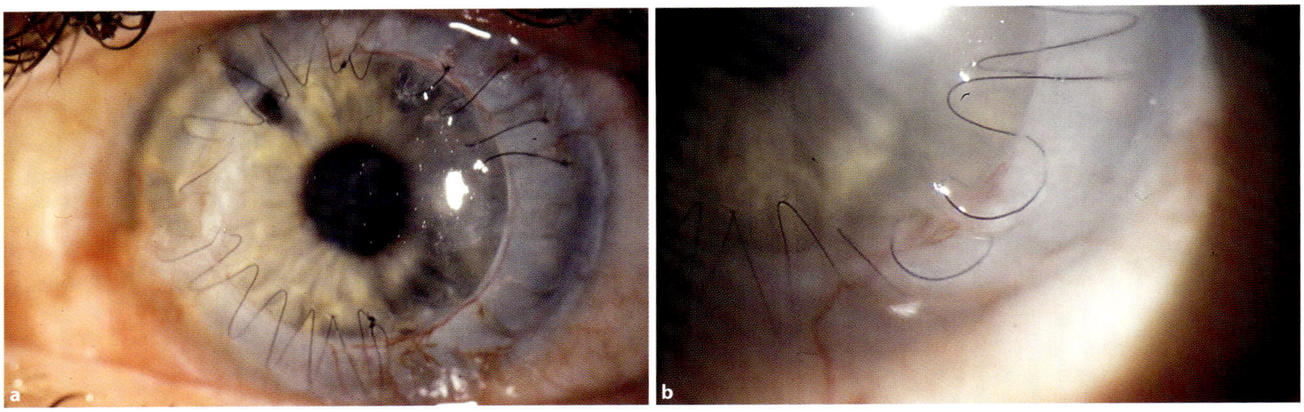

Fig. 2.143 Progressive suture loosening after keratoplasty with a single running suture in a herpes eye necessitating frequent corrections (see text)

## 2.14.E Special Problem: Amebic Keratitis

Chronic interstitial amebic keratitis may deteriorate into a deep amebic ulcer. Both are often mistaken for herpes keratitis. The differential diagnosis has already been discussed (Sect. 2.6). Severe pain is the most important symptom for amebic etiology.

However, the symptom of pain considerably decreases in importance if a differential diagnosis has to be made in keratoplasty eyes. First, corneal pain is no longer reliable after keratoplasty, because all sensory nerves have been circumferentially cut by trephination. Second, the herpes eyes operated on by keratoplasty have already a preoperative sensory defect resulting from herpetic nerve destruction. Consequently, additional nerve damage by entameba organisms looses most of its importance for differential diagnosis.

The two cases presented here were further complicated by the circumstance in which the general pathologists involved were not sufficiently familiar with the microscopic diagnosis of amebic cysts in the corneal stroma. The cysts were simply overlooked, and the ophthalmic surgeon received no warning. It is recommended, therefore, to explicitly ask general pathologists, who have no special training in ophthalmic pathology, to exclude an amebic etiology in all corneal buttons in which amebic keratitis is a possible diagnosis.

### Analysis of Fig 2.144

The features of amebic keratitis were still widely unknown when the patient in Fig. 2.144a presented with an ulcerating interstitial keratitis classified as herpetic. There was significant pain, but this typical amebic symptom was then not correctly appreciated. As the ulcer deteriorated under antiherpetic therapy, keratoplasty à chaud was performed, but the graft quickly clouded again (Fig. 2.144b) from what was thought to be either an immune reaction or a herpes recurrence. The true diagnosis of an amebic recurrence was not detected until the ophthalmic surgeon gave direct notice to the pathologist to also look for entameba cysts. The eye could be saved

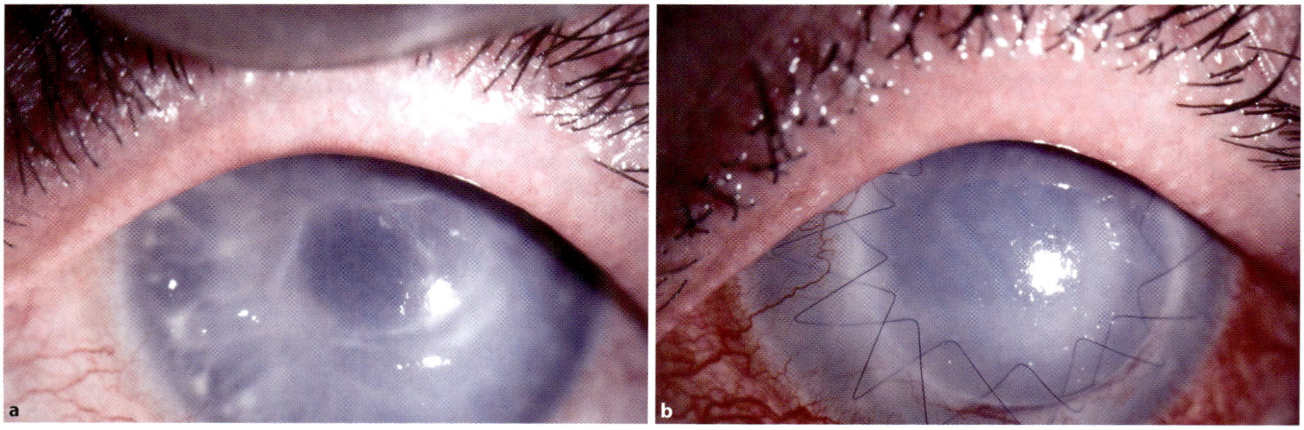

Fig. 2.144a,b Ulcerating amebic keratitis (**a**), with amebic recurrence after keratoplasty (**b**)

morphologically by antiamebic drug therapy plus cryotherapy for the scleral invasion of the organisms. But subsequent blinding from intractable glaucoma could not be prevented.

Retrospectively, Fig. 2.144a and b fit well together. The presurgical picture is so suggestive of an amebic etiology with its central oval ulcer that one wonders why the correct diagnosis was not achieved in time. But the actual situation was such that the surgeon who had to deal with the situation in Fig. 2.144b had been informed that this was a herpes eye, and the diagnostically decisive corneal aspect of Fig. 2.144a was not available to him in time. It was detected in the archives only years later.

## Analysis of Fig 2.145

A preoperative picture of the eye of Fig. 2.145 has unfortunately never been made. Reportedly, the patient suffered for many years from recurrent herpes disease of the cornea, and the correctness of the herpes diagnosis could not be doubted from the records. The last recurrence did no longer respond to antiherpetic therapy as it had been regularly been the case before. Keratoplasty à chaud became necessary with appropriate antiherpetic plus immune suppressive combination therapy thereafter. Nonetheless, already within a few weeks, a rapidly increasing infiltration of the host as well as of the donor cornea was noted, which comprised the whole circumference of the trephination line (Fig. 2.145a). After a week, host as well as donor cornea started to ulcerate in an upper quadrant of the trephination line (Fig. 2.145b). This ulceration slowly became circumferential in spite of all vigorous antiherpetic therapy. This was in striking contrast to positive therapeutic experiences with similar looking but more localized herpes recurrences (see Fig. 2.138). A suspicion of amebic superinfection in a herpes eye arose. This entameba diagnosis could be confirmed by histopathology after re-keratoplasty. Intensive circular cryotherapy in order to damage remaining amebic cysts, together with a years medical antiamebic therapy resulted in a satisfying morphologic and functional rehabilitation. The patient has had good vision with the second transplant for 20 years now, with no recurrence of amebic disease, but some recurrences of HSV disease, which could all treated in time without causing much damage.

Unexplained therapy refractoriness could have alerted already before the first keratoplasty to the possibility of amebic superinfection of a herpes cornea. Additionally, the biomicroscopic features of the recurrence in the graft were not typical for herpes. A herpes recurrence would not primarily comprise the whole circumference but only a limited sector (compare Fig. 2.138). Progression of circular infiltration to circular ulceration is also not a typical feature of a herpes recurrence.

## References


Alino AM, Perry HD, Kanellopoulos AJ, Donnenfeld ED, Rahn EK (1998) Conjunctival flaps. Ophthalmology 105: 1120–1123

Barequet IS, Wasserzug Y (2007) Herpes simplex keratitis after cataract surgery. Cornea 26: 615–617

Beyer CF, Byrd TI, Hill JM, Kaufman HE (1990) Herpes simplex virus and persistent epithelial defects after penetrating keratoplasty. Am J Ophthalmol 109: 95–96

Birnbaum F, Reinhard T, Ulbricht T, Haußer J, Sundmacher R (2004) Funktionelle Ergebnisse nach autologer Rotationskeratoplastik. Eine retrospektive Analyse. Ophthalmologe 101: 54–58

Birnbaum F, Reinhard T, Böhringer D, Sundmacher R (2005) Endothelial cell loss after autologous rotational keratoplasty. Albrecht von Graefes Arch Clin Exp Ophthalmol 243: 57–59

Böhringer D, Reinhard T (2008) Prognosis in repeat keratoplasty: per indication analysis in a large monocentric cohort. Klin Monatsbl Augenheilkde 225: 50–56

Böhringer D, Sundmacher R, Reinhard T (2007) HLA B27 sems to promote graft failure following penetrating keratoplasties for herpetic corneal scars. Ophthalmologe 104: 705–708

Böhringer D, Sundmacher R, Reinhard T (2006) Histocompatibility matching in penetrating keratoplasty. In: T Reinhard, F Larkin (vol-eds): Esssentials in ophthalmology: Cornea and external eye disease. Springer, Berlin – Heidelberg – NY, pp 101–108

Borderie VM, Méritet JF, Chaumeil C, Rozenberg F, Baudrimont M, Touzeau O, Bourcier T, Laroche L (2004) Culture-proven herpetic keratitis after penetrating keratoplasty in patients with no previous history of herpes disease. Cornea 23: 118–124


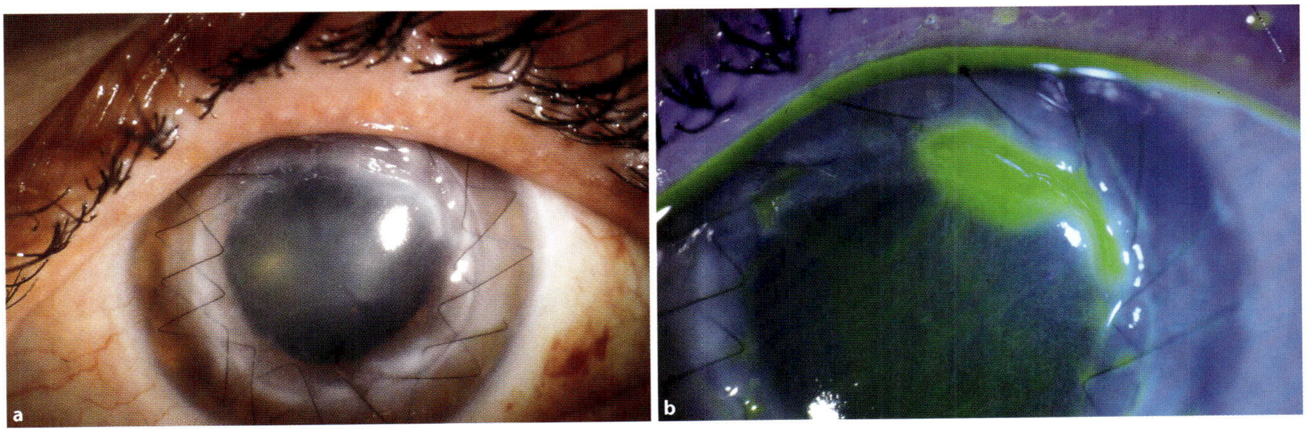

Fig. 2.145a,b "Recurrence of the disease" after keratoplasty for "non-healing interstitial ulcerating heratitis" in a herpes eye (see text)

Cheng C-K, Chang S-W, Hu F-R (1995) Acyclovir treatment for linear endotheliitis on grafted corneas. Cornea 14: 311–315

Dana MR, Streilein JW (1996) Loss and restoration of immune privilege in eyes with corneal neovascularization. Invest Ophthalmol Vis Sci 37: 2485–2494

Engelskirchen U, Sundmacher R (1990) Aufklebung harter Kontaktlinsen als Notfallmaßnahme bei drohender Hornhautperforation. Sitzungsbericht 152. Versammlung Rhein.-Westf. Augenärzte: 247–251

Garweg J, Böhnke M (1996) Slow viral replication of HSV-1 is responsible for early recurrence of herpetic keratitis after corneal grafting. Albrecht von Graefes Arch Clin Exp Ophthalmol 234 Suppl 1: S133–S138

Heiligenhaus A, Li H, Hernandez Galindo EE, Koch JM, Steuhl KP, Meller D (2003) Management of acute ulcerative and necrotizing herpes simplex and zoster keratitis with amniotic membrane transplantation. Br J Ophthalmol 87: 1215–1219

Heiligenhaus A, Li H, Yang Y, Wasmuth S, Bauer D, Steuhl KP (2004) Amniotic membrane transplantation improves experimental herpetic keratitis. Modulation of matrix metalloproteinase-9. Ophthalmologe 101: 59–65

Kersten A, Sundmacher R, Reinhard T (1997) Postoperative Komplikationen nach perforierender Keratoplastik in Herpesaugen. Differentialdiagnose, Therapie und prognostische Bedeutung. Ophthalmologe 94: 889–896

Khodadoust A, Quinter AP (2003) Microsurgical approach to the conjunctival flap. Arch Ophthalmol 121:1189–1193

Kirkness CM, Adams GG, Dilly PN, Lee JP (1988) Botulinum toxin A-induced protective ptosis in corneal disease. Ophthalmology 95: 473–480

Kruse FE, Rohrschneider K, Völcker HE (1999) Multilayer amniotic membrane transplantation for reconstruction of deep corneal ulcers. Ophthalmology 106: 1504–1510

Mackensen G, Haug P, Horn C, Sundmacher R, Witschel H (1978) Nahtlockerung nach Keratoplastik und Korrekturmöglichkeiten. Klin Monatsbl Augenheilk 173: 700–707

Mannis MJ, Plotnik RD, Schwab IR, Newton RD (1991) Herpes simplex dendritic keratitis after keratoplasty. Am J Ophthalmol 111: 480–484

Marx W, Madjlessi F, Reinhard T, Althaus C, Sundmacher R (1999) Mehr als vier Jahre Erfahrung mit der elektronischen intraokularen Nadel-Druckmessung bei irregulären Hornhäuten. Ophthalmologe 96: 498–502

Mayer K, Reinhard T, Reis A, Voiculescu A, Sundmacher R (2003) Synergistic effect of acyclovir and mycophenolate mofetil following keratoplasty in patients with herpetic eye disease. Albrecht von Graefes Arch Clin Exp Ophthalmol 241: 1051–1054

Mietz H, Cassinotti P, Siegl G, Kirchhof B, Krieglstein GK (1995) Detection of herpes simplex virus after penetrating keratoplasty by polymerase chain reaction: correlation of clinical and laboratory findings. Albrecht von Graefes Arch Clin Exp Ophthalmol: 233: 714–716

Reinhard T, Böhringer D, Sundmacher R (2001) Accelerated chronic endothelial cell loss after penetrating keratoplasty in glaucoma eyes. J Glaucoma 10: 446–451

Reinhard T, Kallmann C, Cepin A, Godehardt E, Sundmacher R (1997) The influence of glaucoma history on graft survival after penetrating keratoplasty. Albrecht von Graefes Arch Clin Exp Ophthalmol 235: 553–557

Reis A, Reinhardt T (2006) Current systemic immunosuppressive strategies in penetrating keratoplasty. In: T Reinhard, F Larkin (vol–eds): Esssentials in ophthalmology: Cornea and external eye disease. Springer, Berlin – Heidelberg – NY, pp 109–122

Reis A, Reinhard T, Voiculescu K, Mayer K, Sundmacher R (2001) Hochaktive antivirale und immunsuppressive Kombinationstherapie mit Acyclovir und Mycophenolatmofetil nach Keratoplastik mit herpetischer Grunderkrankung. Klin Monatsbl Augenheilk 218: 183–186

Remeijer L, Doornenbal P, Geerards AJ, Rijneveld WA, Beekhuis WH (1997) Newly acquired herpes simplex virus keratitis after penetrating keratoplasty. Ophthalmology 104: 648–652

Rezende RA, Bisol T, Hammersmith K, Hofling–Lima AL, Webster GF, Freitas JF, Rapuano CJ, Laibson PR, Cohen EJ (2007) Epithelial herpes simplex keratitis recurrence and graft survival after corneal transplantation in patients with and without atopy. Am J Ophthalmol 143: 623–628

Rezende RA, Uchoa UB, Raber IM, Rapuano CJ, Laibson PR, Cohen EJ (2004) New onset of herpes simplex virus epithelial keratitis after penetrating keratoplasty. Am J Ophthalmol 137: 415–419

Richter A, Slowik C, Somodi S, Vick HP, Guthoff R (1997) Corneal reinnervation following penetrating keratoplasty. Correlation of esthesiometry and confocal microscopy. Ger J Ophthalmol 5: 513–517

Sengler U, Spelsberg H, Reinhard T, Sundmacher R, Adams O, Auw-Hädrich C, Witschel H (1999) Herpes simplex virus (HSV-1) infection in a donor cornea. Br j Ophthalmol 83: 1405

Sengler U, Reinhard T, Adams O, Krempe C, Sundmacher R (2001) Herpes–simplex–virus infection in donor corneae during organ culture –frequency and consequences. Eye 15: 644–647

Seitz B (2007) Amnionmembrantransplantation. Eine unverzichtbare Therapieoption bei persistierenden kornealen Epitheldefekten. Ophthalmologe 104: 1075–1079

Shi W, Chen M, Xie L (2007) Amniotic membrane transplantation combined with antiviral and steroid therapy for herpes necrotizing stromal keratitis. Ophthalmology 114: 1476–1481

Shimomura Y, Deai T, Fukuda M, Higaki S, Hooper LC, Hayashi K (2007) Corneal buttons obtained from patients with HSK harbor high copy numbers of the HSV genome. Cornea 26: 190–193

Simon AL, Pavan–Langston D (1996) Long-term oral acyclovir therapy. Effect on recurrent infectious herpes simplex keratitis in patients with and without grafts. Ophthalmology 103: 1399–1404

Spelsberg H, Reichelt JA (2008) Amniotic membrane transplantation in proven ulcerative herpetic keratitis: successful anti-inflammatory treatment in time. Klin Monatsbl Augenheilkde 225: 75–79

Stanojlovic S, Schlickeiser S, Pleyer U (2008) Keratoplasty in HSV keratitis: prevention and therapy for immunologic complications. Klin Monatsbl Augenheilkd 225: 22–29

Sterk CC, Jager MJ, Swart-vd Berg (1995) Recurrent herpetic keratitis in penetrating keratoplasty. Doc Ophthalmol 90: 29–33

Stübinger N, Pleyer U, Erb C, Thiel HJ (1995) Keratoplasty à chaud. Ophthalmologe 92: 427–432

Sundmacher R (1997) Immunreaktionen nach Keratoplastik. Klin Monatsbl Augenheilk 171: 705–722

Sundmacher R (1981) Differential diagnosis of post–keratoplasty complications in herpes patients. In: R Sundmacher (ed) Herpetic eye disease. Bergmann, Munich, pp 439–444

Sundmacher R (1995) Die Vorteile der doppelten fortlaufenden Kreuzstichnaht gegenüber der einfach fortlaufenden Naht bei perforierender Keratoplastik. Klin Monatsbl Augenheilk 207: 342–343

Sundmacher R (ed) (2003) Adequate HLA matching in keratoplasty. Dev Ophthalmol vol 36. Karger, Basel – Sydney, pp 100

Sundmacher R, Ameye C (1989) Keratoplastik und Kapselsacklinseneinpflanzung bei Herpespatienten. In: GK Lang et al (eds): 2. DGII-Kongress. Enke, Stuttgart, pp 106–109

Sundmacher R, Reinhard T, Kersten A: Intraokularlinsen-Implantation bei Herpeserkrankung des Auges. In: 12. Kongress der DGII (Duncker et al, eds) Springer, Berlin – Heidelberg – New York, pp 76–71 (1998)

Sundmacher R, Müller O (1983) Endothelzellverluste nach Keratoplastik. Spiegelmikroskopische Verlaufsbeobachtungen bei Immunreaktionen gegen Transplantatendothel. Klin Monatsbl Augenheilk 182: 86–90

Sundmacher R, Stefansson A, Mackensen G (1983) Verlaufsbeobachtungen nach Keratoplastik. Fortschr Ophthalmol 80: 224–227

Sundmacher R, Wolff M (1993) Four years´ experience with triple procedures in herpes eyes. German J Ophthalmol 2: 65–69

Tei M, Nishida K, Kinoshita S (1996) Polymerase chain reaction detection of herpes simplex virus in tear fluid from atypical herpetic epithelial keratitis after penetrating keratoplasty. Am J Ophthalmol 122: 732–735

Van Gelderen BE, van der Lelij A, Treffers WF, van der Gaag R (2000) Detection of herpes simplex virus type 1, 2 and varicella zoster virus DNA in recipient corneal buttons. Br J Ophthalmol 84: 1238–1243

Van Rooij J, Rijneveld WJ, Remeijer L, Völker-Dieben HJ, Eggink CA, Geerards AJ, Mulder PG, Doornenbal P, Beekhuis WH (2003) Effect of oral acyclovir after penetrating keratoplasty for herpetic keratitis: a placebo-controlled multicenter trial. Ophthalmology 110: 1916–1919

Völker-Dieben HJ, Claas FH, Schreuder GM, Schipper RF, Pels E, Persijn GG, Smits J, D´Amaro J (2000) Beneficial effect of HLA-DR matching on the survival of corneal allografts. Transplantation 70: 640–648

Zheng X, Marquart ME, Loustch JM, Shah P, Sainz B, Ray A, O´Callaghan RJ, Kaufman HE, Hill JM (1999) HSV-1 migration in latently infected and naive rabbits after penetrating keratoplasty. Invest Ophthalmol Vis Sci 40: 2490–2497

# Prophylaxis of HSV Recurrences

Section

2.15

## Core Messages

- A *systemic* prophylaxis of endogenous HSV recurrences is possible by ACV 200 mg 5–4 qd or ACV 400 mg 3–2 qd.
- Systemic prophylaxis is indicated for all periods with increased risks of recurrences. This comprises iatrogenic therapeutic triggers (steroid therapy) as well as spontaneous situations with increased danger of herpes recurrences (e. g., fever, sunburn, emotional stress).
- Systemic prophylaxis may also be used for a prolonged period of time without identified triggers, if a patient shall be given a longer physical and emotional recovery time without anxiously expecting new recurrences.
- *Topical* antiviral prophylaxis is also possible. However, its reliable protective potency is restricted to the corneal epithelium.

Common questions of herpes patients are:

- What can I do against the frequent recurrences?
- Must I change my life?
- How can I enforce antiherpetic immunity?
- What else can be done?

It must then be explained that:

- Insufficient immunity is normally *not* operative as the primary trigger for HSV recurrences
- "Immune stimulating" measures, including vaccinations, will therefore not help and that the opposite is sometimes true
- The general trigger for herpes recurrences is *stress in its various forms*

Having come so far with explanation, some patients will become thoughtful and comment: "Well, I have been thinking that myself before. But I really cannot see where my stress comes from and, if I could, I would certainly not be able to control it."

Others will frankly deny any stress in their life, although their professional or family life contains lots of stress situations, as judged from the outside.

Therefore, educational talks about the etiologic role of stress for herpes recurrences often have no or only little practical prophylactic consequences, although some herpes patients may be helped in identifying and reducing their specific stress situations. They may then indeed benefit from a change in life attitude. The great majority of herpes patients, however, can only be helped by medical means, and medical prophylaxis of herpes recurrences is only operative as long as it is given.

A mostly efficient *systemic* prophylaxis against endogenous HSV recurrences is by ACV 200 mg 5–4 qd (ACV 400 mg 3–2 qd). This prophylaxis has already been recommended in the chapter on surgery in herpes eyes as the minimum dose of ACV in all combinations with steroids. This concomitant ACV prophylaxis suppresses the clinical manifestation of new HSV recurrences.

The indication comprises first of all identified triggers for recurrences (e. g., steroids, fever, sunburn, surgery, emotional stress). If children are known to react with herpes recurrences on infectious fever, the parents can be provided with a dose of prophylactic ACV tablets for a week, together with the advice to administer it to the children as soon as temperature starts to rise in the course of infection. Another example which enlightens the role of psychologic stress is that of an old lady living alone and coming only once a year with recurrent herpes, and that is always some days before Christmas Eve. Evidently, her personal situation puts too much emotional stress on her during this time of the year. ACV prophylaxis for 3 weeks takes away her fear of the otherwise invariably recurring herpes at Christmas time.

ACV prophylaxis can also be indicated in patients *without* an identified trigger. If a patient with frequently recurring HSV disease anxiously awaits the next recurrence and is so sure that it will come soon, then this anxiety causes so much stress that the prophecy of soon-recurring herpes disease becomes self-fulfilling – unless made impossible by systemic ACV prophylaxis.

*Topical* prophylaxis with antiviral agents is also possible, but only to a rather limited degree. If deep herpetic eye disease is treated with topical steroids only, then dendritic keratitis often arises as a complication of steroid-monotherapy. These complicating dendrites can reliably be prohibited by concomitant topical antiviral therapy, e. g., by trifluorothymidine eye drops or by ACV ointment. The reliable protective potency of topical

TFT eye drops is mostly restricted to the corneal epithelium, however, as TFT does not sufficiently penetrate an intact epithelial surface. Therefore, for deeper tissues, TFT offers no safe protection. The corneal penetration of ACV from ointment may lead to a relatively higher concentration of the antiviral agent in the cornea and in the anterior chamber. But with topical application alone, the high protective level of systemic ACV prophylaxis also cannot be achieved.

For curiosity, the experiences with interferon prophylaxis shall also be reported. Systemically applied interferon has side effects which are far too severe to be considered as a potential prophylactic agent against herpes recurrences. It was hoped a while, however, that interferon eye drops 1 qd would be able to at least inhibit dendritic recurrences in the course of steroid therapy, as does TFT. But even these much reduced expectations turned out to be wrong. The antiviral peptide interferon was unable to prevent the complication of dendritic lesions. The explanation is given in Fig. 2.146. When planning the study, the pathophysiologic details of recurrent dendritic keratitis were not adequately appreciated: The viruses causing epithelial disease are set free endogenously from sensory nerve ramifications ending between the basal epithelial cells. Cell infection and viral cytolysis therefore start in the basal cell layer, and expand then upwards through the multilayered epithelium. However, the superficial epithelial layer, which is then still normal, is impermeable for water soluble molecules at that time, and interferon molecules can only protect the superficial epithelial cells. This is insufficient to prevent recurrent dendritic keratitis. It makes its way upwards from the basal cells and finds enough unprotected epithelium in the deeper layers to expand and then break up.

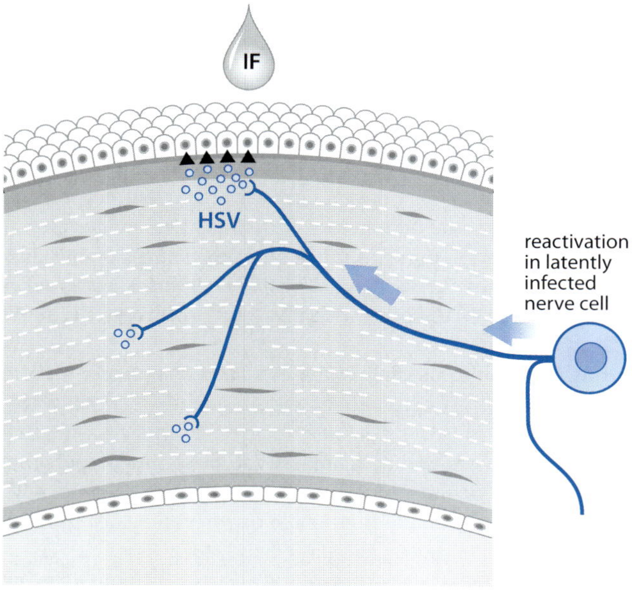


Fig. 2.146 Interferon eye drops cannot penetrate an intact epithelial corneal surface and thus cannot inhibit recurring dendritic keratitis (see text)

## References

Freeman ML, Sheridan BS, Bonneau RH, Hendricks RL (2007) Psychological stress compromises CD8+ T cell control of latent herpes simplex type 1 infections. J Immunol 179: 322–328

Herpetic Eye Disease Study Group (1997) A controlled trial of oral acyclovir for the prevention of stromal keratitis or iritis in patients with epithelial keratitis. The epithelial keratitis trial. Arch Ophthalmol 115: 703–712

Herpetic Eye Disease Study Group (1998) Acyclovir for the prevention of recurrent herpes simplex virus eye diseases. N Engl J Med 339: 300–306

Herpetic Eye Disease Study Group (2000) Oral acyclovir for herpes simplex virus eye disease: effect on prevention of epithelial keratitis and stromal keratitis. Arch Ophthalmol 118: 1030–1036

Herpetic Eye Disease Study Group (2001) Predictors of recurrent herpes simplex virus keratitis. Cornea 20: 123–128

Lairson KR, Begley CE, Reynolds TF, Wilhelmus KR (2003) Prevention of herpes simplex virus eye disease: a cost effectiveness analysis. Arch Ophthalmol 121: 108–112

Mascola JR (1999) Herpes simplex virus vaccines – why don´t antibodies protect? (editorial). JAMA 282: 379–380

Nesburn AB, Wiley DE, Trousdale MD (1983) Effect of intensive acyclovir therapy during artificial reactivation of latent herpes simplex virus. Proc Soc Exp Biol Med 72: 316–320

Pepose JS, Keadle TL, Morrison LA (2006) Ocular herpes simplex: changing epidemiology, emerging disease patterns, and the potential of vaccine prevention and therapy. Am J Ophthalmol 141: 547–557

Rezende RA, Bisol T, Hammersmith K, Rapuano CJ, Lima AL, Webster GF, Freitas JF, Laibson PR, Cohen EJ (2006) Efficacy or oral antiviral prophylaxis in preventing ocular herpes simplex virus recurrences in patients with and without self-reported atopy. Am J Ophthalmol 142: 563–567

Rodriguez A, Power WJ, Neves RA, Foster CS (1995) Recurrence rate of herpetic uveitis in patients on long-term oral acyclovir. Doc Ophthalmol 90: 331–340

Shuster JJ, Kaufman HE, Nesburn AB (1981) Statistical analysis of the rate of recurrence of herpesvirus ocular epithelial disease. Am J Ophthalmol 91: 328–331

Simon AL, Pavan-Langston D (1996) Long-term oral acyclovir therapy. Effect on recurrent infectious herpes simplex keratitis in patients with and without grafts. Ophthalmology 103: 1399–1404

Sundmacher R (1978) Trifluorthymidinprophylaxe bei der Steroidtherapie herpetischer Keratouveitiden. Klin Monatsbl Augenheilk 173: 516–519

Sundmacher R, Cantell K, Haug P, Neumann-Haefelin D (1978) Interferon Prophylaxe von Dendritica-Rezidiven bei lokaler Steroidtherapie. Ber Dtsch Ophthalmol Ges 75: 569–570

Sundmacher R, Neumann-Haefelin D, Cantell K (1981) Therapy and prophylaxis of dendritic keratitis with topical human interferon. In: R Sundmacher (ed): Herpetic eye disease. Bergmann, Munich, pp 401–407

Uchoa UB, Rezende RA, Carrasco MA, Rapuano CJ, Laibson PR (2003) Long term acyclovir use to prevent recurrent ocular herpes simplex virus infection. Arch Ophthalmol 121: 1702–1704

# Varicella Zoster Virus (VZV) Diseases of the Anterior Segment and the Adnexes

*Rainer Sundmacher*

Chapter 3

Diseases caused by the alpha herpes viruses VZV and HSV have so many clinical features in common that the classification for HSV, as depicted in Fig. 2.1, is principally valid also for VZV diseases. This sometimes makes clinical differential diagnosis between them difficult, although many differences, which facilitate differentiation, do exist.

Differential diagnosis is so important, because the sensitivity against antiviral agents and the therapeutic strategies often differ considerably in the two disease groups. In Sects. 3.2–3.9, the typical features of VZV diseases of the anterior segment and the adnexes are presented with special emphasis on differential diagnosis to the corresponding HSV diseases. A summary of the most important differences is compiled in Sect. 3.10.

# Zoster Pathophysiology and Therapy

Section

3.1

## Core Messages

- The basic pathophysiology of ophthalmic zoster and recurrent HSV eye disease is similar.
- In detail, there are multiple clinically important differences between the two viral diseases.
- Basic therapy of ophthalmic zoster is with systemic antiviral agents, e.g., ACV.
- In the beginning of zoster, a monotherapy with antiviral agents is recommended.
- In the later course of ophthalmic zoster, low-dosed steroids may become additionally necessary.
- Peripherally persistent VZV infections are relatively resistant to therapy.

## Pathophysiology

The basic facts of zoster pathophysiology are identical with those of recurrent HSV disease. After primary infection, which is mostly clinically manifest as varicella, VZV remains dormant in a latent state in neuronal tissues. From there, it may be re-activated by adequate triggers, and then may cause secondary peripheral disease, i.e., zoster, via endoneuronal spread.

The detailed differences to HSV disease are multiple, however. They start with the *virus properties*. In contrast to HSV, VZV particles are physically more labile, and VZV grows much slower in tissue culture than HSV.

*Primary infection* is typically clinically apparent with VZV, while with HSV it is typically unapparent (see Sects. 2.12 and 3.2).

For HSV disease, the *site of primary infection* is of utmost importance because it is identical with the site of recurring peripheral disease. This is different in VZV disease, where primary infection site and site of zoster disease are not identical.

Also, the importance of *viremia* is different in both infections. In VZV primary infection, viremia causes dissemination with cutaneous varicella eruptions and transportation of VZV to the sensory ganglia, where the virus hides thereafter in latency. On the contrary, HSV normally gains primary access to its latency sites by the endoneuronal axoplasmatic route only. Primary and recurrent infection site are strictly bound to each other by the connecting sensory axons. HSV normally involves just one or a rather limited number of ganglionic latency sites, while VZV becomes latent in many dorsal root and cerebral sensory ganglia. Viremia is also regularly present in zoster disease, although not always clinically manifest. Associated varicella-like skin rashes, however, are not rare in conjunction with typical sectoral zoster disease. As in primary infection, also in recurrent HSV disease, viremia plays no role.

In the sensory ganglia, VZV seems to be able to establish true latency, not only in the ganglia cells as HSV, but also in the satellite cells.

Which mechanisms exert *latency control* on the cellular and molecular level is still mostly unknown, especially with HSV. With VZV, it is much clearer that cellular anti-VZV immunity is of central importance. A critical lowering of specific anti-VZV cellular immunity goes along with a loss of latency control of VZV, while in HSV disease, fluctuations in anti-HSV immunity cannot be identified as primary triggers for recurrences. The most important primary trigger for HSV recurrences is stress in its various forms.

After HSV infection, endogenous recurrences – subclinical and clinical ones – are relatively frequent, which leads to recurrent boostering and a continuously high level of cellular anti-HSV immunity. After VZV primary infection, subclinical endogenous recurrences may also occur, but much more rarely. In consequence, if no repeated contact is made with external infection sources, above all with varicella patients, and if immunity cannot be boostered by this external route, specific anti-VZV cellular immunity tends to gradually go down with age until it falls below a critical level, and zoster disease becomes possible. This natural decline in immunity is dramatically enhanced by all diseases which go along with severe reduction in immunity. AIDS patients are just one especially afflicted group.

While for most people immunologic latency control of VZV is currently still sufficient for their lifetime, a future increase in zoster incidence has to be expected just by general expansion of life span.

The fact that zoster in "normal" immune-competent persons is experienced only once in life is explained by the booster effect, which increases anti-VZV immunity so much again, that a sufficiently high level can be maintained for the rest of life. The patient is immunologically quasi turned back to the time when he was first infected with VZV decades ago. With young zoster patients, the prospects are different, of course. They have a higher statistical risk to experience disease a second time. Severely immune-compromised patients, who are unable to reach full immunologic protection, e.g., AIDS patients, are permanently at high risk of recurrent or even persistent zoster.

While secondary HSV disease is characterized best by the phenomenon of *neuronal recurrence*, secondary VZV disease, especially eye disease, is *additionally* characterized by the phenomenon of *peripheral persistence*. Others have termed this phenomenon "peripheral latency", which must not be mixed up with true neuronal latency. It describes a persistence of VZV in peripheral cells, in which the virus replicates so slowly that the host cells are barely affected by the virus replication alone. However, the host cells express VZV antigens, and these elicit cellular immune reactions, which lead to chronic inflammatory disease. Such disease can easily be "pseudo-cured" by steroids. After tapering of the steroids, however, the virus is mostly *still persistent* and clinical disease recurs. Therefore, such recurrences should be differentiated from endoneuronally recurring new herpes disease. They are, in fact, only pseudo-recurrences. Subclinically persisting viral disease flares up and becomes clinically visible again, as soon as immune cells are free again to attack VZV antigens. Peripheral persistence is a much more difficult therapeutic problem in VZV eye infections than in HSV infections, where it can also be observed.

## Therapy

Different to antiviral therapy of HSV disease, which can often be topical, *therapy of VZV eye disease is basically systemic*. Topical zoster therapy is at most supportive.

Both, HSV and VZV, can effectively be inhibited by ACV and related drugs (see Pavan-Langston, 2008). VZV diseases call for much higher doses of ACV, however, and for more prolonged therapeutic strategies. This is not only explained by different binding characteristics of ACV to its respective target enzymes. It is above all explained by a much slower virus replication in VZV disease. As a rule, the activity of antiviral agents goes down if the replication cycle of the target virus becomes longer. This is much more the case with peripherally persistent VZV and its presumed minimal replication. It follows that VZV disease goes along with a relative refractoriness in therapeutic response, which may be further enhanced if the virus is allowed to stay in a state of peripheral persistence. The only way to counteract is to treat zoster as efficient and as *long* as possible.

Therapy of VZV eye disease has not been scientifically evaluated for as many clinical situations as would be desirable. That has to do with the many different clinical situations, each of which is relatively rare. This makes controlled prospective clinical trials difficult and often impossible. It is to be expected that this lack of evidence based therapy will be a lasting one for many zoster complications in ophthalmology. Therefore, the detailed therapeutic recommendations in the clinical sections hereafter can often only be *experienced-based*.

As just one basis for systemic therapy of zoster disease in general, the recommendations of a consensus conference of the German Paul-Ehrlich Institute from 2002 are included (Table 3.1). Another recent review of the general therapeutic

Table 3.1 Antiviral therapy of zoster

| Antiviral agent | Dose | Duration of treatment |
|---|---|---|
| Aciclovir iv infusion | Adults*<br>5–10 mg/kg body weight, 3 qd | 7 days |
| | Children<br>10(–15) mg/kg body weight, 3 qd<br>maximally 2.500 mg qd | 7 days |
| Aciclovir orally | Adults<br>800 mg, 5 qd | 7 days |
| | Children and adolescents<br>15 mg/kg body weight, 5 qd<br>(maximally 4.000 mg qd) | |
| Brivudine (BVDU) orally | Immune competent adults<br>125 mg, 1 qd | 7 days |
| | Children and adolescents<br>2 mg/kg body weight, 1 qd<br>(maximally 125 mg, 1 qd) | |
| Famciclovir orally | Immune competent adults<br>250 mg, 3 qd | 7 days |
| | Adults with ophthalmic zoster<br>500 mg, 3 qd | 7 days |
| | Immune suppressed patients of over 25 years<br>500 mg, 3 qd | 7 days |
| | Children and adolescents**<br>125–250 (–500) mg, 3 qd | 7 days |
| Valaciclovir orally | Immune competent adults<br>1.000 mg, 3 qd | 7 days |

* Recommended for patients with severe disease, especially for immune-suppressed individuals, possibly not extending 10 days of application.

** Brivudine and famciclovir are not yet licensed for use in children; they may be used under study conditions only with appropriate consent of the patients.

Adapted from: Wutzler et al (2003)

possibilities is given by Pavan-Langston (2008). While the recommended doses of the various antiviral agents in Table 3.1 are a generally accepted basis for zoster, *the recommended duration of treatment may suffice for dermal zoster, but is often far too short for ophthalmologic indications.* This will be addressed in the clinical sections.

The most important factor for therapeutic success of systemic zoster therapy is an early initiation of therapy. Best results are obtained with antiviral monotherapy starting no later than 72 hours after beginning of the first *symptoms*. Thereafter, therapy is still partly successful and necessary, of course, but the chances for quick and complete recovery decrease.

Different to the treatment of deep HSV disease, which is always with a combination of antiviral agents plus steroids, the *application of steroids in zoster is generally undesired* because of the much greater stabilizing role of immunology in VZV disease, as compared with HSV disease. Nonetheless, in *ophthalmic* zoster, therapeutic compromises then must always be made when the optic media are critically threatened by infiltration and destruction. Then, additional steroids often become inevitable. However, the general therapeutic policy must always be to apply as little as necessary.

Two topics, postherpetic neuralgia (PHN) and vaccination, had to be omitted because they are outside the scope of this atlas. In spite of all therapeutic progress, it has not been possible to treat all zoster patients in such a way that PHN loses all of its horrors. It is agreed, therefore, that the best way to handle this severe complication would be to prophylactically inhibit all zoster disease. This is a project which is based on the possibilities which are offered by VZV vaccination with a life vaccine. Vaccination is currently recommended in early childhood and beyond the age of 60, which is easily understood from the immunologic peculiarities after VZV infection, as shortly presented above. Experiences with vaccination have mostly been positive and encouraging. It is too early, however, for a final judgement (see recent summaries by Liesegang, 2008, and Gelb, 2008).

## References


Arvin A (2005) Aging, immunity, and the varicella-zoster virus. N Engl J Med 352: 2266–2267

Aylward GW, Claoué CM, Marsh RJ, Yasseem N (1994) Influence of oral acyclovir on ocular complications of herpes zoster ophthalmicus. Eye 8: 70–74

Cobo M, Foulks GN, Liesegang T, Lass J, Sutphin J, Wilhelmus K, Jones DB (1987) Observations on the natural history of herpes zoster ophthalmicus. Curr Eye Res 6: 195–199

Cooper M (1987) The epidemiology of herpes zoster. Eye 1: 413–421

De Freitas D, Martins EN, Adan C, Alvarenga LS, Pavan-Langston D (2006) Herpes zoster ophthalmicus in otherwise healthy children. Am J Ophthalmol 142: 393–399

Devlin ME, Gilden DH, Mahalingam R, Dueland AN, Cohrs R (1992) Peripheral blood mononuclear cells of the elderly contain varicella-zoster virus DNA. J Infect Dis 165: 619–622

Gelb LD (2008) Preventing herpes zoster through vaccination. Ophthalmology 115 Suppl: S35–S38

Gilden DH, Devlin M, Wellish M, Mahalingam R, Huff C, Hayward A, Vofai A (1988) Persistence of varicella-zoster virus DNA in blood mononuclear cells of patients with varicella or zoster. Virus Genes 2: 299–305

Harding SP, Lipton JR, Wells JCD (1986) Natural history of herpes zoster ophthalmicus: predictors of postherpetic neuralgia and ocular involvement. Br J Ophthalmol 71: 353–358

Hayward AR, Herberger M (1987) Lymphocyte responses to varicella zoster virus in the elderly. J Clin Immunol 7: 174–178

Hedges TR III, Albert DM (1982) The progression of the ocular abnormalities of herpes zoster. Histopathologic observations of nine cases. Ophthalmology 89: 165–177

Herbort CP, Buchi ER, Piguet B, Zogafos L, Fitting P (1991) High dose oral acyclovir in acute herpes zoster ophthalmicus: the end of the corticosteroid era. Curr Eye Res 10 (Suppl.): S171–S175

Hope-Simpson R (1965) The nature of herpes zoster: a long-term study and a new hypothesis. Proc R Soc Med 58: 9–20

Kaufman SC (2008) Anterior segment complications of herpes zoster ophthalmicus. Ophthalmology 115 Suppl: S24–S32

Kezuka T, Sakai J, Minoda H, Takeuchi M, Keino H, Streilein JW, Usui M (2002) A relationship between varicella-zoster virus-specific delayed hypersensitivity and varicella-zoster virus-induced anterior uveitis. Arch Ophthalmol 120: 1183–1188

Liesegang TJ (1999) Varicella-zoster virus eye disease. Cornea 18: 511–531

Liesegang TJ (2004) Herpes zoster virus infection. Curr Opinion Ophthalmol 15: 531–536

Liesegang TJ (2008) Herpes zoster ophthalmicus. Natural history, risk factors, clinical presentation, and morbidity. Ophthalmology 115 Suppl: S3–S12

Mahalingam R, Wellish M, Wolf W, Dueland AN, Cohrs R, Vafai A, Gilden D (1990) Latent varicella-zoster viral DNA in human trigeminal and thoracic ganglia. N Engl J Med 323: 627–631

Margolis TP, Milner MS, Shama A, Hodge W, Seiff S (1998) Herpes zoster ophthalmicus in patients with immunodeficiency virus infection. Am J Ophthalmol 125: 285–291

Marsh RJ (1973) Herpes zoster keratitis. Trans Ophthalmol Soc UK: 93: 181–192

Marsh RJ, Cooper M (1991) Double-masked trial of topical acyclovir and steroids in the treatment of herpes zoster ocular inflammation. Br J Ophthalmol 75: 542–546

Marsh RJ, Cooper M (1993) Ophthalmic herpes zoster. Eye 7: 350–370

Maudgal PC, Dieltiens M, De Clercq E, Missotten L (1985) Oral bromovinyldeoxyuridine treatment of herpes zoster ophthalmicus. In: PC Maudgal, L Missotten (eds) Herpetic Eye Diseases. Doc Ophth Proc Ser 44. Dr. W Junk, Dordrecht, pp 403–411

Meier JL, Holman RO, Croen KD, Smialek JE, Strauss SE (1993) Varicella-zoster virus transcription in human trigeminal ganglia. Virology 193: 193–200

Mietz H, Eis-Hubinger AM, Sundmacher R, Font RL (1997) Detection of varicella-zoster virus DNA in keratectomy specimens by use of polymerase chain reaction. Arch Ophthalmol 115: 590–594

Miller AE (1980) Selective decline in cellular immune response to varicella-zoster in the elderly. Neurology 30: 582–587

Mitchell BM, Bloom DC, Cohrs RJ, Gilden DH, Kennedy PG (2003) Herpes simplex virus-1 and varicella-zoster virus latency in ganglia. J Neurovirol 9: 194–204

Naseri A, Good WV, Cunningham ET (2003) Herpes zoster virus sclerokeratitis and acute anterior uveitis in a child following varicella vaccination. Am J Ophthalmol 135: 415–417

Naumann GOH, Gass JDM, Font RL (1968) Histopathology of herpes zoster ophthalmicus. Am J Ophthalmol 65: 533–541

Neoh C, Harding SP, Saunders D, Wallis S, Tullo AB, Nylander A, Nelson ME (1994) Comparison of topical and oral acyclovir in early zoster ophthalmicus. Eye 8: 688–691

Pavan-Langston D (2008) Herpes zoster, antivirals and pain management. Ophthalmology 115 Suppl: S13–S20

Pepose JS (1997) The potential impact of the varicella vaccine and new antivirals on ocular disease related to varicella-zoster virus. Am J Ophthalmol 123: 243–251

Piebenga LW, Laibson PR (1973) Dendritic lesions in herpes zoster ophthalmicus. Arch Ophthalmol 90: 268–270

Starr CE, Pavan–Langston D (2002) Varicella-zoster virus: mechanisms of pathogenicity and corneal disease. Ophthalmol Clin North Am 15: 7–15

Straus SE (1989) Clinical and biological differences between recurrent herpes simplex virus and varicella-zoster virus infections. JAMA 262: 3455–3458

Sundmacher R (1981) Trials with interferon in ophthalmic zoster. In: R Sundmacher (ed): Herpetic eye disease. Bergmann, Munich, pp 465–467

Wenkel H, Rummelt C, Rummelt V, Jahn G, Fleckenstein B, Naumann GOH (1993) Detection of varicella zoster virus DNA and viral antigen in human cornea after herpes zoster ophthalmicus. Cornea 12: 131–137

Wenkel H, Rummelt V, Fleckenstein B, Naumann GOH (1998) Detection of varicella zoster virus DNA and viral antigen in human eyes after herpes zoster ophthalmicus. Ophthalmology 105: 1323–1330

Wood MJ, Johnson RW, McKendrick MW, Taylor J, Mandal BK, Crooks J (1994) A randomized trial of acyclovir for 7 days or 21 days with and without prednisone for treatment of acute herpes zoster. N Engl J Med 330: 896–900

Wutzler P, De Clercq E, Wutke K, Färber I (1995) Oral brivudin vs intravenous acyclovir in the treatment of herpes zoster in immunocompromised patients. A randomized double-blind trial. J Med Virol 46: 252–257

Wutzler P, Gross G, Doerr HW (2003) Antivirale Therapie des Zoster. (Results of a consensus conference), Dtsch Arztebl 100: A858–860 (Heft 13)

Yamada K, Hayasaka S, Yamamoto Y, Setogawa T (1990) Cutaneous eruption with or without ocular complications in patients with herpes zoster involving the trigeminal nerve. Albrecht von Graefes Arch Clin Exp Ophthalmol 228: 1–4

Zaal MJW (2000) Herpes zoster ophthalmicus. Clinical studies on virus–host interactions. (Doctoral thesis, Vrije Universiteit Amsterdam)

Zaal MJM, Maudgal PC, Rietveld E, Suir EPE (1991) Chronic ocular zoster responsive to antiviral treatment with oral BVDU. Curr Eye Res 10 (Suppl.): S125–130

Zaal MJW, Völker-Dieben HJ, D´Amaro J (2003) Prognostic value of Hutchinson´s sign in acute herpes zoster ophthalmicus. Albrecht von Graefes Arch Clin Exp Ophthalmol 241: 187–191

Zaal MJW, Völker-Dieben HJ, Wienesen M, D´Amaro J, Kijlstra A (2001) Longitudinal analysis of varicella–zoster virus DNA on the ocular surface associated with herpes zoster ophthalmicus. Am J Ophthalmol 131: 25–29

# Ocular Disease in the Course of Primary VZV Infection (Varicella)

Section

3.2

## Core Messages

- Ocular involvement in the course of varicella is rare. Therapy must aim at the earliest possible onset of systemic ACV therapy and at refraining from all steroids.
- Dendritic complications are no problem. They heal spontaneously.
- VZV interstitial keratitis and VZV endotheliitis may necessitate additional therapy with low-dosed topical steroids in the later course if the corneal transparency is seriously threatened.
- Steroid monotherapy of VZV interstitial keratitis and endotheliitis is strictly contraindicated because of the great risk of promoting peripheral persistent VZV disease.

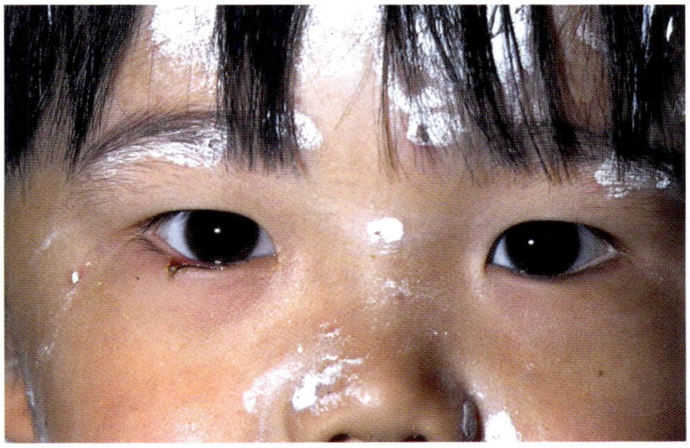

Fig. 3.1 Varicella with intermarginal VZV blepharitis

Ocular disease in the course of primary VZV infection (varicella) does not seem to be a frequent problem, as judged from the sparse reports in the literature.

The following case descriptions are examples of ocular disease after primary infection with VZV.

## Analysis of Fig 3.1

The child in Fig. 3.1 exhibits an intermarginal VZV blepharitis, which is barely visible from the distance and, therefore, easily overlooked. Both eyes are white, from which the ophthalmologist may take the message "no danger for the eyes". This message is correct. The small erosive intermarginal area in the middle of the right lower lid resembles exactly that of *recurrent* intermarginal HSV blepharitis (see Fig. 2.12) and *not* that of *primary* intermarginal HSV blepharitis, as one could expect (see Fig. 2.105). The probable explanation is that VZV has less attraction than HSV to the intermarginal epithelium of the lids. It replicates much slower than HSV. That leads to a rarer incidence and a milder form of intermarginal blepharitis in the course of primary infection. If it develops, it does not expand as rapidly as in HSV primary disease, and in the immune-competent individual, it heals quickly spontaneously. No antiviral therapy is needed.

## Detailed analysis of fig 3.2

***Clinic:*** The young lady in Fig. 3.2a exhibited a moderately severe serous unilateral conjunctivitis (Fig. 3.2b) a couple of days after initiation of a varicella rash. The corneal epithelium was normal at that time, but in the corneal stroma, some flecks of very subtle infiltrations were visible with the slit-lamp. These infiltrations were so faint that photographic documentation failed to unequivocally show them. The aqueous humor was clear with no precipitates on the endothelium. Intraocular pressure was normal.

***Diagnosis:*** Serous conjunctivitis and beginning interstitial keratitis in the course of primary VZV infection (varicella).

***Differential diagnosis:*** None. The older a person at primary infection with VZV, the more severe varicella may develop – ocular complications included. Such acute edematous swelling of the conjunctiva is normally not seen with secondary VZV conjunctivitis in zoster, but only with primary disease. Biomicroscopically, there was no doubt as to the development of interstitial VZV keratitis.

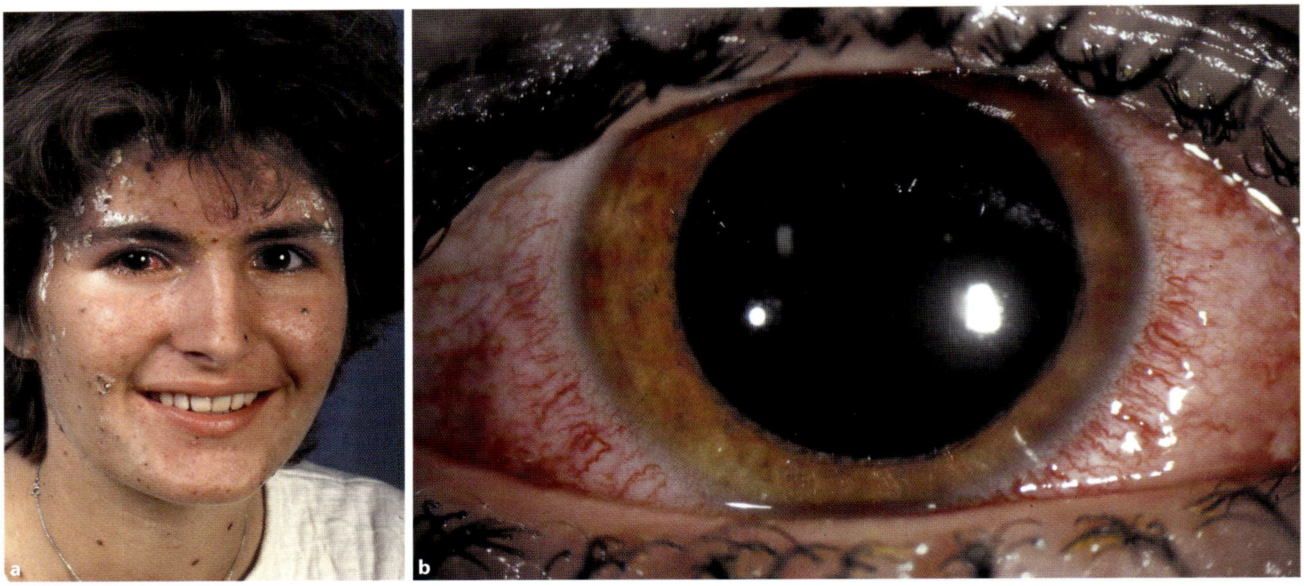


Fig 3.2a,b Varicella with VZV conjunctivitis and barely visible macular interstitial corneal infiltrations (see text)

The primary, exogenous infection must have affected the corneal epithelium prior to expanding into the corneal stroma. Probably, at the time of first ophthalmological investigation (Fig. 3.2b), the epithelial disease had already spontaneously healed without sequelae (see Sect. 3.4).

***Therapy:*** When this case was observed, systemic ACV therapy of varicella was not yet available. No steroids were given. The patient recovered spontaneously without ocular sequelae. The faint macular infiltrations resolved within a few months. It is reassuring to know that interstitial VZV keratitis may heal completely without antiviral therapy, provided no steroids have ever been applied. In so far, the clinical situation with deep corneal disease in varicella resembles that of nummular keratitis in the course of adenovirus infection. From the latter disease, we also know that it mostly spontaneously heals in the long run, provided no steroids are ever given.

Nowadays, with ACV available, we would prefer not to completely rely on spontaneous healing, but to support the healing process by an as rapidly as possible instituted systemic ACV regime with 800 mg 5 qd for 2–3 weeks. As ACV is well tolerated by most patients, one should not content oneself with a 7 day regime, as recommended for VZV dermal disease. Systemic therapy should be at least extended until the eye has turned completely white again. If at this time there are still notable amounts of interstitial infiltrations, it is advisable to prolong systemic ACV therapy by another 1–3 weeks. Steroids should, if possible, be avoided. With only minimal infiltrations left after these weeks of systemic ACV monotherapy, one may rely on complete spontaneous healing of the remaining keratitis without antiviral agents and without any steroid therapy. The risk of development of peripheral persistent VZV keratitis is minimal with such a cautious therapeutic policy.

## Detailed analysis of Fig 3.3

***Clinic:*** The boy presented 2 weeks after dermal healing of varicella, claiming reduced vision in one eye. A clearly red eye had never been observed in conjunction with varicella. It could not be excluded, however, that a slight conjunctivitis might have occurred for a couple of days together with the skin rash. Ophthalmological investigation revealed relatively densely packed interstitial nummuli in one eye (Fig. 3.3a), and only two peripheral nummuli without visual impairment in the fellow eye (not shown).

***Diagnosis:*** Bilateral interstitial VZV keratitis in the course of primary VZV infection (varicella).

***Differential diagnosis:*** None. Nummular keratitis from adenovirus infection may look identical. This differential diagnosis was excluded, however, by the virologically proven diagnosis of concomitant varicella.

***Therapy:*** Starting with systemic ACV therapy so late after varicella disease was not really promising. Therapeutic success with systemic ACV is lower the later the therapy is started. Waiting for spontaneous healing would have been an alternative. That would have taken months, however. As the boy´s parents were extremely motivated to shorten the healing course, it was decided to try a long-term treatment with a *topical* combination therapy of ACV ointment 5 qd with very small amounts of steroids added (steroid ointment 2 qd). This was applied for the visually impaired eye only. The visually unimpaired eye with the peripheral nummuli was left untreated. The topical combination therapy was expected to shorten the healing time without enhancing the risk of peripherally persistent VZV infection. It took 8 weeks for the center of the severely affected cornea to clear. Peripherally, faint remnants of the nummuli were still seen. Therapy was prolonged for another month, and then withdrawn. As a final result, both corneas had cleared perfectly after half a year, and kept clear thereafter. There was no recurrent disease from peripherally persisting VZV in the

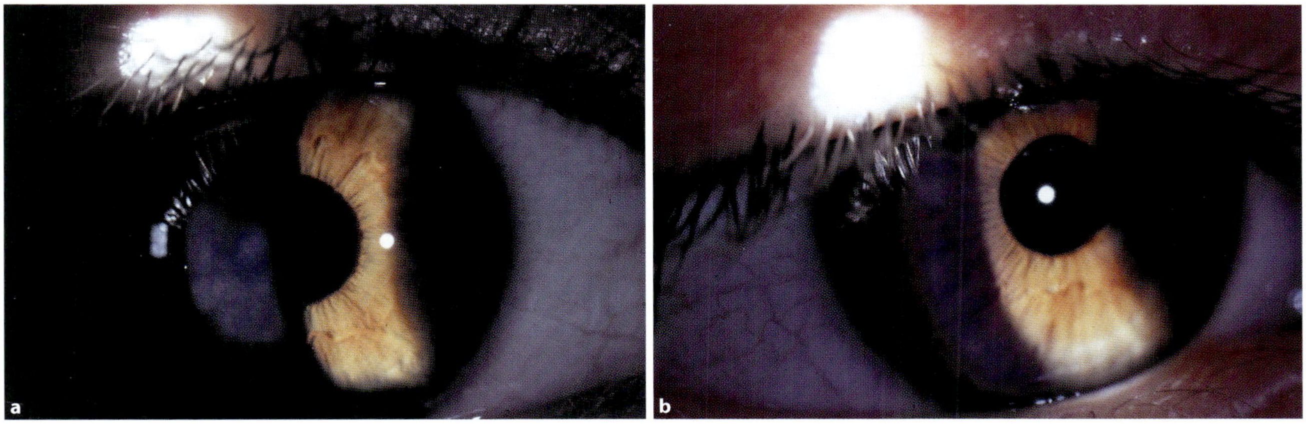

Fig. 3.3 Primary interstitial VZV keratitis **a** at beginning of therapy, **b** 3 months later

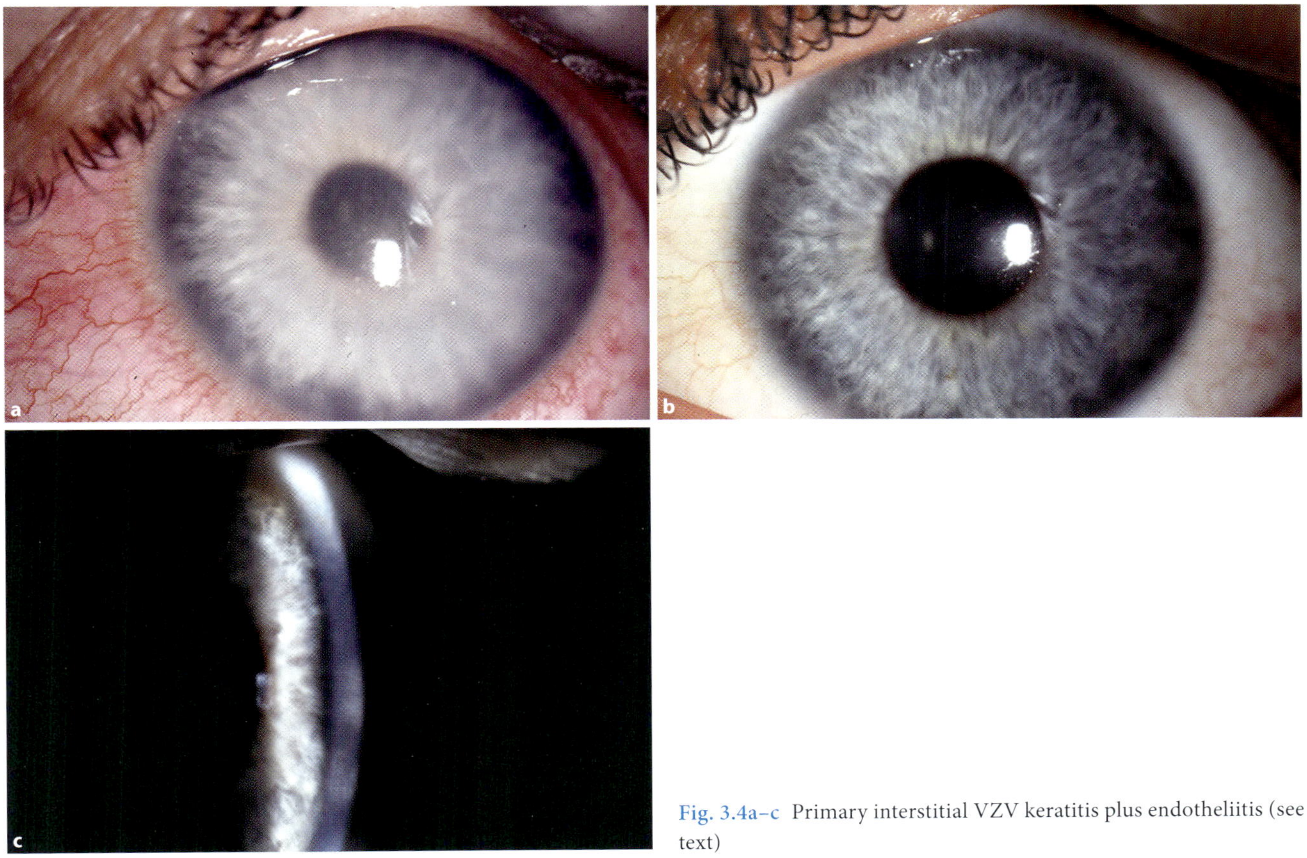

Fig. 3.4a–c Primary interstitial VZV keratitis plus endotheliitis (see text)

steroid treated eye. Such minor amounts of topical steroids may thus help quicker resolution of infiltrations without simultaneously enhancing the risk of peripheral persistent VZV infection, provided they are always covered by a full topical dose of ACV.

## Analysis of Fig 3.4

The case of a young girl in Fig. 3.4 is presented as an example of the danger of steroid monotherapy of primary VZV keratitis. It dates back to the time, when ACV was not yet available and when topical steroid monotherapy was routine with severe corneal involvement. The cornea was not only affected by VZV interstitial infiltrates, as in Fig. 3.3, but also by a diffuse corneal edema from primary VZV endotheliitis (Fig. 3.4a). This severe deep VZV disease started to develop when the dermal rash healed already, and it did not reach its maximum before the rash had completely gone. This time course is typical for varicella and for zoster, and it must be observed for the timing of ophthalmological controls and the duration of therapy. The girl then had intensive treatment with topical steroids only. Corneal edema as well as most of the interstitial infiltrations cleared quickly within 7–10 days (Fig. 3.4b). Every time it was tried to get the patient off the topical steroids, however, interstitial infiltrates (Fig. 3.4c) and also areas of circumscribed endotheliitis with edema recurred and led to frequent re-institution of steroid therapy. In the end, the cornea was so scarred and its surface so irregularly distorted that perforating keratoplasty became necessary to restore vision. Retrospectively, it can be taken for very probable that a spontaneous healing course without any therapy would have been better than such an ever re-instituted steroid monotherapy. Nowadays, such severe corneal and intraocular complications would be answered with a systemic full-dose therapy of ACV (800 mg 5 qd) for 3–6 weeks, with a concomitant *low-dose topical* steroid therapy of only 3 qd for 2 weeks and 2 qd for the rest of the ACV treatment. Topical ACV therapy (ointment 5 qd, without reduction) would also have been given as an adjunct therapy where available. If 6 weeks of such a combination therapy were not sufficient to restore the eye to normal again, one would prolong at least the topical combination regime as long as possible.

## References


Borit A, Pentelei-Molnar J, Lazaro R (1974) Varicella dendritic keratitis. Invest Ophthalmol 13: 764–770

Magone MT, Nasser RE, Cevallos AV, Margolis TP (2005) Chronic recurrent varicella-zoster virus keratitis confirmed by polymerase chain reaction testing. Am J Ophthalmol 139: 1135–1136

Naseri A, Good WV, Cunningham ET (2003) Herpes zoster virus sclerokeratitis and acute anterior uveitis in a child following varicella vaccination. Am J Ophthalmol 135: 415–417

Pepose JS (1997) The potential impact of the varicella vaccine and new antivirals on ocular disease related to varicella-zoster virus. Am J Ophthalmol 123: 243–251

Sanke RF, Welham RAN (1982) Lacrimal canalicular obstruction following chickenpox. Brit J Ophthalmol 66: 71–74

Sundmacher R, Strunck-Kortenbusch B (1991) Varizellenkeratitis, ein wenig bekanntes Krankheitsbild. Sitzungsbericht 153. Versammlung Rhein.-Westf. Augenärzte: 89–90

Uchida Y, Kanedo M, Hayashi K (1980) Varicella dendritic keratitis. Am J Ophthalmol 89: 259–262

# Zoster Blepharitis, Conjunctivitis, and General VZV Dissemination

Section

3.3

## Core Messages

- Vesicles in the dermatome V/1 usually precede eye disease by several days.
- Hutchinson's sign is predictive for eye disease in the course of ophthalmic zoster, but it is not absolutely reliable.
- There is also *no* reliable correlation between the severity of Hutchinson's sign or of dermal disease with the severity of subsequent eye disease.
- VZV eye disease rarely develops without typical preceding dermal disease (zoster sine herpete). This can be then suspected from the features of the eye affections only. A PCR analysis of eye material may be necessary for a definite diagnosis.
- General dissemination of VZV in the course of zoster may manifest itself in varicella-like dermal and various neuronal and visceral diseases.

Ophthalmic zoster may affect:

- The dermatome V/1 *plus* the anterior segment of the eye
- The dermatome V/1 only, *without* any eye disease
- Rarely the eye only, without any dermal disease, or with very subtle atypical dermal disease (zoster sine herpete)

The time course of dermal and ocular disease is always such that dermal disease comes first, and eye disease follows some days later. That probably has to do with the different times required for the replication cycles of VZV in the involved tissues. The time lag between onset of dermal and eye disease may be longer than a week. In consequence, one can never be sure that the eye will be spared by zoster unless at least 10 days have elapsed since appearance of the first vesicles in the skin and no eye disease has developed up to this time.

Fortunately, we dispose of a potent clinical predictor whether or not eye involvement must be awaited, i. e., *Hutchinson´s sign*. Its anatomical basis is the nasociliary nerve, a major ramification of V/1, which splits up again to serve two areas, the anterior segment of the eye and an area of the lateral nasal dermis up to the tip of the nose. If this lateral nasal dermis – and especially the lateral tip of the nose – show vesicles in the beginning of zoster, then it becomes very probable, that VZV had been endogenously set free also in the anterior segment of the eye and that eye disease is already about to develop. However, it will stay subclinical for some more days, because replication of VZV in the eye is slower than in the dermis.

Unfortunately, Hutchinson´s sign fails in a small percentage of zoster cases. If we deal with a false positive Hutchinson's sign, i. e., no eye disease follows, although we waited for it to arise, that is no problem. If we deal with a false negative Huchinson´s sign, i. e., severe eye disease develops after a week without preceding typical involvement of the nasal dermis, the sequelae can be very unpleasant. The most important first 3 days for starting efficient systemic ACV treatment have elapsed then already, and if systemic ACV therapy had not been instituted for therapy of dermal disease or pain, permanent eye damage may result from delay in the onset of therapy.

## Analysis of Fig 3.5

Figure 3.5 demonstrates the variable expression of Hutchinson´s sign. It also shows that the *severity* of Hutchinson´s *does not correspond* with the severity of associated eye disease.

The patient in Fig. 3.5a shows a severe vesicular eruption along the whole dermatome of the nasal ramification of the nasociliary nerve with involvement of the lateral side and frontal tip of the nose. Both lids are severely edematous and the lid fissure can hardly be opened for inspection at that time. Surprisingly, in this case, there was only harmless monosymptomatic conjunctivitis associated with some conjunctival bullae from impeded lymph drainage (Fig. 3.7).

The disease of the patient in Fig. 3.5b looks far less dramatic. The upper lid is barely swollen and allows a free view at an eye with only a mild conjunctival redness. There are, however, two circumscribed groups of vesicles, which give a positive Hutchinson´s sign: one group in the dermis of the inner lid angle, and another separated one on the lateral tip of the nose. The latter can easily be overlooked if the doctor´s attention is distracted by the more severe disease on the forehead. Although Hutchinson´s sign was relatively discrete in this case, the patient experienced a rather recalcitrant course of interstitial keratitis, which healed only after months of consequent therapy.

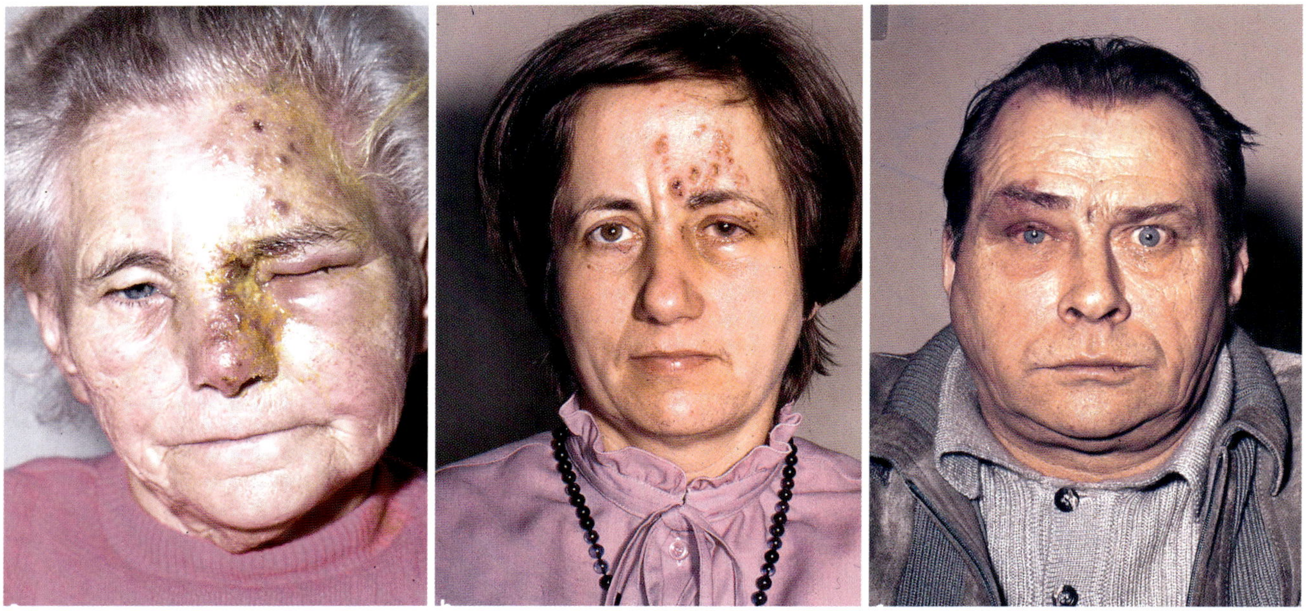

Fig. 3.5 Ophthalmic zoster with Hutchinson's sign, **a** pronounced, **b** discrete, **c** minimal

Finally, the patient in Fig. 3.5c exhibits only three circumscribed small areas of skin disease, one in the brow area, one supranasally, and a third in the skin of the inner lid angle. When he first presented with then even more minor skin affections (not shown here), the eye was still perfectly white and clinically normal, and the rudimental Hutchinson´s sign with two areas at the base of the nose was unfortunately not identified as such. Zoster was suspected but not unequivocally diagnosed, and if it was zoster, ocular involvement was not expected to develop. No systemic zoster therapy was instituted, and the patient controlled 1 week later. Then (Fig. 3.5c) the diagnosis of ophthalmic zoster was clear, and also evident was beginning ocular involvement. The ocular situation had dramatically changed to the worse with interstitial and endothelial involvement. The ocular VZV disease turned out to be extremely resistant to systemic plus topical anti-VZV therapy – possibly because of the late onset of therapy. It took many months of treatment before finally healing could be achieved, however, with corneal scars.

## Analysis of Fig 3.6

Figure 3.6 shows a zoster case from the pre-ACV era. It documents the amount of damage that can be brought about if VZV is allowed to cause severe arterial vasculitis in immunologically compromised persons without efficient antiviral therapy. This patient developed hemorrhagic dermal zoster after cytostatic therapy for malignancy. When she first showed-up 10 days after beginning of zoster (Fig. 3.6a), the frontal dermis was covered with black crusts as was the upper lid (Fig. 3.6b), which proved to be thickened, hard, and unmovable. The eye itself was affected with interstitial corneal infiltrations and a slight endotheliitis. Ocular involvement was relatively mild as compared with the severe necrotizing skin disease. The black necrotic areas sequestered within some weeks and left wounds which had to heal "per secundam" (Fig. 3.6c). The loss of lid substance and the shrinking lid scars led to progressive traction ectropion of the upper lid, which finally was firmly fixed to the brow, and the conjunctiva permanently exposed (Fig. 3.6d). The resulting permanent lagophthalmus necessitated reconstructive lid surgery with mobilisation of the tarsal remnants, interposition of a tarsal transplant, and transplantation of a free dermal flap. Thereafter, the lids could be closed again, and the eye, which had survived all these complications with stunningly little permanent damage, could be preserved with useful function (Fig. 3.6e). It can also be seen from Fig. 3.6e, that permanent ocular motor nerve palsies were another complication of this severe zoster (see also Fig. 3.9). Such a bad course should no longer be possible with modern antiviral therapy. It is presented here to document what kind of severe permanent damage may arise, if we do not or cannot make adequate use of all diagnostic and therapeutic progress which has been achieved in the last decades.

## Analysis of Fig 3.7

Conjunctivitis in ophthalmic zoster is mostly of no major therapeutic interest. It may occur as the only sign of associated eye disease, as in Fig. 3.7, which belongs to the patient in Fig. 3.5a and demonstrates that the severity of dermal and eye disease must not necessarily be the same. It is also to be noted, that the conjunctival bullae, which are frequently seen in early ophthalmic zoster, are no sign of severity of conjunctivitis. Instead, these bullae are a sequelae of momentarily impeded lymph drainage (see the massively swollen lower lids in Fig. 3.5a). Edema disappears quickly as soon as sufficient lymph flow becomes possible again.

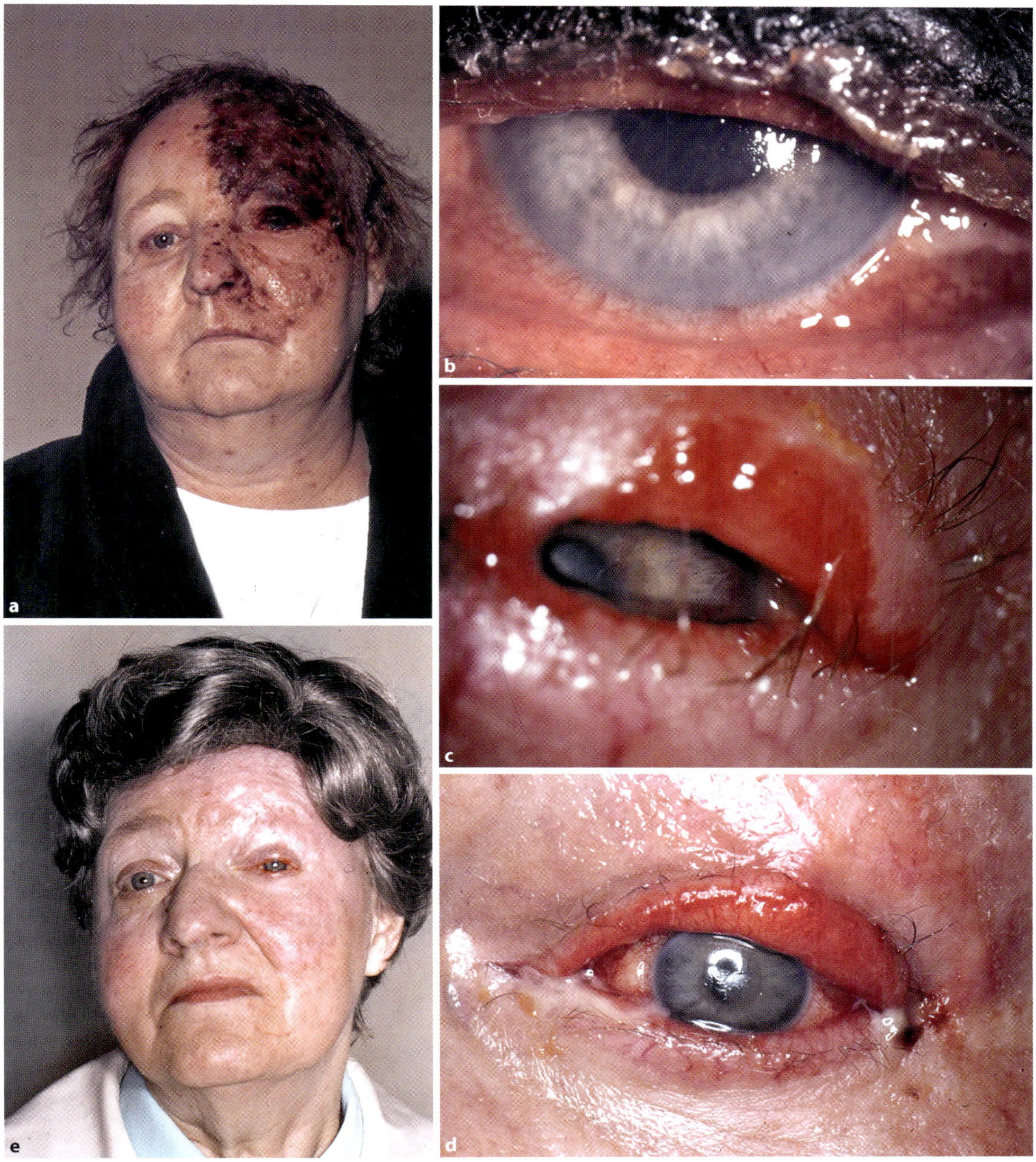


Fig. 3.6 Severe zoster V/1 plus V/2 with necrotizing blepharitis (**a, b**), substantial loss of upper lid tissues (**c**), and fixed secondary ectropion (**d**), aspect after healing and reconstructive lid surgery (**e**) (see text)

## Analysis of Fig 3.8

In the course of typical segmental zoster, VZV can spread by the endoneuronal route and hematogenous spread can also occur, as has already been mentioned (Sect. 3.1). Such hematogenous spread affects above all the dermis. It mostly causes only single disseminated vesicles, which quickly heal and are often overlooked (Fig. 3.8a). Sometimes, the associated dermal rash is so dense and severe, however (Fig. 3.8b), that a "second varicella disease" may be suspected. This is impossible, of course. The term varicella is reserved for primary VZV infection *without* pre-existing anti-VZV immunity. In cases like the one shown here, we deal with hematogenous VZV spread in the presence of *reduced* anti-VZV immunity. Such dermal disease differs from varicella, and we can at most speak of *varicelliform* eruptions in the course of zoster. The possibility of VZV spreading not only to the dermis, but also to the nervous system or the viscera, is an important reason to *always* treat segmental dermal zoster *systemically as early as possible*, irrespective of how mild or severe it may appear initially.

## Analysis of Fig 3.9

We use to look at zoster as a segmental disease of sensory neurons. General hematogenous spread and associated cutaneous

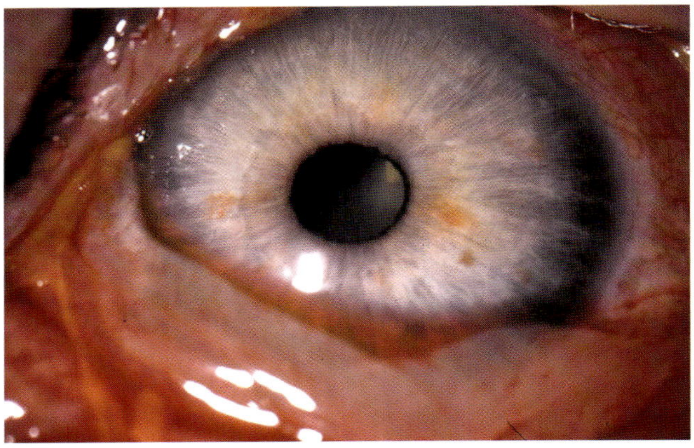

Fig. 3.7 Monosymptomatic serous zoster conjunctivitis (same patient as in Fig. 3.5a)

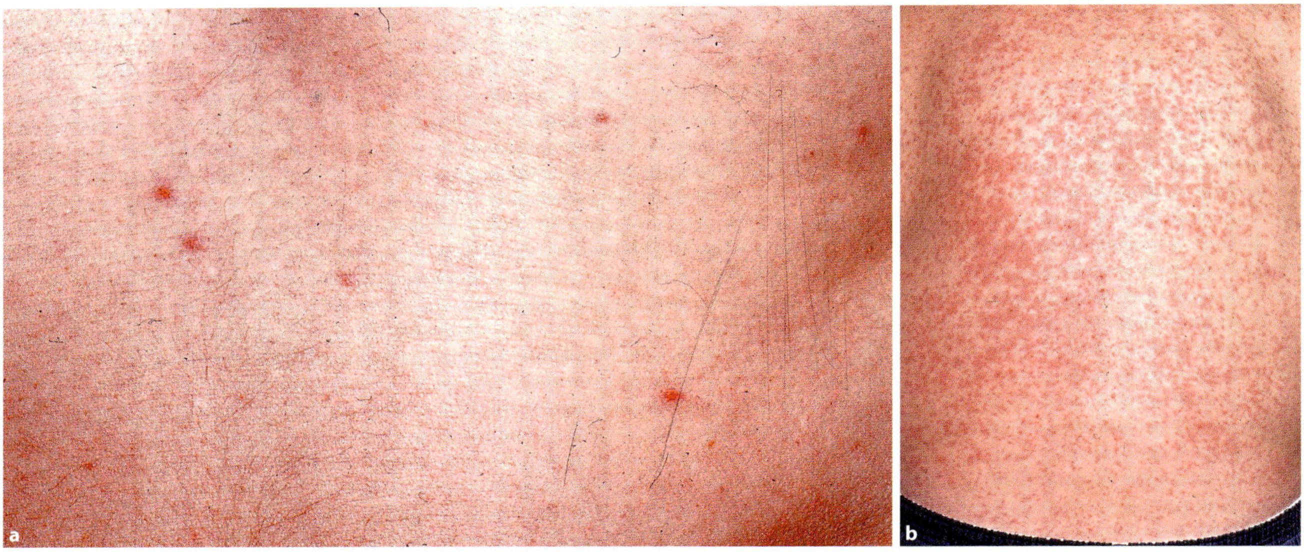

Fig. 3.8 Hematogenous cutaneous spread of VZVin the course of ophthalmic zoster, **a** minimal, **b** severe

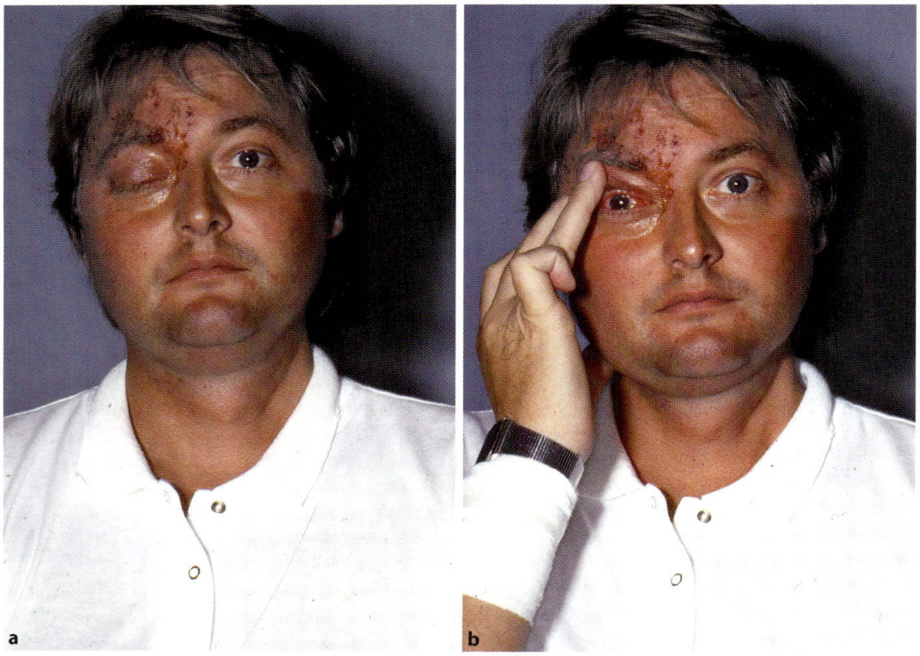

Fig. 3.9a,b Complete oculomotor palsy in the course of ophthalmic zoster

disease are another clinical manifestation, as shown above. In addition, various other neuronal affections may occur. Among these are the rare ocular motor palsies as shown in Fig. 3.9. The eye itself did *not* disease in the course of this zoster case, although the affection of nasal dermis at the inner lid angle could be understood as a minimal Hutchinson´s sign.

Rarely, other neural sites develop secondary VZV disease with or without obvious correlation with ophthalmic zoster, e.g., the retina (see Chap. 6). All these rare events may be subsumed one way or another under "general dissemination".

## References


Beards G, Graham C, Pillay D (1998) Investigation of vesicular rashes for HSV and VZV by PCR. J Med Virol 54: 155–157

Forrest WM, Kaufman HE (1976) Zosteriform herpes simplex. Am J Ophthalmol 81: 86–88

Im M, Kim BJ, Seo YJ, Park JK, Lee JH (2007) Complete ophthalmoplegia after herpes zoster. Clin Exp Dermatol 32: 162–164

Kalman CM, Laskin OL (1986) Herpes zoster and zosteriform herpes simplex virus infections in immunocompetent adults. Am J Med 81: 775–778

Kattah JC, Kennerdell JS (1978) Orbital apex syndrome secondary to herpes zoster ophthalmicus. Am J Ophthalmol 85: 378–382

Marsh RJ, Dulley B, Kelly V (1977) External ocular motor palsies in ophthalmic zoster: a review. Br J Ophthalmol 61: 677–682

Nahass GT, Goldstein BA, Zhu WY, Serfling U (1992) Comparison of Tzanck smear, viral culture and DNA diagnostic methods in detection of herpes simplex and varicella-zoster infection. JAMA 268: 2541–2555

Singal A, Mehta S, Pandhi D (2006) Herpes zoster with dissemination. Indian Pediatr 43: 353–356

Tamura T, Yoshida M, Tezuka T (1994) Detection of varicella-zoster virus DNA in conjunctivas of patients with herpes zoster. Ophthalmologica 208: 41–43

Thiel MA, Bossart W, Bernauer W (1998) Clinical evaluation of impression cytology for the diagnosis of superficial viral eye diseases. Klin Monatsbl Augenheilkd 212: 388–391

Waring GO, Ekins MB (1981) Corneal perforation in herpes zoster ophthalmicus caused by eyelid scarring with exposure keratitis. In: R Sundmacher (ed) Herpetic Eye Diseases. Bergmann, Munich, pp 469–478

Waring GO, Ekins MB (1983) Corneal perforations secondary to exposure keratitis. Ophthalmic Surg 15: 153

Yamada K, Hayasaka S, Yamamoto Y, Setogawa T (1990) Cutaneous eruption with or without ocular complications in patients with herpes zoster involving the trigeminal nerve. Albrecht von Graefes Arch Clin Exp Ophthalmol 228: 1–4

Yamamoto S, Shimomura Y, Kinoshita S, Tano Y (1994) Differentiating zosteriform herpes simplex from ophthalmic zoster. Arch Ophthalmol 112: 1515–1516

Zaal MJW, Völker-Dieben HJ, D´Amaro J (2003) Prognostic value of Hutchinson´s sign in acute herpes zoster ophthalmicus. Graefe´s Arch Clin Exp Ophthalmol 241: 187–191

# Epithelial Zoster Keratitis

Section 3.4

## Core Messages

- *Early* epithelial viral efflorescences in ocular zoster heal spontaneously and quickly. They need no therapy.
- Their real importance is a prognostic one: their presence indicates that more severe deep zoster disease will invariably follow within some days.
- It is advisable, therefore, to start with maximal systemic and topical anti-VZV therapy as soon as these early epithelial efflorescences have been detected.
- The pathophysiology of *late* dendritiform efflorescences is still debated. Therapeutically, these pseudodendrites do not need antiviral agents for healing (see Sect. 3.8).

## Analysis of Fig 3.10 and Fig 3.11

While every ophthalmologist has personal experience with the diagnosis of HSV dendritic keratitis, this is not the case with epithelial viral efflorescences in ophthalmic zoster. The reason is that these efflorescences arise so early in the course of zoster and heal spontaneously so quickly, that they have already mostly disappeared at the time when the first eye examination takes place.
These efflorescences are also widely unknown for the reason that they often do not grow beyond the state of coarse punctate lesions. Their presence is easily overlooked if the cornea is not thoroughly checked, also with fluorescein stain (Fig. 3.10). If they grow further, they first elongate to plump linear lesions (Fig. 3.11a), and if they branch, the branching results in short plump stellate or dendritic figures (Fig. 3.11b,c). These have formal similarities with HSV viral epithelial lesions, but they lack the microdestruction pattern, which is pathognomonic for epithelial HSV disease (see Sect. 2.5). Therefore, the differential diagnosis from HSV epithelial disease is easy with the branched lesions. With the punctate lesions, a differential diagnosis is impossible from biomicroscopy alone. In conjunction with typical dermal zoster, there should be no doubts in diagnosing VZV disease. Without characteristic dermal VZV disease (zoster sine herpete), however, PCR tests from epithelial material may be needed to differentiate VZV etiology from other causes of punctate keratitis.

From the pre-ACV era, we know that the early epithelial zoster lesions of the cornea not only heal spontaneously – often already within 1–2 days – they heal even in the presence of topical or systemic steroid-monotherapy. They do not enlarge under steroids and they never form geographic viral lesions like in HSV disease. In so far, they are no therapeutic problem. The ophthalmologist must know them well, however, and carefully check for their presence in early ophthalmic zoster, because they have a clear prognostic value: if these lesions are detected, deep zoster disease of the eye will invariably develop some days later. This, again, is sufficient reason not only to start immediately with high-dosed systemic antiviral agents, but also to start immediately with adjunctive topical ACV therapy, where available.

Sometimes, peculiar *late* dendritiform efflorescences arise many months after zoster. Formally, they sometimes have stunningly gross similarity with HSV dendrites (Fig. 2.34). Biomicroscopically, however, there are no signs of viral epithelial destruction. They are usually addressed as peudodendrites, i.e., as non-viral lesions. However, viral involvement and a role for antiviral treatment have also been claimed. This will be further addressed in Sect. 3.8.

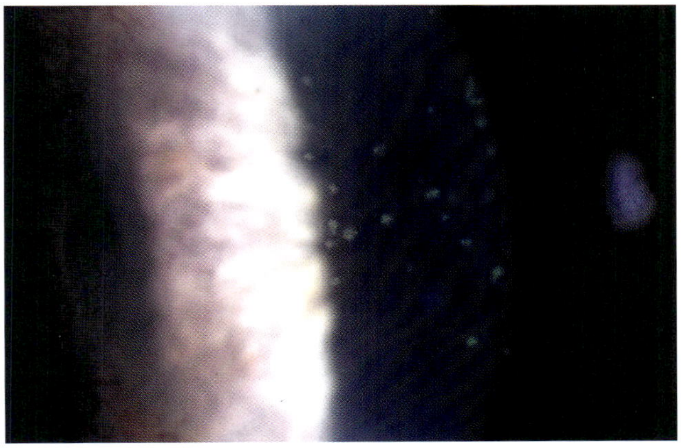

Fig. 3.10 Coarse punctate epithelial zoster efflorescences (fluorescein)

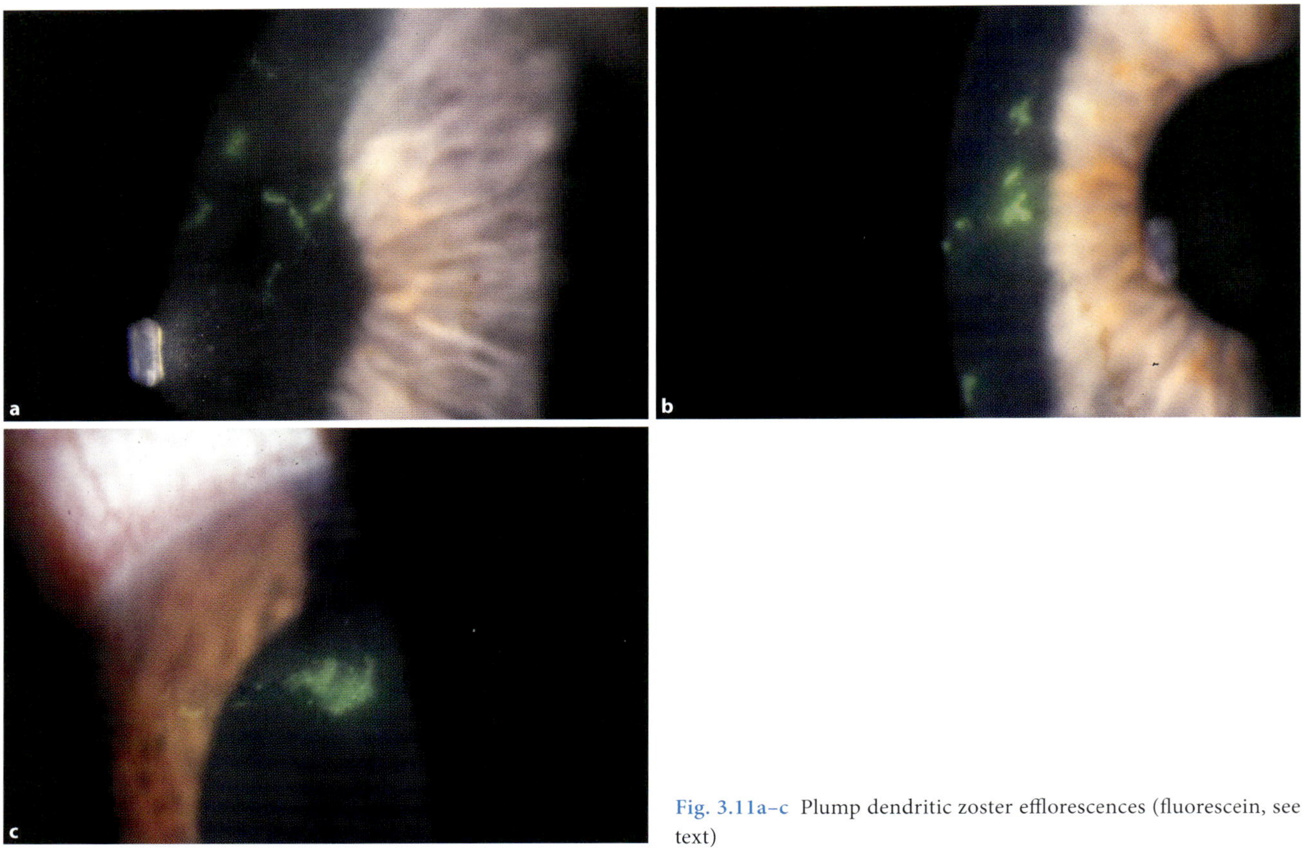


Fig. 3.11a–c Plump dendritic zoster efflorescences (fluorescein, see text)

## References


Chern KC, Conrad D, Holland GN, Holsclaw DS, Schwartz LK, Margolis TD (1998) Chronic varicella-zoster virus epithelial keratitis in patients with acquired immunodeficiency syndrome. Arch Ophthalmol 116: 1011–1017

Pavan-Langston D, McCulley JP (1973) Herpes zoster dendritic keratitis. Arch Ophthalmol 89: 25–29

Pavan-Langston D, Yamamoto S, Dunkel EC (1995) Delayed herpes zoster pseudodendrites. Polymerase chain reaction detection and a role for antiviral therapy. Arch Ophthalmol 113: 1381–1385

Piebenga LW, Laibson PR (1973) Dendritic lesions in herpes zoster ophthalmicus. Arch Ophthalmol 90: 268–270

Zaal MJ, Völker-Dieben HJ, Wienesen M, D´Amrao J, Kijlstra A (2001) Longitudinal analysis of varicella-zoster virus DNA on the ocular surface associated with herpes zoster ophthalmicus. Am J Ophthalmol 131: 25–29

# Interstitial Zoster Keratitis and Endotheliitis

Section

3.5

## Core Messages

- Functionally, the most important VZV eye diseases in the anterior segment are interstitial zoster keratitis and endotheliitis. They often occur together.
- Disease development and response to treatment are slower than with HSV disease and there is a dangerous tendency for the establishment of persistent infections.
- Vigorous antiviral therapy without steroids is the best way to avoid severe complications in early disease states.
- If the function of the optic media become seriously threatened, however, the additional application of low-dosed steroids is mostly inevitable.
- A unique form of chronic demarcating immune keratitis is possibly also caused by VZV. It is demonstrated in the addendum to this section.

## Detailed analysis of Fig 3.12

***Clinic:*** If the eye becomes involved in ophthalmic zoster, first notice of disease is often made as late as 5–7 days after manifestation of the first cutaneous zoster eruptions. The previously clear corneal stroma shows one or several separated fluffy areas of faint infiltration. The aqueous humor appears to be normal. Vision is only slightly affected, dependent on the distribution of the infiltrations. A zoster dendritic keratitis will mostly have preceded this interstitial keratitis and could have served as an indicator of subsequently arising deep disease (see Sect. 3.4), but, mostly, it has already healed at this time, which gives the impression that interstitial zoster keratitis develops without preceding epithelial disease. In Fig. 3.12a, two separated areas are visible in the pupil, but there are more of them. They are too faint for photographic documentation. A careful slit lamp screening is necessary, therefore, to detect and document all foci (Fig. 3.12b)

***Diagnosis:*** Early stage of interstitial zoster keratitis.

***Differential diagnosis:*** None with coexisting typical dermal zoster and with the typical time lag of appearance. Without dermal signs, HSV disease could not be differentiated. On an average, for VZV keratitis, multiple separated foci are typical, while with HSV, expanding single infection sites are more often encountered. But this difference does not really help for differential diagnosis in the individual case.

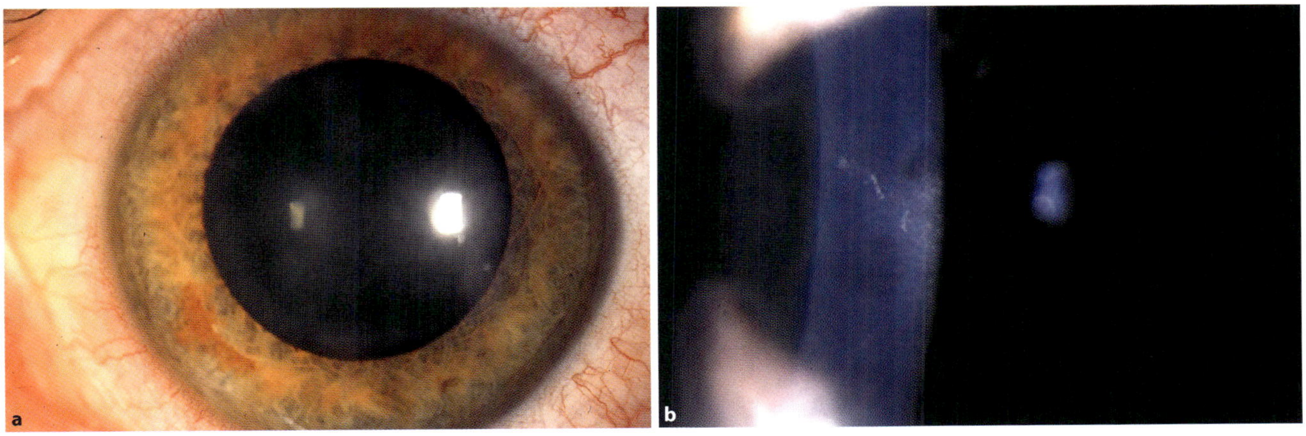

Fig. 3.12a,b Early stage of interstitial zoster keratitis

***Therapy:*** Most patients will already receive systemic ACV treatment (800 mg 5 qd) at the time when the corneal involvement is first detected. This basic systemic therapy must be continued not only for 1 week as recommended for cutaneous zoster, but for at least 3 weeks, irrespective of how faint and harmless the infiltrations may initially look. That can rapidly worsen. Additional topical ACV therapy is advisable where available (ACV ointment 5 qd). Mydriasis is not absolutely necessary without notable inflammation in the anterior chamber, but it facilitates slit lamp control of the cornea. Steroids are forbidden in this early state and with such subtle infiltrations.

After 2–3 weeks of intensive ACV monotreatment, depending on the actual findings, a decision has to be made whether or not this therapy must go on, whether it can be reduced to topical therapy only, or whether steroids must cautiously be added, if infiltrations which are too dense so require.

## Detailed analysis of Fig 3.13

***Clinic:*** After some time, the fluffy infiltration areas of interstitial zoster keratitis become denser and more circumscribed. Often, a typical "nummular" keratitis develops. In Fig. 3.13a, the outlines are still fluffy, giving an impression of ongoing acute inflammation. These nummuli are about 3 weeks old. The nummuli in Fig. 3.13b are older, about 5 weeks old. They are chalky white now with a sharper outline, and they reflect the light more intensely.

***Diagnosis:*** Nummular stage of interstitial zoster keratitis.

***Differential diagnosis:*** None with typical preceding dermal zoster. Without preceding dermal signs, HSV and adenovirus diseases could not be differentiated. HSV disease should exhibit a reduced corneal sensitivity as differential criteria to adenovirus disease.

***Therapy:*** Assuming that the eye in Fig. 3.13a had received full systemic and topical antiviral treatment for 3 weeks and nonetheless still shows active zoster infiltrations, it becomes improbable that antiviral therapy alone will bring about quick functional recovery. The additional therapy with low-dosed steroids then becomes an option. Nonetheless, prolongation of high-dosed antiviral monotherapy by 1 or 2 more weeks would certainly not be wrong.

With the denser zoster nummuli in Fig. 3.13b, an ongoing ACV monotherapy offers no prospects for quick visual rehabilitation, and if the patient is not extremely *patient* in the original sense of the word, then time has come to change from ACV monotherapy to a combination therapy of ACV plus steroids. As a rule, only a full ACV dose, which must never be tapered, is combined with low-dosed steroids (2–3 drops qd suffice to begin with). The patient must be informed that the necessary treatment time will presumably be not weeks but months, and that the patient must never change the regime himself or abruptly end it. It is advisable not to stop with therapy immediately after clearing of the cornea but to treat some 3–4 weeks longer in order to minimize the risk of recurring nummular keratitis. The worst scenario is recurrence of nummuli after discontinuing therapy too early. That can confront us with the same problem as with ever recurring adenovirus nummuli. We will barely get rid of them and will often be forced to treat symptomatically for years or a lifetime with minor steroid doses (e.g., 1 drop qd) in order to keep the cornea clear. The great advantage of zoster nummuli over adenovirus nummuli is that, in former, we afford about active antiviral therapy as a basic measure, while in the latter, this is unfortunately not the case to date.

## Detailed analysis of Fig 3.14

***Clinic:*** At 5 o'clock, a shallow stromal ulcer is seen in an area of dense interstitial infiltrations, which are much denser than those in Fig. 3.13. A vascular front is already invading the cornea between 3 and 6 o'clock. Intraocularly, some inflammation has taken place as exhibited by the pigment near the pupillary margin. Apart from the infiltrated areas, the cornea is clear without edema. There are no precipitates and no aqueous humor inflammation.

***Diagnosis:*** Ulcerating interstitial zoster keratitis.

***Differential diagnosis:*** None with preceding typical dermal zoster. Without zoster history, microbial etiologies are fairly improbable because the aqueous humor does not show enough inflammatory material. A differential diagnosis between HSV and VZV etiology based on ocular biomicroscopy alone would be speculative. But the rather circumscribed infiltration areas, with the rest of the cornea being clear and unaffected, would be more typical for VZV than for HSV etiology.

***Therapy:*** The complication of ulcerating interstitial zoster keratitis can only develop if no or no sufficient antiviral treatment was

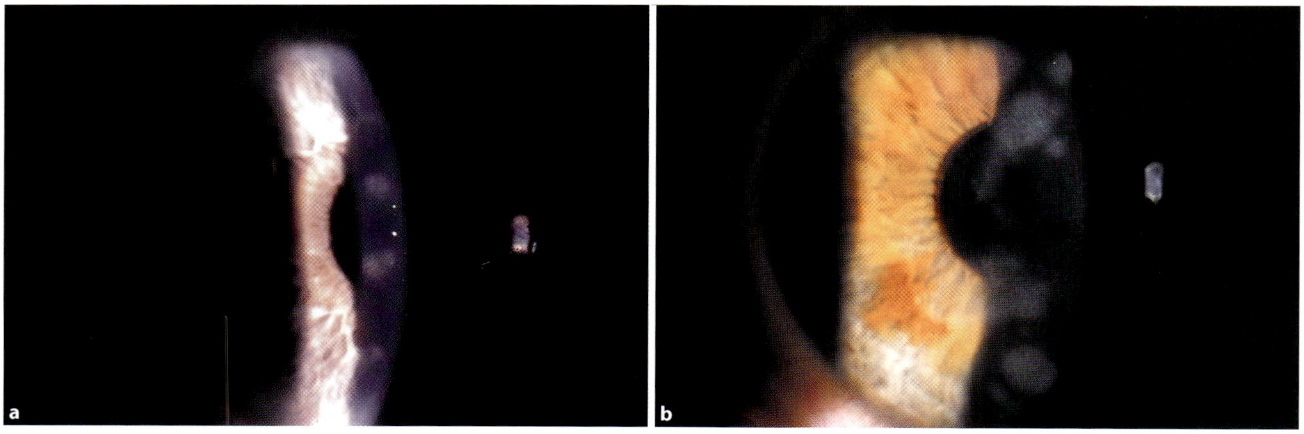


Fig. 3.13a,b Later stages of interstitial zoster keratitis (see text)

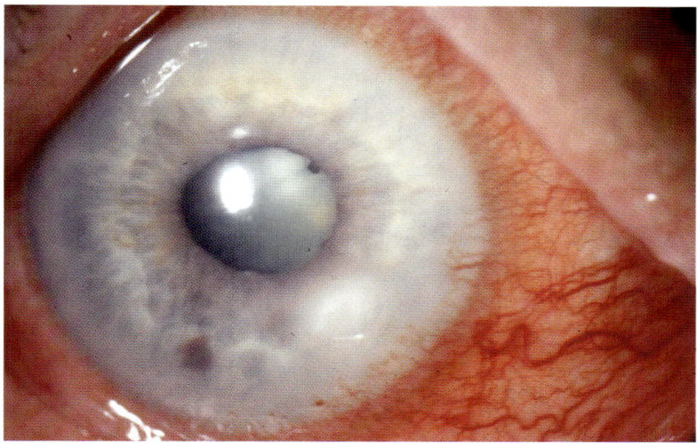

Fig. 3.14 Ulcerating interstitial zoster keratitis

given. It is important, therefore, to institute immediately maximal systemic and, where available, also topical antiviral therapy, e.g., with 800 mg ACV 5 qd plus ACV ointment 5 qd. Steroids should be cautiously added from the beginning in order to reduce the severe infiltration and limit cellular and extra-cellular stromal lysis. One injection of a microcrystalline steroid depot preparation can be given subconjunctivally, and the resorption of infiltrations and the development of the ulcer can be carefully observed thereafter. A second steroid injection may follow 1 week later, if progress of healing has been satisfying up to that time. It is also possible to start exclusively or additionally with small amounts of systemic steroids (20–10 mg ultracortenol qd). However, topical steroids should be strictly avoided as long as the ulcer has not been again covered by corneal epithelium. In case the ulcer dangerously deepens, an amnion cover – eventually multi-layered – should be sutured in time on the ulcer (compare Sect. 2.14).

## Analysis of Fig 3.15

Figure 3.15 shows that proper combination treatment of ulcerating interstitial zoster keratitis is successful in reducing infiltrations (a: before, b: after combination therapy), but it cannot always prevent melting of the stroma quickly enough. That may have to do with an especially compromised trophic situation in zoster corneas, where corneal sensitivity is often about zero. In Fig. 3.15b, a semi-flexible therapeutic contact lens was fitted on top of the ulcer in an attempt to stop further melting and help the spontaneous closure of the deep defect. We would not recommend such attempts any longer today. Instead, one should quickly proceed to amnion surgery as long as Descemet´s and some deep stroma layers are still intact. Medical therapy, as described above, must invariably go on, of course, also after amnion surgery.

## Analysis of Fig 3.16

Relatively rarely in zoster, interstitial keratitis does not develop with multiple separated foci but with a larger central area topographically correlated with underlying endotheliitis, giving the typical "sandwich" disease of disciform keratitis. Biomicroscopically, a differential diagnosis between HSV and VZV etiology is impossible. Both look perfectly identical. Treatment is the same as for any other deep corneal zoster. The relative "advantage" of the coexisting endotheliitis is that the presence or absence of endotheliitic precipitates can be used as a marker to decide about the duration and intensity of therapy (compare Sect. 2.7). In Fig. 3.16, the endotheliitic precipitates cannot be directly seen at such a low magnification. However, the gross appearance is very typical of a swollen corneal disc (compare Fig. 2.71).

## Analysis of Fig 3.17

Zoster endotheliitis does not announce itself with spectacular clinical signs. It mostly develops insidiously. In the beginning (Fig. 3.17a), cornea and aqueous humor may even appear normal with the slit lamp. But at this time, VZV already starts to replicate in the endothelial cells. The affected endothelia swell gradually, but overall endothelial pump action is still sufficient to keep the cornea clear. Immune precipitates have not yet assembled, and the only chance to detect developing endotheliitis is by investigation with a specular microscope. Then, pathologic endothelial *cell* edema would become clearly visible in the affected areas. As soon as sufficient numbers of primed immune cells have come to

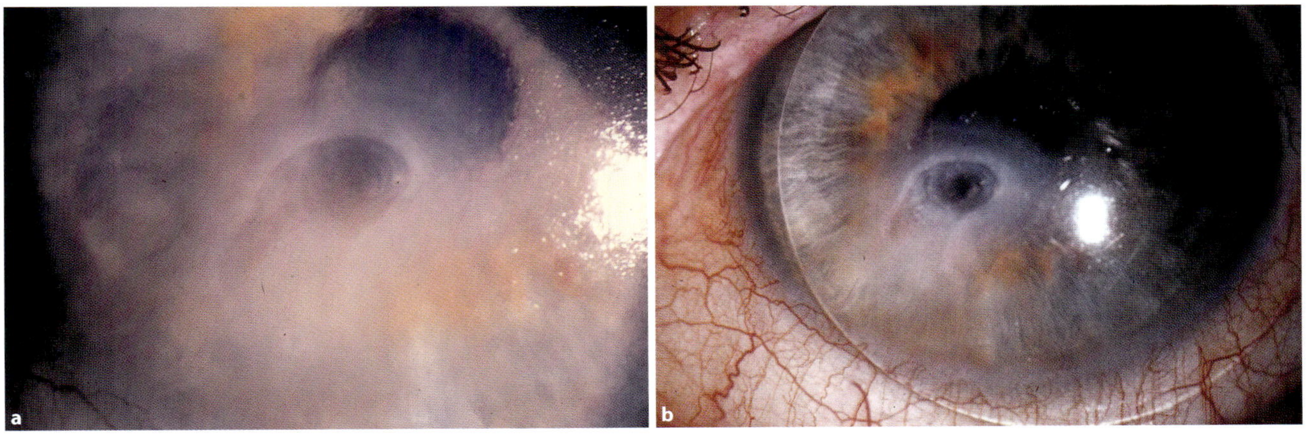


Fig. 3.15 Ulcerating interstitial zoster keratitis progressing to perforation (see text) **a** before, **b** after combination therapy

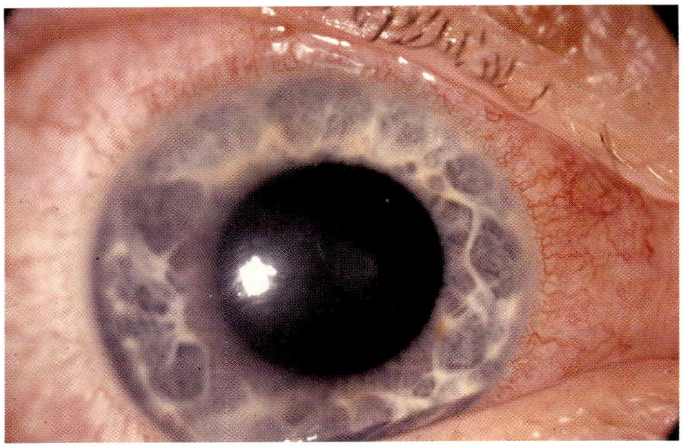

Fig. 3.16 Central interstitial zoster keratitis plus endotheliitis (disciform zoster keratitis)

the scene, these cells attack the marked endothelial cells. From then on, the endothelial pump fails with subsequent rapid development of *corneal* edema in the area affected by endotheliitis. In Fig. 3.17b, two thirds of the cornea have turned edematous within two days only. Numerous immune precipitates can now be seen in spite of the massively swollen cornea. The swelling makes further specular microscopic investigation of the endothelium impossible. Only after the cornea has become clear again under proper combination therapy, specular microscopic investigation of the endothelium discloses how many cells are still involved and still massively swollen (Fig. 3.17c).

Rapid breakdown of the endothelial pump comes nearly exclusively from the destructive action of the immune cells. The immune cells in the anterior chamber must, therefore, as quickly and as efficiently as possible, be impeded and destroyed by addition steroids. In such a severe case, one can dare to prescribe steroids a bit more vigorously in the beginning than with interstitial keratitis (e.g., 30 mg fluorocortolone qd plus 1 subconjunctival injection of a crystalline steroid depot). Additionally, a short-term course with higher dosed topical steroids (5 applications qd, quickly reduced over 4–3–2 qd) will help the stop the immune attack quickly and thus preserve endothelial function. As always, treatment with full ACV dose and low dose steroids should be carried on for about 3 weeks longer than the last endotheliitic precipitate disappeared (see the same rules for HSV endotheliitis, Sect. 2.7).

## Analysis of Fig 3.18

Figure 3.18 shows the follow-up by specular microscopy of a slight zoster endotheliitis. Compared with Fig. 3.17, this disease course was much milder and the patient was above all immediately treated. Consequently, with quick blockade of immune destruction by steroids and with an optimal simultaneous antiviral treatment, nearly all endothelial cells recovered and the overall loss of endothelial cells was minimal with full functional recovery.

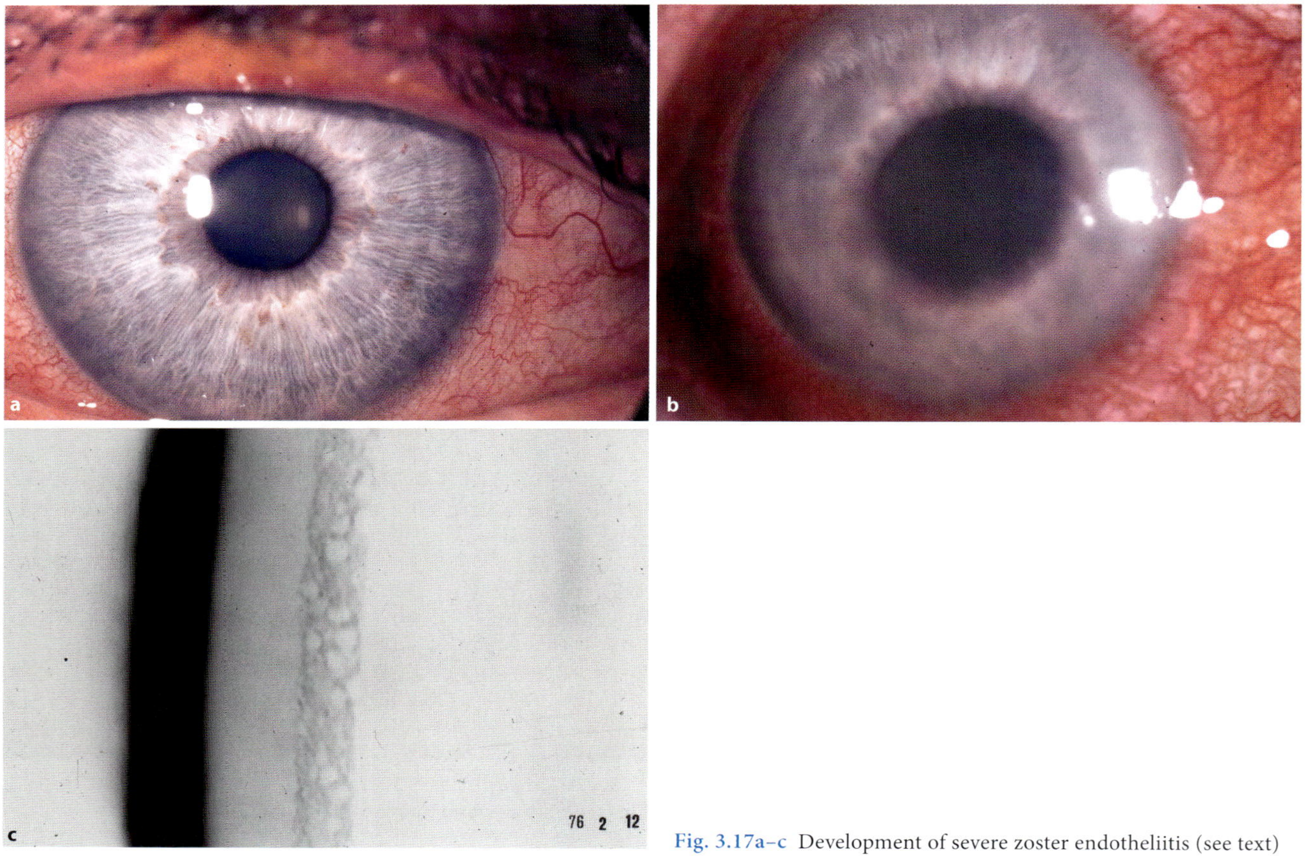


Fig. 3.17a–c Development of severe zoster endotheliitis (see text)

## Analysis of Fig 3.19

At the beginning of treatment, at day 10 of zoster (Fig. 3.19a), a large area of circumscribed corneal edema is visible on the left (i.e., endotheliitis) with adjacent clear cornea on the right. The large pigmented precipitates behind the clear, unaffected cornea at 6 o´clock at the pupillary margin are iritic precipitates. Another sign of focal zoster iritis (see Sect. 3.6) is the swollen iris sector visible through the corneal edema from 7 to 8 o'clock, and the disfigured pupil in this area. Endotheliitic immune precipitates are not microscopically distinguishable from iritic precipitates, but they must be present behind the circumscribed edematous corneal area. The additional presence of interstitial infiltrates is also not discernible in the corneal edema. The location of infiltrates becomes apparent, however, after the edema has disappeared (Fig. 3.19c).

This photographic sequence shows that not all manifestations of ocular zoster must be clearly discernible at any time, but an experienced investigator will mostly be able to give a complete description of the diseased tissues, also from indirect signs in the early course of disease. The sequence shows further how healing is slow in ocular zoster, even with therapy. In this case, the anterior segment of the eye looked "quiet" with only two small circumscribed areas of previous interstitial keratitis after 22 days of treatment. It would have been a failure, however, to stop treatment at this time already. In spite of full corneal transparency, there was still massive endothelial cell edema present (Fig. 3.19d), indicating a need for ongoing therapy.

## Analysis of Fig 3.20

Apart from acute endotheliitis with rapidly progressing corneal edema (Fig. 3.17), chronic endotheliitis may also occur either primarily chronic or chronically persistent after treatment of acute endotheliitis had been stopped too early. In Fig. 3.20, the immune precipitates are clearly visible behind the circumscribed affected corneal area. Such chronic cases have a double-edged aspect. On one hand, they may be slow in progressing to more damage. On the other hand, their treatment requires even more patience and persistence than is required for the acute cases. While a topical combination therapy with ACV ointment 5 qd plus steroid ointment 2 qd may suffice for many such cases, the time period required for definite healing is mostly at least four months and often longer.

## Analysis of Fig 3.21

The circumscribed severe bullous keratopathy in Fig. 3.21 exhibits the sequels of insufficiently or untreated chronic VZV endotheliitis. Endotheliitic precipitates are still visible through the swollen cornea in the pupillary area. The relatively clear stromal edema shows that infiltrations from interstitial VZV keratitis did not play a significant role in that case. In such final stages of disease, even intensive long-term medical therapy has become functionally useless, and early keratoplasty should be considered in order to accelerate healing, restore function, and spare time and therapy costs.

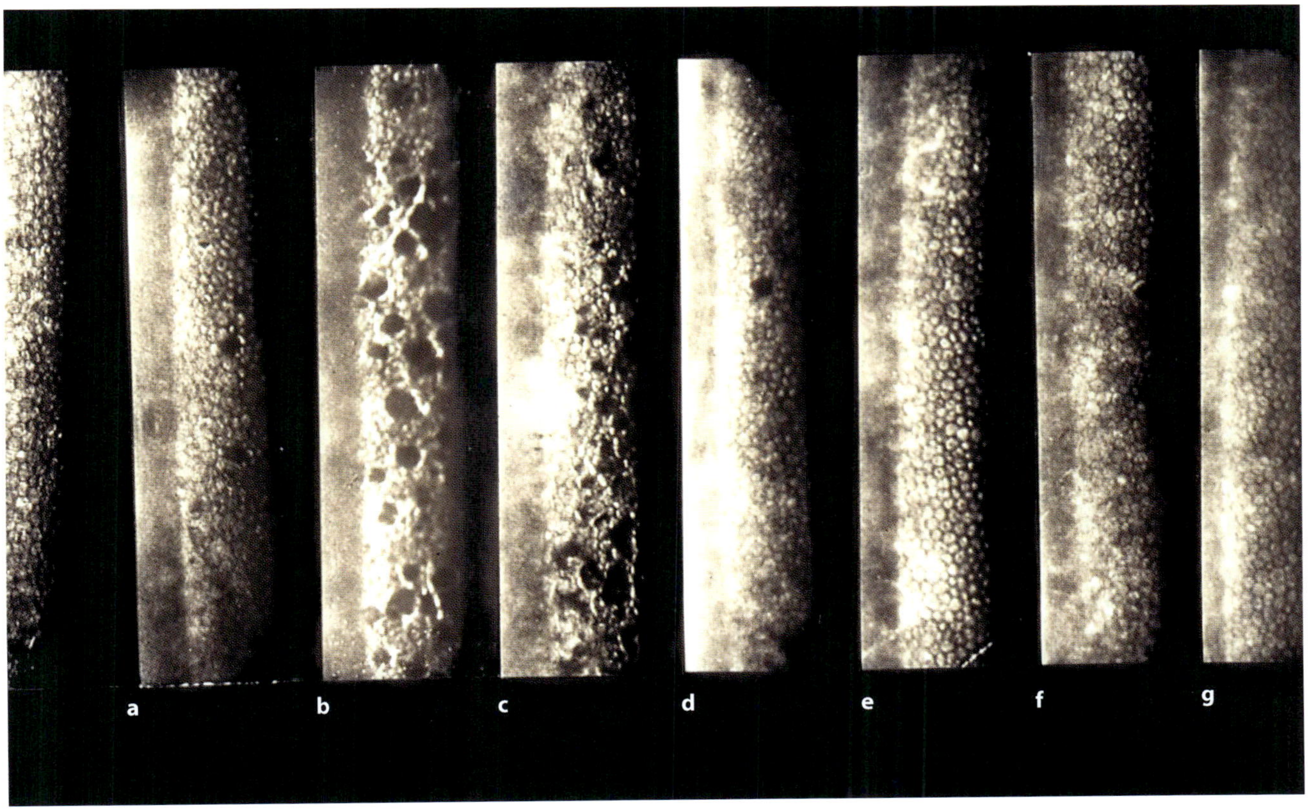


Fig. 3.18 Specular micrococoscopic follow-up of a case with slight zoster endotheliitis (from: Sundmacher R., Müller O., 1982)

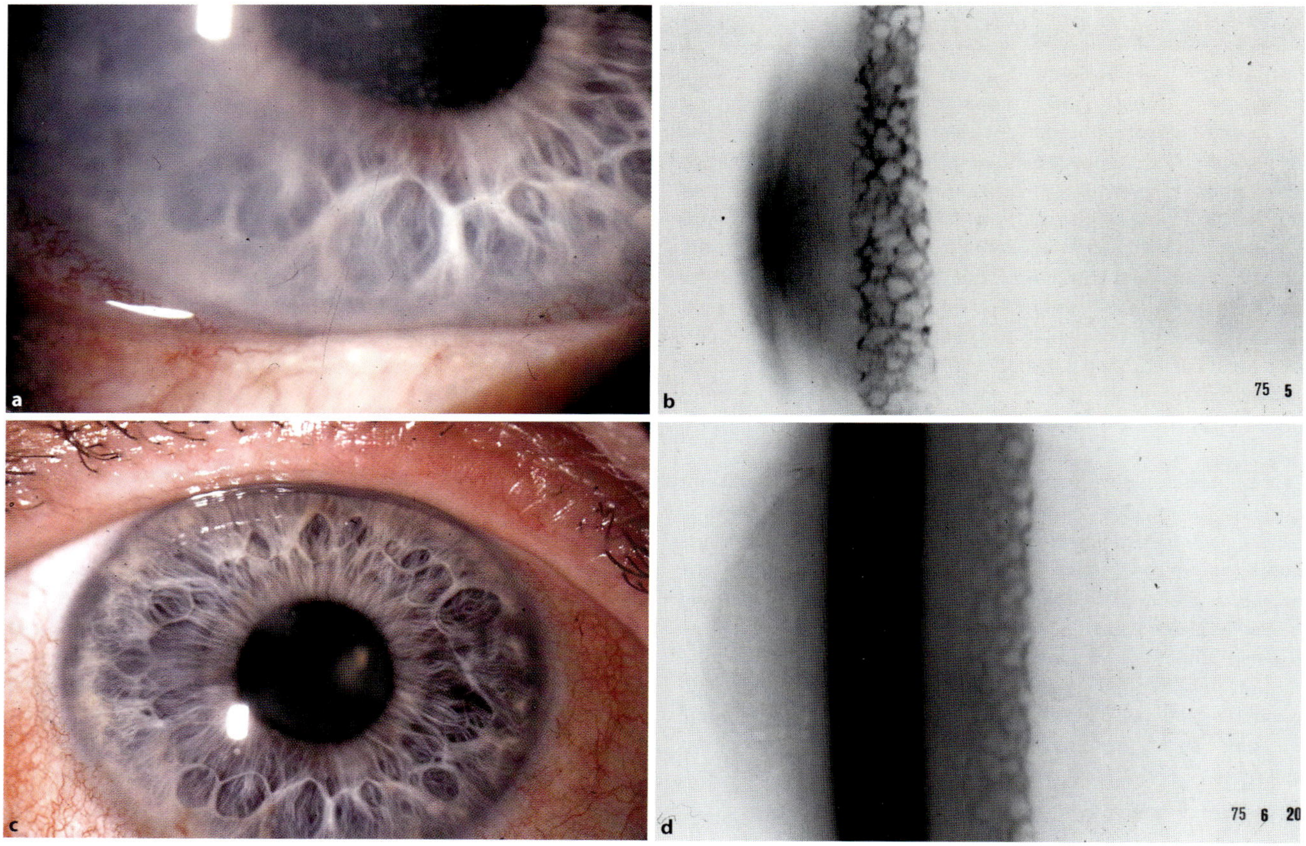


Fig. 3.19 Zoster endotheliitis and interstitial keratitis plus iritis on disease day 10, when treatment started (**a**). On follow-up day 22 (**b**). On follow-up day 58 (**c, d**)

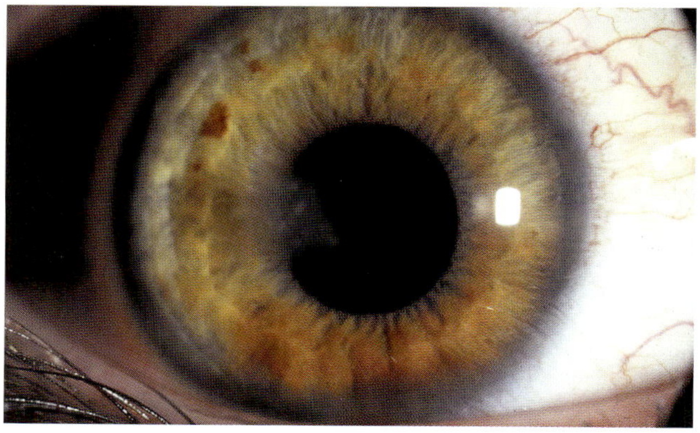

Fig. 3.20 Chronic zoster endotheliitis plus interstitital keratitis

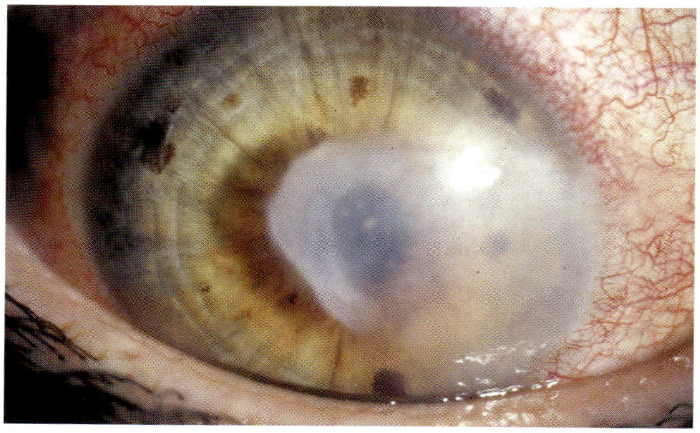

Fig. 3.21 Circumscribed bullous keratopathy from chronic zoster endotheliitis

## Analysis of Fig 3.22

Severe clinical states, like that shown in Fig. 3.22, should no longer occur with proper ACV therapy started early enough. Once such complex disease of the cornea, iris, and sclera has developed, however, functionally satisfying healing can often no longer be brought about by medical therapy alone. Intensive long-term combination therapy with 800 mg ACV 5 qd and 10 mg fluorocortolone qd can at best "quieten" the eye and "prepare" it for subsequent perforating keratoplasty (often together with cataract surgery and IOL implantation). But this time is not lost. As after surgery, trophic insufficiencies may cause grave problems and may considerably reduce the success rate of keratoplasty, it is wise to take one's time in such cases. When the eye

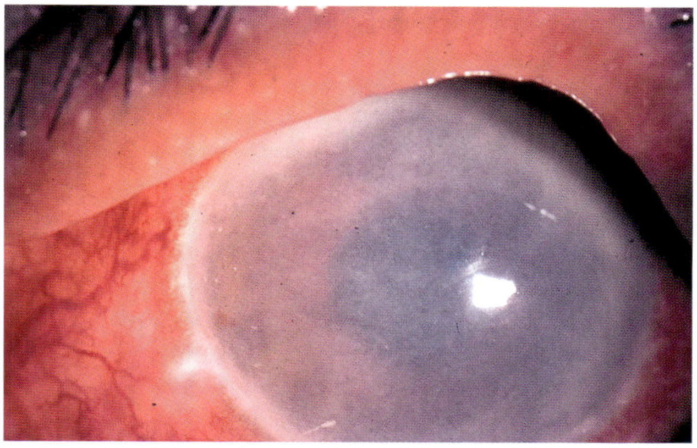

Fig. 3.22 Complex severe zoster disease of the anterior segment

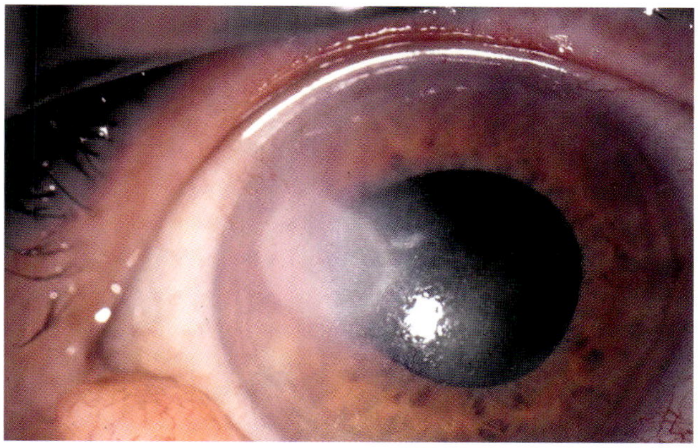

Fig. 3.23 Acute form of interstitial demarcating immune keratitis in the course of zoster (see text)

has calmed down, there is a good chance for partial spontaneous recovery of the trophic functions. Secondary glaucoma must also be excluded or efficiently treated. Meanwhile, one can organize HLA-matched transplantation, if this is desired. With all these measures taken together, the prognosis of planned keratoplasty in a clinically quiet eye will on average be better than operating immediately à chaud, as would be possible in similar HSV cases (see Sect. 3.9).

## Addendum

The following pictures show a unique form of *interstitial demarcating keratitis*, which I believe to be caused by VZV. I have occasionally observed such inflammations as an acute form in the course of ophthalmic zoster. However, much more frequently, similarly shaped primarily chronic progressive forms were found in eyes *without* a reliable zoster history. Nonetheless, my suspicion is that all these rounded or arcuate forms of immunologically demarcated keratitis with a slowly progressing immune ring border are caused by the same infectious agent which persists in keratocytes. In my opinion, the most likely candidate is VZV. The morphological similarity between the *acute infiltrative cases* observed *in the course of zoster* (Fig. 3.23) and the much more often observed *primarily chronic cases without* a direct history link to *zoster* is obvious. However, unequivocal proof of VZV etiology is not yet available. For proof, VZV genetic material should have been demonstrated in corneal biopsies or on occasion of keratoplasty from typical chronic lesions. That has not yet been done. PCR tests on such corneal materials have to comprise *all* herpes viruses, of course, and an evidence of VZV etiology can only be accepted if VZV genetic material is invariably present in the lesions while the genetic material of other viruses is absent.

The pathophysiological hypothesis for these cases would be that VZV becomes peripherally persistent in circumscribed areas of the corneal stroma, where it is attacked, "suppressed", and topographically "fixed" by the host's cellular immune defence. This battle is more dramatic and more evident in the acute zoster-associated cases with a dense demarcating ring of immune cells (Fig. 3.23). It is less evident but still visible in the primarily chronic cases, where over many months and years, we observe a progression and enlargement of the affected areas with finally even occlusion of the pupillary area (Figs. 3.24 to 3.27). If the hypothesis of a VZV etiology for these types of keratitis proves correct, we have no difficulties to imagine VZV becoming persistent in keratocytes, especially with a steroid monotherapy without efficient antiviral treatment in zoster (see Sect. 3.1). On what occasion VZV would get access to the infectious foci in the primarily chronic forms is unclear. A possible speculation would be that VZV, like HSV, occasionally escapes latency but causes only *subclinical* peripheral viral shedding. In the cornea, this may lead to peripheral viral persistence. The immediate clinical sequels are so minor, and the affected areas grow so slowly, that it takes a long time for the patient and the ophthalmologist to realize that something infectious is unexpectedly progressing. This delay in notice and diagnosis is further enhanced by the fact that the majority of the chronically progressive lesions develops at or near the corneal limbus and from there expands centrally. Therefore, not all of them are circularly rounded. About half of them base at the limbus and develop arcuate forms.

The experiences with medical therapy are only partly positive. Topical low dose steroid therapy always efficiently clears the lesions from visible immune infiltrations, as one would expect. Once the steroids are tapered, however, the disease invariably slowly recurs with its borders again moving progressively towards the pupillary area.

Attempts to eradicate the presumed VZV persistence by long-term therapy with ACV or BVDU have as yet been unsuccessful in my experience. This does not come as a surprise and is no argument against a VZV etiology. The therapeutic refractivity of peripherally persistent viral infections has already been addressed several times.

Therefore, currently, the only means to stop the insidious progression is the continuous application of low-dosed topi-

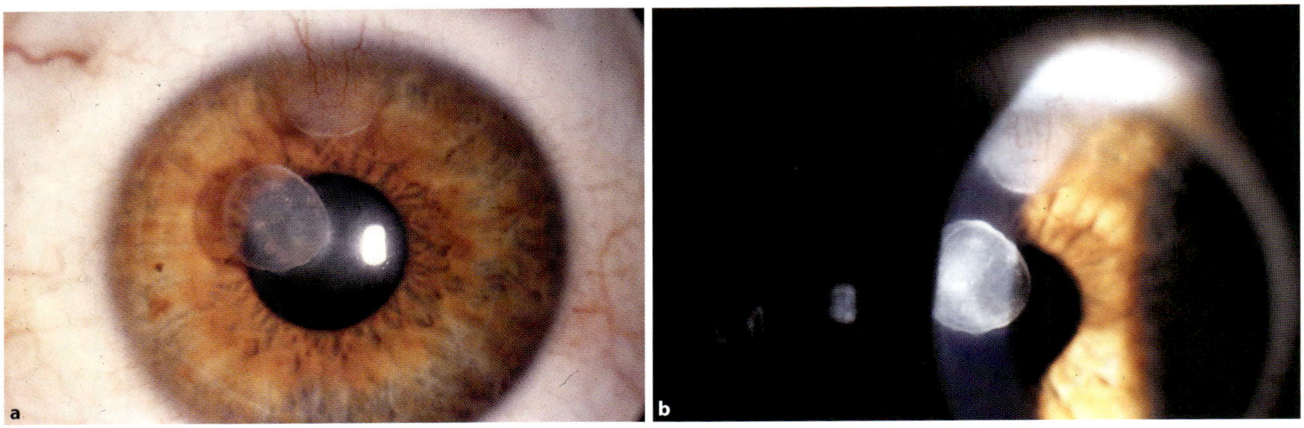

Fig. 3.24a,b Primarily chronic form of interstitial demarcating immune keratitis with one paracentral circumscribed area and one limbus-based area with arcuate central borders (see text)

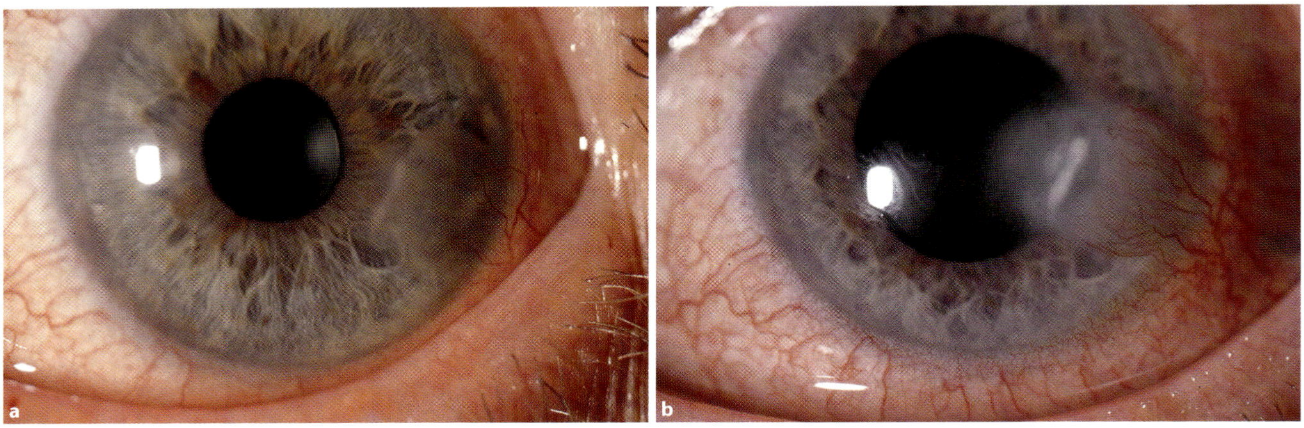

Fig. 3.25a,b Exceptionally aggressive form of primarily chronic interstitial demarcating immune keratitis. **a** After topical steroid therapy. **b** One month after withdrawal of steroids (see text)

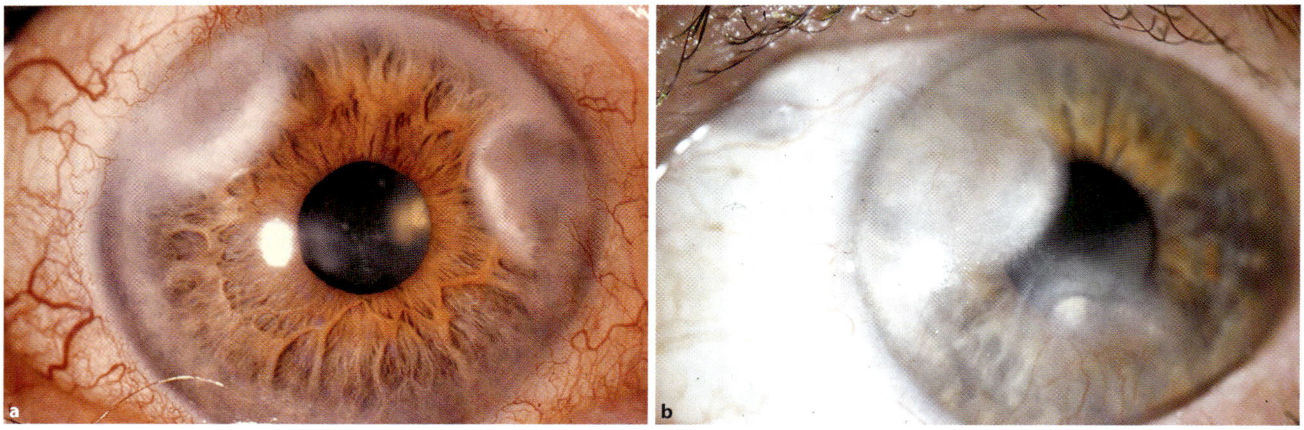

Fig. 3.26a,b Two cases of „pseudo-quiet" primarily chronic interstitial demarcating immune keratitis without steroid therapy. They progress centrally within months or a couple of years (see text)

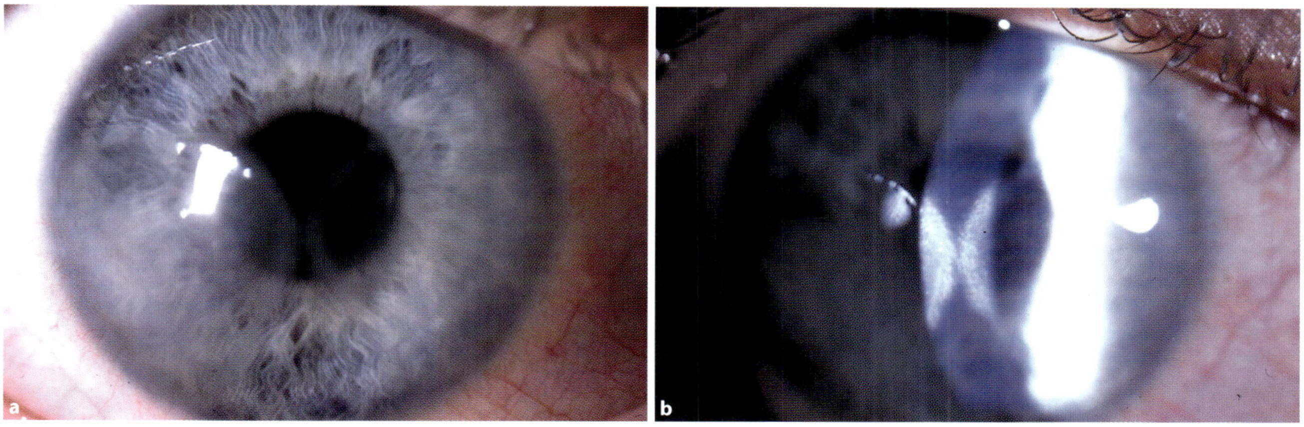

Fig. 3.27a,b Primarily chronic interstitial demarcating immune keratitis, which was noted by the patient only after the two foci met in the pupillary area (see text)

cal steroids. Fortunately, often as little as 1 drop qd suffices to control progression.

## References


Ahonen R, Vannas A, Mäkitie J (1983) Endothelial cell loss in herpes zoster keratouveitis. Br J Ophthalmol 67: 751–754

Ameye C, Sundmacher R, de Clercq E (1989) Topical BVDU plus low-dosage steroids in the treatment of chronic relapsing zoster keratouveitis. A pilot study. Albrecht von Graefes Arch Clin Exp Ophthalmol 227: 118–122

Heiligenhaus A, Li H, Hernandez Galindo EE, Koch JM, Steuhl KP, Meller D (2003) Management of acute ulcerative and necrotizing herpes simplex and zoster keratitis with amniotic membrane transplantation. Br J Ophthalmol 87: 1215–1219

Mietz H, Eis-Hubinger AM, Sundmacher R, Font RL (1997) Detection of varicella-zoster virus DNA in keratectomy specimens by use of polymerase chain reaction. Arch Ophthalmol 115: 590–594

Reijo A, Antti V, Jukka M (1983) Endothelial cell loss in herpes zoster keratouveitis. Brit J Ophthalmol 67: 751–754

Silverstein BE, Chandler D, Neger R, Margolis TP (1997) Disciform keratitis. A case of herpes zoster sine herpete. Am J Ophthalmol 123: 254–255

Sundmacher R, Müller O (1982) Das Hornhautendothel bei Zoster ophthalmicus. Klin Monatsbl Augenheilk 180: 271–274

Wenkel H, Rummelt C, Rummelt V, Jahn G, Fleckenstein B, Naumann GOH (1993) Detection of varicella zoster virus DNA and viral antigen in human cornea after herpes zoster ophthalmicus. Cornea 12: 131–137

Yu DD, Lemp MA, Mathers WD, Espy M, White T (1993) Detection of varicella-zoster virus DNA in disciform keratitis using polymerase chain reaction. Arch Ophthalmol 111: 167–168

# Zoster Iritis

Section

3.6

## Core Messages

- Zoster iritis closely resembles HSV iritis (see Sect. 2.9) with some peculiarities which may help in differential diagnosis.
- *Recurrent* focal serous iritis is normally not of VZV but of HSV origin.
- The functional sequelae of zoster iritis are of limited importance.
- Similar to HSV, which does not so rarely cause monosymptomatic focal serous iritis without accompanying other herpes affections, zoster iritis has also been reported as "zoster sine herpete".

Zoster iritis is very similar to HSV iritis with two peculiarities:

- Like HSV, VZV has a predilection for the cells deriving from the embryonic cup of the eye (iris pigment epithelium and iris muscles), but in addition it has a predilection for vascular endothelium, which is not the case to this extent with HSV.
- VZV normally causes just one recurrent disease in life (i.e., one bout of zoster), while HSV may cause many recurrences.

In consequence:

- VZV causes definitely more and more severe iris *stromal defects* from *vascular necrosis.*
- On an average, the amount of focal *pigment epithelium defects*, however, is less than with HSV disease. The reason is simply that with HSV recurrences, more than one attack may damage the pigment epithelium, which leads to extensive defects, while VZV normally has but one chance for causing damage.

Practically, the following can be noted:

- Secondary acute glaucoma, which is so typical for intraocular HSV replication, does not have the same incidence and importance in intraocular VZV diseases, although secondary glaucoma may also develop.
- Neither HSV nor VZV seem to be able to persist in iris tissues.
- Therapy of VZV iritis is the same as for all deep ocular zoster diseases, e.g., with 800 mg ACV 5 qd plus 20–10 mg fluorocortolone qd as long as inflammatory signs are present in the anterior chamber.
- The overall sequelae of VZV iritis for ocular function are of limited importance.
- Similar to HSV, which does not so rarely cause monosymptomatic focal serous iritis without accompanying other herpes affections, zoster iritis has also been reported as "zoster sine herpete".
- A clear cut *clinical* differential diagnosis between the monosymptomatic forms of HSV and VZV disease does not seem to be possible. The differential diagnosis has to be made by PCR tests. If monosymptomatic focal serous iritis recurs after previous unequivocal healing, VZV becomes very unlikely as the causative agent, and one rather deals with HSV disease.

## Analysis of Fig 3.28 and 3.29

The photo of the early stage of zoster iritis (Fig. 3.28a) shows only sectorial involvement of the iris in the lower right quadrant, as expressed by the relative discrete dysfunction of the iris dilator muscle and the slight dysfiguration of the pupil in this area. 5 weeks later, pigment epithelium defects have developed (not shown here, compare Sect. 2.9 for HSV iritis). But additionally, iris *stromal* defects have become visible, which can be explained by VZV-specific vaso-occlusive sequelae of arterial endotheliitis. Once healed, these iris defects will be stationary without recurrence of VZV disease. Fig. 3.29 documents a similar course with subsequent stromal defects. In addition, a dilator muscle deficit is to be seen from the pupil dysfiguration.

## Analysis of Fig 3.30 and 3.31

Precipitates in zoster iritis (Fig. 3.30 and Fig. 3.31) are on average more pigmented than precipitates in the course of a first attack of HSV iritis. This shows the principally more pronounced destructive potency for the pigment epithelium layer of VZV in comparison to HSV. However, because VZV "strikes" only once and HSV poten-

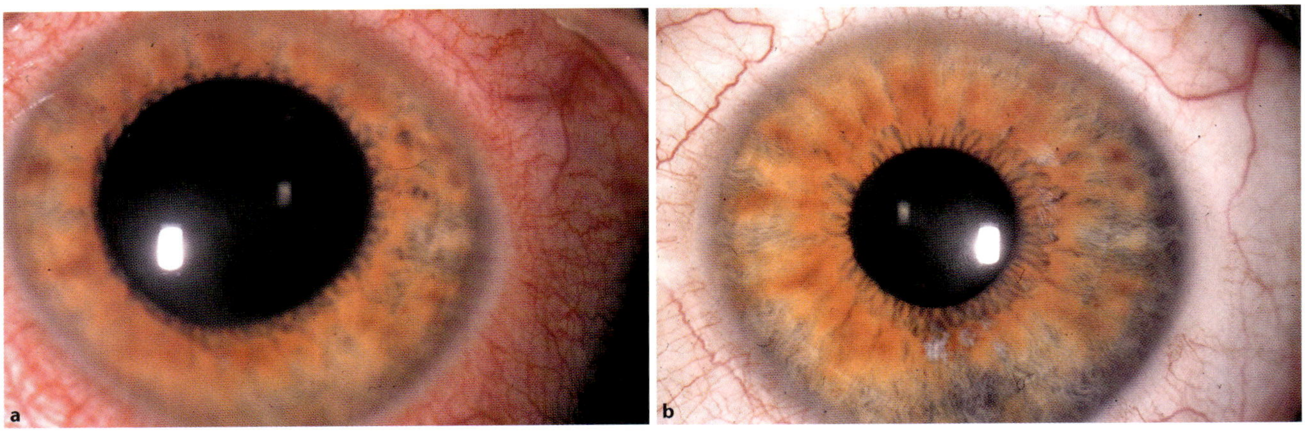


Fig. 3.28 Early zoster iritis (**a**), with stromal defects 5 weeks later (**b**)

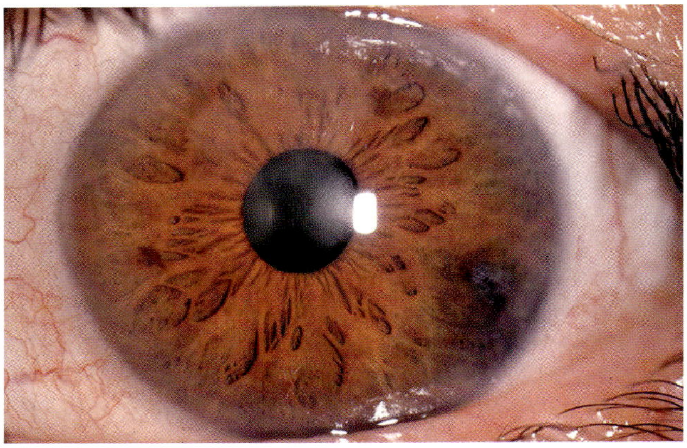

Fig. 3.29 Another example of a deep *stromal* defect after zoster iritis at 4 o'clock

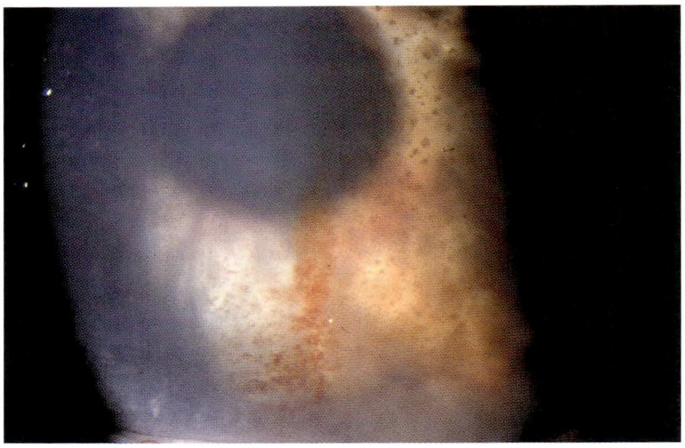

Fig. 3.30 Bleeding iris vessel as a sequela of arterial endotheliitis in zoster iritis

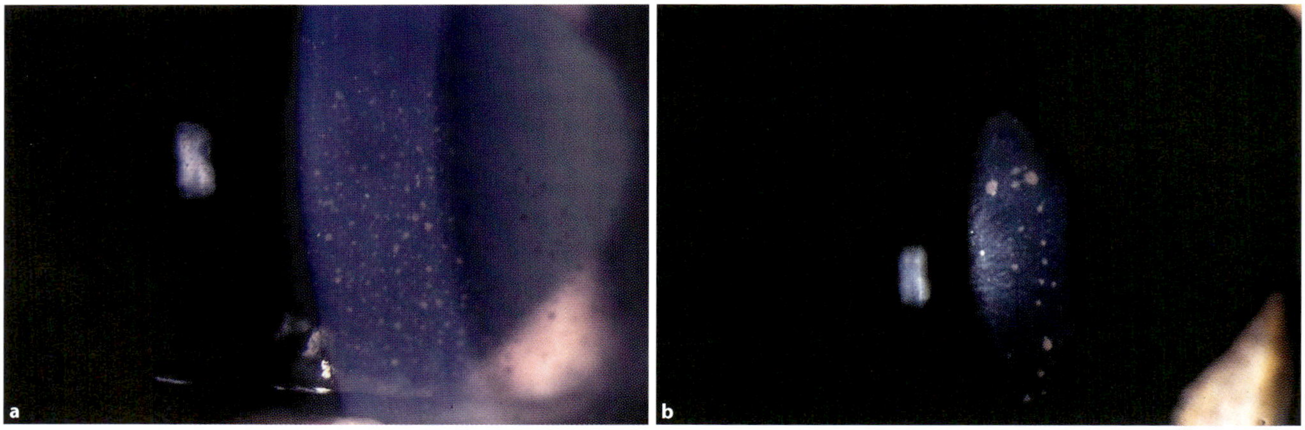


Fig. 3.31a,b Large pigmented endothelial precipitates in zoster iritis

tially strikes many times, the iris defects in HSV disease tend to be more severe than those after zoster iritis.
Bleeding of an iris vessel (Fig. 3.30) indicates associated vasculitis, which is found much more regulary in zoster than in HSV disease (see Fig. 2.91).

## References


Chan CC, Shen D, Tuo J (2005) Polymerase chain reaction in the diagnosis of uveitis. Int Ophthalmol Clin 45: 41–55

Kido S, Sugita S, Horie S, Miyanaga M, Miyata K, Shimizu N, Morio T, Mochizuki M (2008) Association of varicella zoster virus load in the aqueous humor with clinical manifestations of anterior uveitis in herpes zoster ophthalmicus and zoster sine herpete. Br J Ophthalmol 92: 505–508

Marsh RJ, Easty DL, Jones BR (1974) Iritis and iris atrophy in herpes zoster ophthalmicus. Am J Ophthlmol 78: 255–261

Miserocchi E, Waheed NK, Dios E, Christen W, Merayo J, Roque M, Foster CS (2002) Visual outcome in herpes simplex virus and varicella zoster virus uveitis. Ophthalmology 109: 1532–1537

Nakamura N, Tanabe M, Yamada Y, Azumi A (2000) Zoster sine herpete with bilateral ocular involvement. Am J Ophthalmol 129: 809–810

Naumann GOH, Gass JDM, Font RL (1968) Histopathology of herpes zoster ophthalmicus. Am J Ophthalmol 65: 533–541

Schwab IR (1997) Herpes zoster sine herpete: a potential cause of iridoplegic granulomatous iridocyclitis. Ophthalmology 104: 1421–1425

Stavrou P, Mitchell SM, Fox JD, Hope-Ross MW, Murray PI (1994) Detection of varicella-zoster virus DNA in ocular samples from patients with uveitis but no cutaneous eruption. Eye 8: 684–687

Sundmacher R (1981) Die fokale Iritis durch Herpes simplex- und Varizellen-Zoster-Virus. Ber Dtsch Ophthalmol Ges 78: 73–76

Thean JH, Hall AJ, Stawell RJ (2001) Uveitis in herpes zoster ophthalmicus. Clin Experiment Ophthalmol 29: 406–410

Yamamoto S, Tada R, Shimomura Y, Pavan-Langston D, Dunkel EC, Tano Y (1995) Detection of varicella-zoster virus DNA in iridocyclitis using polymerase chain reaction – a case of zoster sine herpete. Arch Ophthalmol 113: 1358–1359

# Zoster Scleritis

Section

3.7

## Core Messages

- Zoster scleritis is rare in spite of VZV's affinity for vascular endothelium.
- With close chronological correlation to zoster, scleritis should primarily be treated as a deep infectious disease with high-dosed systemic antiviral agents plus low-dosed systemic steroids or alternate immune-suppressive agents.
- With increasing time interval between zoster and first manifestation of scleritis, the probability rises that VZV-induced autoimmunological mechanisms are operative and that an infectious pathophysiology becomes of minor or of no importance.

The incidence of zoster-associated scleritis is low. Its pathophysiology remains mostly speculative on the basis of analogous assumptions from the pathophysiology of scleritis in general.

As the vast majority of general scleritis cases is thought to be caused by vasculitis, and as VZV has a predilection for vascular endothelium, it is not surprising that occasionally a serous scleritis is observed some weeks after the beginning of zoster disease elsewhere in the eye (Fig. 3.32). Sometimes, scleritis arises together with peripheral keratitis, i. e., as sclerokeratitis (Fig. 3.33). This close chronological and topographical correlation to established VZV disease suggests that the pathophysiology of scleritis in these situations is an infectious one. Consequently, therapy should primarily consist of maximally dosed systemic antiviral agents, e. g., ACV 800 mg 5 qd, given long enough, 6 weeks as a minimum. Because partially damaging immune reactions are always involved in deep viral disease of the eye, an additional cautious therapy with *low-dosed* systemic steroids is certainly no mistake and can be recommended (e. g., 20 mg fluocortolone qd). With such a combination therapy, the few cases of early scleritis after zoster, which we had to treat, healed quickly and permanently which is perhaps an indication that the hypothesis of an infectious pathophysiology of these early cases is correct.

The crucial question is whether VZV does only directly cause infectious scleritis, or if it serves also – and may be much more in the long run – as an inducing agent for autoimmunological vasculitis. Once established, this runs its own pathophysiological path, and is no longer controllable by antiviral agents, but needs a totally different therapy with high-dose immunosuppresssion. This open question cannot be answered today. One has to rely on therapeutic trial and error. If the systemic combination of high-dosed antiviral agent plus low-dosed steroid does not provide satisfying results within about a month, and scleritis is severe enough, then the steroids have to be increased step by step while the antiviral therapy is maintained until the desired therapeutic response is achieved.

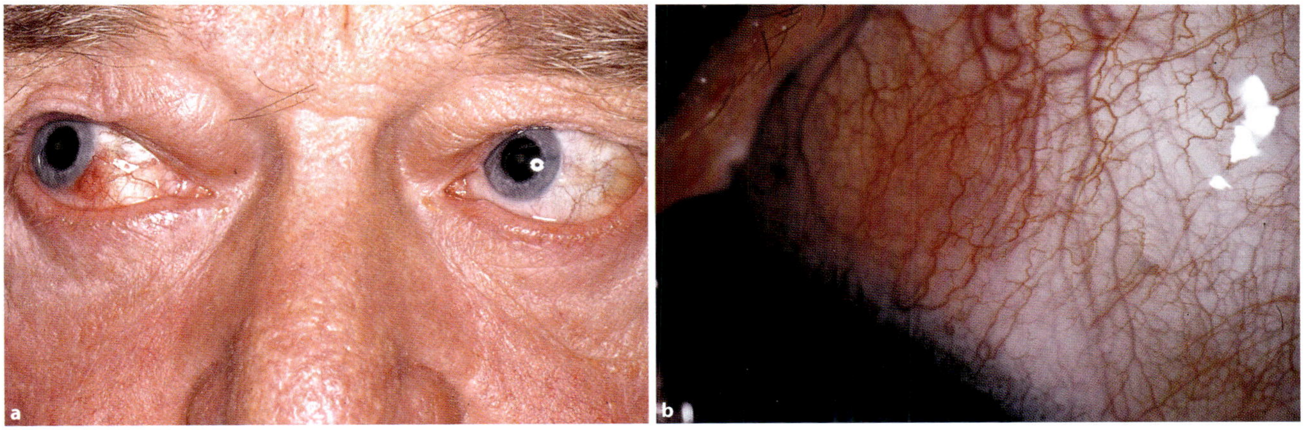

**Fig. 3.32a,b** Serous scleritis (two different patients) in close chronological correlation with ophthalmic zoster (see text)

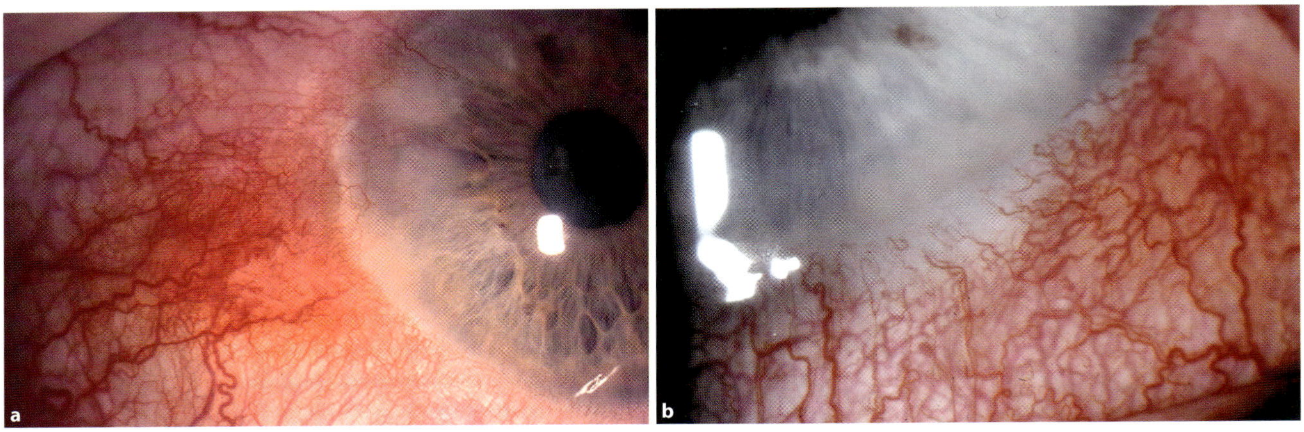


Fig. 3.33a,b Sclero-keratitis, which developed in the course of zoster (see text)

## References

Ahmed TY, Carrim ZI, Diaper CJ, Wykes WN (2007) Spontaneous intraocular lens extrusion in a patient with a scleromalacia secondary to herpes zoster ophthalmicus. J Cataract Refract Surg 33: 925–926

Berry-Brincat A, von Lany H, Evans N (2003) Scleromalacia as a complication of herpes zoster ophthalmicus. Eye 17: 449–451

Dugmore W (1997) Intercalary staphyloma in a case of herpes zoster ophthalmicus. Br J Ophthalmol 51: 350–351

Gilden DH, Kleinschmidt-DeMasters BK, Wellish M, Hedley-Whyte HD, Rentier B, Mahalingam R (1996) Varicella-zoster virus, a cause for waxing and waning vasculitis. Neurology 47: 1441–1446

Gungor IU, Ariturk N, Beden U, Darka O (2006) Necrotizing scleritis due to varicella zoster infection: a case report. Ocul Immunol Inflamm 14: 317–319

Hedges TR, Albert DM (1982) The progression of the ocular abnormalities of herpes zoster – histopathologic observations of nine cases. Ophthalmology 89: 165–177

Livis-Rallatos C, El-Shabrawi Y, Zatirakis P, Pellet PE, Stamey FR, Foster CS (1998) Recurrent nodular scleritis associated with varicella zoster virus. Am J Ophthalmol 126: 594–597

Naseri A, Good WV, Cunningham ET (2003) Herpes zoster virus sclerokeratitis and acute anterior uveitis in a child following varicella vaccination. Am J Ophthalmol 135: 415–417

Womack LW, Liesegang TJ (1983) Complications of herpes zoster ophthalmicus. Arch Ophthalmol 101: 42–45

Yoeruek E, Deuter CME, Szurman P, Tatar O, Zierhut M (2008) Scleromalacia associated with varicella-zoster virus. Ophthalmologe 105: 480–484

# Late Corneal Complications After Zoster

Section

3.8

## Core Messages

- Chronic corneal complications after zoster have a complex trophic etiology.
- Their therapy is mostly a difficult long-time task.
- They can severely reduce the prognosis of keratoplasty.
- The peculiar complication of late pseudodendritic efflorescences after zoster is given special consideration. Late pseudodendrites are therapeutically classified as trophic.

Chronic corneal complications after zoster can be infectious (Sect. 3.5) or non-infectious.

In this section, we present *non-infectious* corneal complications, which are caused by *trophic deficiencies* associated with the severe sensory neural damage, which develops in the course of zoster. While it must be admitted that many details and interactions of the pathophysiological pathways to trophic diseases of the cornea are still unclear and debatable, some sequelae can be described as follows:

- Corneal sensitivity is severely reduced, sometimes to zero.
- The blink reflex lacks its corneal feedback resulting in rare spontaneous blinking and easy drying of the epithelial surface.
- If the tarsal plate of the upper lid has lost its proper shape by necrosis (see Sect. 3.3), the "wiping" of the corneal surface with proper distribution of the tear film and proper lid closure no longer functions.
- Even minor corneal trauma leads to irritation or loss of compromised superficial epithelium.
- Epithelial regeneration is reduced in comparison with normal eyes.
- Therefore, trophic epithelial ulcers develop easily. They tend to persist and deepen if not treated properly and quickly enough.
- Also stromal repair seems to be impeded after zoster (see Sect. 3.9).
- An especially dangerous variant of trophic corneal ulcers is neuroparalytic ulcer, which is more typical, however, for complete destruction of the ophthalmic nerve, which is not regularly the case in zoster.
- The tear film lacks the normal stimulation which renders it insufficient in terms of quantity and quality.
- Quantity and quality of the tear film are further affected by infectious sequelae in its major production sites, above all in the conjunctiva. Pathologic mucous may be produced in excess.
- Defective tear film plus defective corneal epithelial surface plus reduced blinking rate result in a severely reduced stability of the tear film on the cornea.
- The tear film tends to partially decompose with frequent break-up and with adhesion of single components, especially mucous, to lesions in the epithelial surface. This makes the epithelium additionally mechanically vulnerable.

The list is probably far from being complete, but it gives an impression of the multitude of influences and interactions, which we tend to simplify as "trophic disturbances". Such a list also helps to understand which therapeutic interventions are needed. They are by no means practically easy:

- *Surface protection* of the corneal epithelium *from mechanical trauma*:
  To achieve this, anatomically correct lid position, physiologically correct blinking with complete lid closure, and correct "wiping" of the corneal surface are required. If necessary, lids must be surgically corrected or closed for a while.
- Surface protection of the corneal epithelium by *a sufficiently stable tear film:*
  If artificial tears, or single component preparations, or surface protecting ointments are insufficient, a trial can be made with daily wear of movable highly hydrophilic contact lenses *plus hourly substitution of conservative-free fluids*. The contacts serve as a protecting fluid reservoir. They regularly have to be removed at night, and the eye then protected by ointments only. If the fluids are not often enough substituted, the lens dries and lens therapy becomes quite dangerous.
- Removal or inhibition of mucous adhesions (Fig. 3.37):
  Mucus solving agents (e.g., acetyl-cysteine) can be tried in filiform keratitis in addition to dry eye therapy. If these are unavailable or inefficient, fluid-substituted contact lenses

sometimes also help in removal of adherent mucous threads. Personal positive anecdotal experience exists with an experimental symptomatic anti-inflammatory therapy by topical CS-A eye drops.

- Surgical measures:
  If trophic melting has led to persistent deep corneal ulcers, a surgical therapy (starting with an amnion cover) is necessary in addition to conservative medical measures. Sometimes, even emergency perforating keratoplasty becomes inevitable in order to save the eye (see Sect. 3.9).

## Analysis of Fig 3.34

The case in Fig. 3.34 could show the late trophic complications of that in Fig. 3.22. In fact, they are different cases, but they illustrate perfectly the development of trophic disturbances after severe ocular zoster. In this case, regeneration of the whole corneal epithelial layer is pathologic, as shown by its grey-white colors with diffuse punctate keratopathy. At six o´clock, a deep persistent corneal ulcer has developed, the margins of which are steep and sharp. The incoming epithelium is always abraded anew or simply falls off, because it cannot firmly enough attach to the ulcer base. On the limbal side of the ulcer, a regenerative buckle of partially vascularized epithelium has piled up, which is unable to transgress the peripheral ulcer margin. Its prominent configuration is another cause for insufficient wiping of the corneal surface by the upper lid. This is partly destructed (as evidenced by the lid margin), so that it can no longer provide the necessary protective and tear distributing functions. The severe limbal injection with circular progressive corneal neovascularization is primarily a reaction to the chronically defective epithelial surface and its invasion by inflammatory cells. But secondarily, the reproductive activity of the limbal stem cells, which is probably reduced by VZV infection anyway, is further severely depressed by the chronic inflammatory milieu. One could say that a vicious cycle of inflammation, disturbed regeneration, and lid dysfunction together with severe dry eye problems (see Fig. 3.36) continuously enforces itself. The therapeutic task is to break this vicious cycle in order to allow for solid scarring and quietening of the eye (Fig. 3.35). Only after this has been achieved, a decision should be made whether or not keratoplasty can follow (see Sect. 3.9). Different to HSV disease, where keratoplasty à chaud can often be advocated in order to shorten the overall course of severe disease, such trophic zoster cases are better not operated à chaud, if anyway avoidable.

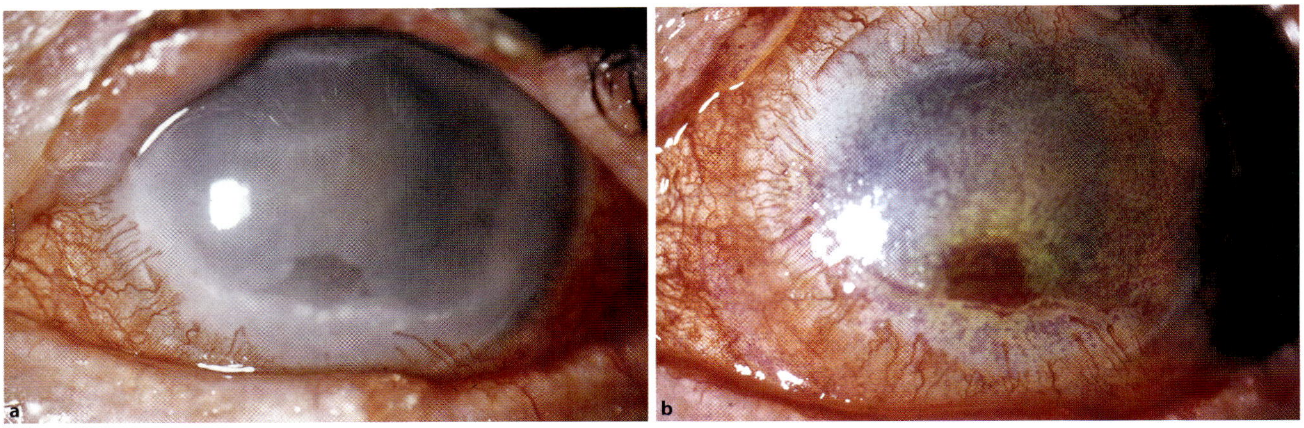

Fig. 3.34a,b Persistent trophic ulcer in the course of severe ophthalmic zoster, with a questionable prognosis of keratoplasty if operated à chaud. **a** Unstained. **b** Fluorescein and Bengal rose

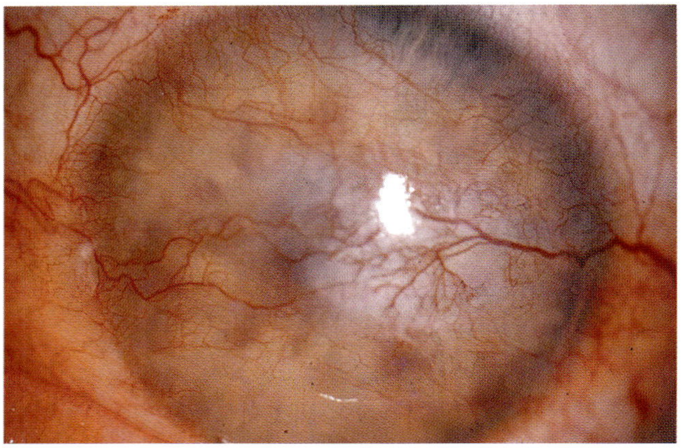

Fig. 3.35 Scarred and vascularized cornea after zoster with a good prognosis of perforating keratoplasty under CS-A or mycophenolate protection

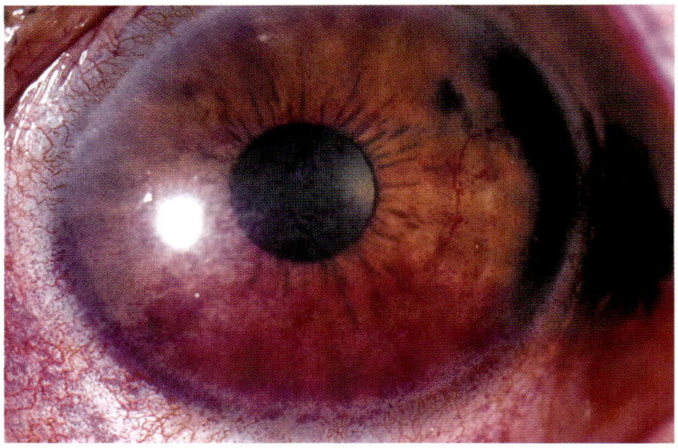

Fig. 3.36 Severe dry eye disease with massive punctate staining of conjunctiva and cornea after zoster (Bengal rose, see text)

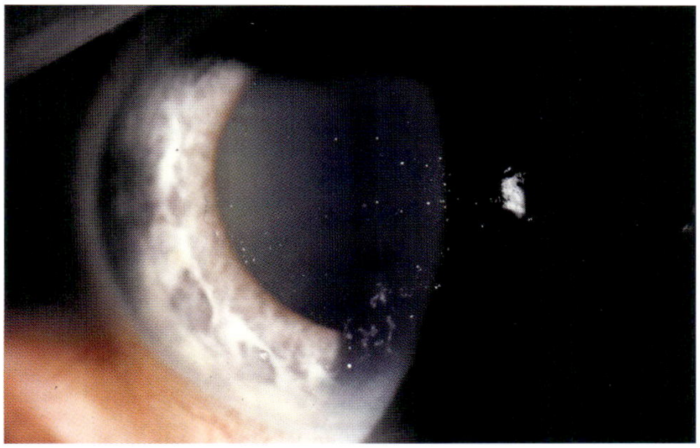

Fig. 3.37 Filiform keratopathy after ophthalmic zoster (see text)

The case in Fig. 3.34 could be treated as follows:
*Medical therapy* with 800 mg ACV 5 qd to treat a potentially persistent VZV infection, 20 mg fluorocortolone qd to reduce symptomatically the nocious inflammation, and mydriasis.
*Surgical therapy:* The lower 1/3 of the corneal epithelium are removed including the piled-up masses at the lower limbus and the new vessels imbedded in the epithelium. The ulcer is cleaned, and an amnion is sutured on the ulcer and on the cleaned corneal surface down to the limbus. In the ulcer, the amnion may be multilayered. As failure of lid closure will persist as long as the destructed lid margins are swollen so much, the lids can be surgically closed by temporary mattress sutures through the lid margins, and the patient is instructed to keep this eye intentionally "closed" as permanently as possible to reduce eye movements and stress on the sutures. The inner lid angle can still be opened by the investigator for eye inspection and for additional topical therapy with lubricants.
After an estimated 2–3 week period, it is often possible to remove the lid sutures and thereafter proceed to a continuous intensive topical dry eye therapy, while the systemic combination therapy is invariably carried on until the eye has turned quiet and the corneal surface has stabilized.

## Analysis of Fig 3.38

The two late peudodendrites in Fig. 3.38 stem from two different cases (a: case one, unstained, bc: case two, unstained and stained with Bengal rose). They usually develop months after healing of acute zoster disease, thus the designation "late". At that time, no viral activity is any longer suspected in the anterior segment of the eye. Their gross appearance sometimes stunningly resembles that of HSV dendritic efflorescences (see also Fig. 2.34). The biomicroscopic criterion of a typical destruction pattern, however, is missing. The efflorescences are build-up of prominent uniformly grey layers of epithelium, covered by a reflecting mucus layer. There is also no similarity with true viral VZV dendrites, as described in Sect. 3.4. Mostly, these late dendrites are understood as purely trophic pseudodendrites. But VZV involvement has also been suspected. Their pathophysiology may be more complex

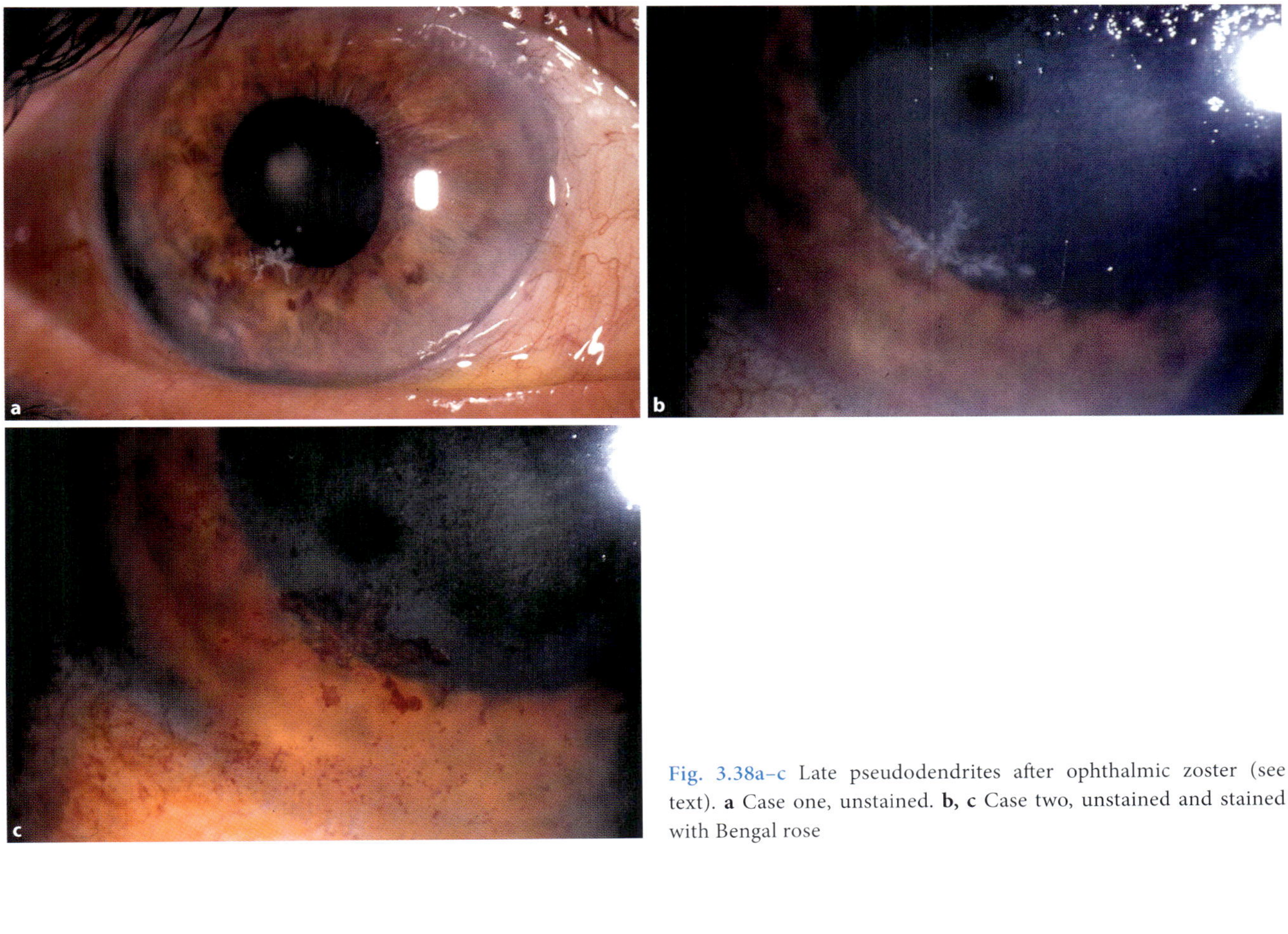

Fig. 3.38a–c Late pseudodendrites after ophthalmic zoster (see text). **a** Case one, unstained. **b, c** Case two, unstained and stained with Bengal rose

than currently recognizable. However, as these late dendritic efflorescences invariably heal with consequent dry eye therapy only, their clinical character is clearly trophic. Reports that topical steroids are sometimes needed to successfully treat such conditions are in accordance with my own positive experiences with Cs-A eye drops in recalcitrant severe filiform keratitis: By symptomatically reducing the grade of inflammation in the conjunctiva, the pathologic conjunctival mucous production is reduced. Mucous production seems to be the most important cause for the late pseudodendritic efflorescences. Consequent therapy with mucosolvents, sufficient tear substitution without preservatives and potentially in addition a cautious anti-inflammatory therapy with minimally dosed steroids or potent non-steroidal anti-inflammatory substances, e.g., Cs-A eye drops, will probably be a good combination to get rid of these chronic epithelial efflorescences after zoster.

## References


Al-Muammar A, Jackson WB (2004) Management of ophthalmic zoster mucous plaques keratopathy: report of three cases. Can J Ophthalmol 39: 74–76

Chen HJ, Pires RT, Tseng SC (2000) Amniotic membrane transplantation for severe neurotrophic ulcers. Br J Ophthalmol 84: 826–833

Cobo LM (1988) Corneal complications of herpes zoster ophthalmicus. Prevention and treatment. Cornea 7: 50–56

Engstrom RE, Holland GN (1988) Chronic herpes zoster virus keratitis associated with the acquired immunodeficiency syndrome. Am J Ophthalmol 105: 556–558

Hedges TR, Albert DM (1982) The progression of the ocular abnormalities of herpes zoster: histopathologic observations of nine cases. Ophthalmology 89: 165–176

Kaufman SC (2008) Anterior segment complications of herpes zoster ophthalmicus. Ophthalmology 115 Suppl: S24–S32

Liesegang TJ (1985) Corneal complications of herpes zoster ophthalmicus. In: PC Maudgal, L Missotten (eds) Herpetic Eye Diseases. Doc Ophth Proc Ser 44, pp 395–402

Marsh RJ (1973) Herpes zoster keratitis. Trans Ophthalmol Soc UK: 93: 181–192

Marsh RJ, Cooper M (1987) Ophthalmic zoster: mucous plaque keratitis. Br J Ophthalmol 71: 725–728

Mondino BJ, Brown SI, Mondzelewski JP (1978) Peripheral corneal ulcers with herpes zoster ophthalmicus. Am J Ophthalmol 86: 611–614

Pavan-Langston D, Yamamoto S, Dunkel EC (1995) Delayed herpes zoster pseudodendrites. Polymerase chain reaction detection and a role for antiviral therapy. Arch Ophthalmol 113: 1381–1385

Piebenga LW, Laibson PR (1973) Dendritic lesions in herpes zoster ophthalmicus. Arch Ophthalmol 90: 268–270

Waring GO, Ekins MB (1981) Corneal perforation in herpes zoster ophthalmicus caused by eyelid scarring with exposure keratitis. In: R Sundmacher (ed) Herpetic Eye Diseases. Bergmann, Munich, pp 469–478

Womack LW, Liesegang TJ (1983) Complications of herpes zoster ophthalmicus. Arch Ophthalmol 101: 42–45

Zaal MJW, Maudgal PC, Rietveld E, Suir P (1991) Chronic ocular zoster. Curr Eye Res 10 (Suppl): S125–130

# Keratoplasty in Zoster Eyes

Section

3.9

## Core Messages

- Different to keratoplasty in HSV eyes, recurrences of VZV disease in the graft are normally *not* to be expected, and a systemic antiviral prophylaxis is therefore unnecessary.
- Because trophic problems cause a good deal of complications after keratoplasty in zoster eyes, if possible, it is not recommended to perform systemic immune prophylaxis as usual with steroids, but with non-steroidal agents, above all with cyclosporine A or mycophenolatemofetile.

Many common aspects, problems, complications, and available solutions for perforating keratoplasty have already been presented in detail in Sect. 2.14 on surgery in HSV eyes. In this section, emphasis can be laid, therefore, on the major differences between keratoplasty in VZV disease as compared with keratoplasty in HSV disease:

- The *immunological problems* and the risk of immune reactions and immunologic graft failure are *identical* in both groups, as are the chances and indications for using HLA matched donor material.
- The risk of recurring viral disease is high in HSV infection, and it is normally zero in zoster eyes. Except for the special situation in severely immune compromised individuals, and except for the rare event of zoster in children or young adults, which make a second bout of zoster theoretically possible after many decades, zoster does not recur a second time in a patient. Therefore, *antiviral prophylaxis* is *unnecessary*. This is an important advantage of keratoplasty in zoster eyes.
- This advantage is counteracted, however, by much more trophic problems after severe zoster than after recurrent HSV disease. These trophic disturbances often persist in the time period after keratoplasty, and they may dangerously interfere with the integrity and function of the graft. A special danger comes from the circumstance where severe trophic disease is mostly incompatible with high-dosed steroid prophylaxis of immune reactions, especially with topical steroids. If the surgeon refrains from steroids in an attempt not to allow trophic disease to establish, the battle for survival of the corneal graft has already been lost in many cases. The solution of this problem is to administer non-steroidal systemic immunosuppressive agents, above all cyclosporine A or mycophenolate mofetil, for the time period of the highest immune threat, i. e., for 1–1.5 years. If this is done not only for immunologically especially compromised zoster cases but for all zoster keratoplasties (!), and if simultaneously the risk of trophic disturbances is consequently reduced by efficient dry eye prophylaxis, then the prognosis of keratoplasty in zoster eyes may approach the excellent prognosis of keratoplasty in HSV eyes.
- In contrast to severe HSV disease, where keratoplasty à chaud can often shorten the course of disease and reduce the overall need for systemic therapy, costs included, keratoplasty à chaud in zoster eyes can not be recommended. Severe *trophic* problems are the most frequent reason for emergency situations in zoster, and these severe trophic problems continue to be operative also after keratoplasty à chaud. If it is possible to defer keratoplasty up to a time when a sufficient percentage of the trophic problems has resolved or at least ameliorated, the chances for successful graft survival become much better. It is always worthwhile, therefore, to try to defer keratoplasty in zoster eyes until the eye has become clinically quiet.

## Analysis of Fig 3.39

The zoster patient in Fig. 3.39 was treated at a time, when non-steroidal immune suppression was not yet available for keratoplasty. Thus, he was given systemic and topical steroids "as usual" together with dry eye prophylaxis. When he returned to his surgeon for a control 6 weeks after surgery, the lower half of the cornea had become dramatically opaque in a half-moon shaped area. The graft epithelium had fallen off and no host epithelium had come in to cover the defect (Fig. 3.39a). The Bengal rose stain (Fig. 3.39b) discloses that the area of diseased epithelium is even larger than the epithelial ulcer. As no immune reaction was detectable and the miserable state of the graft had exclusively been attributed to trophic reasons, it was decided to carry on for some months with a moderate systemic steroid prophylaxis, to refrain of all topical steroids, and, instead, to enhance the topical dry eye therapy. The success of these simple measures was stunning. 12 weeks later (Fig.3.39c), the defect had closed. The pupillary area had become

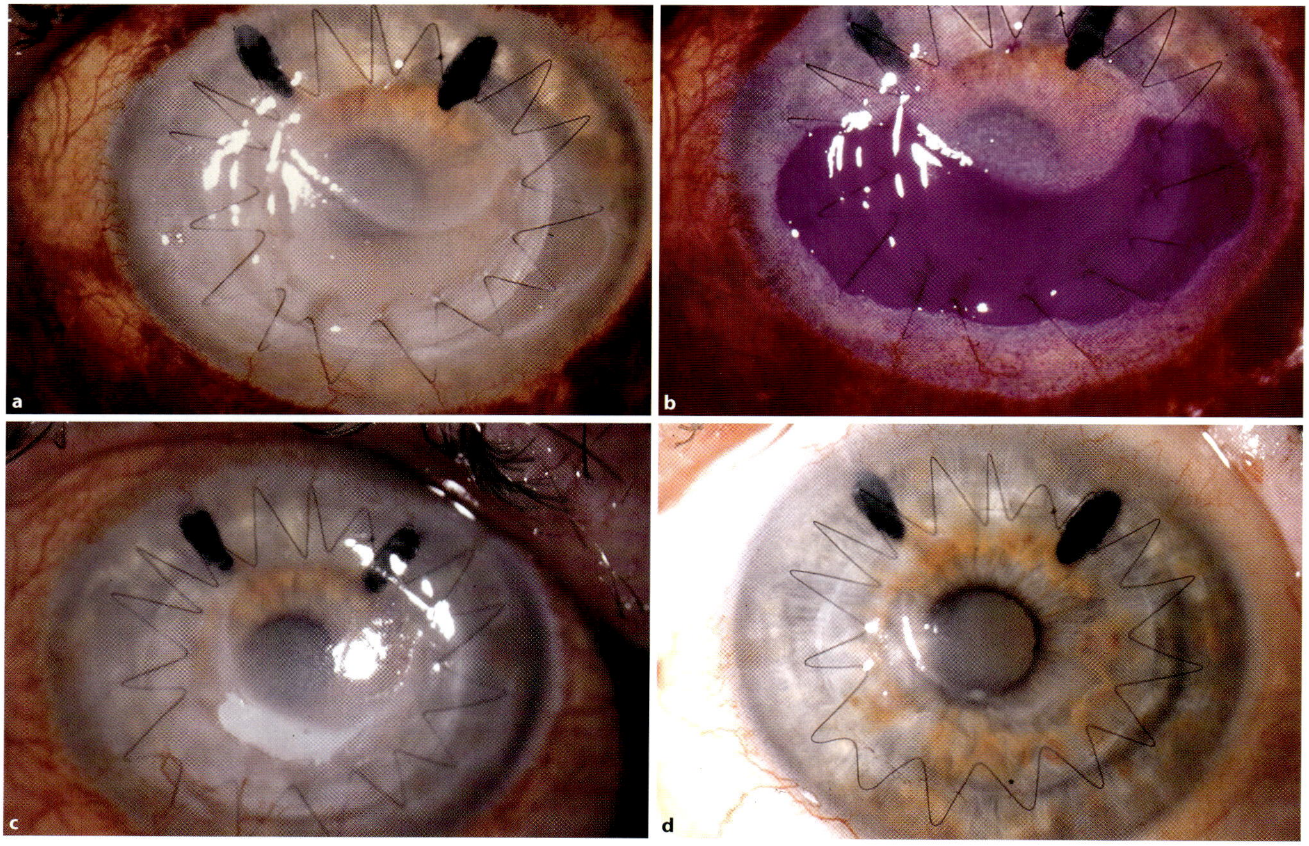


Fig. 3.39a–d Trophic graft complications after keratoplasty in a zoster eye. **a**, **b** 6 weeks. **c** 12 weeks. **d** 18 months after kp

much more transparent, and only a dense superficial calcification from the intensified application of phosphate-containing eye drops was a new unpleasant complication. 1.5 years after keratoplasty, the graft had functionally again become crystal clear in the center. The calcifications had spontaneously been resorbed after reduction of artificial eye drop application from every 0.5 hr to 7 qd. Immune reactions had not interfered, and new trophic problems did not interfere either.

## Analysis of Fig 3.40

The treatment of the 77-year-old zoster patient in Fig. 3.40 also dates back to the time when neither ACV nor non-steroidal systemic immune-suppressive agents were available. When he showed-up first 10 days after beginning of zoster, the cornea was already superficially ulcerated, and the ulceration quickly proceeded to comprise nearly the whole inferior cornea. The lids did not close tightly, and the ulceration was judged to be enforced by intermittent lagophthalmus, i. e., by exposure. In spite of antibiotic therapy, a hypopyon developed (Fig. 3.40a). Shortly after, a paralimbal pinpoint perforation was detected (Fig. 3.40b), and the cornea was covered with an oxygen-permeable silicon contact lens, which was then "en vogue" for sealing of corneal perforations. The perforation broadened, however, under the silicon lens, and emergency surgery became inevitable (Fig. 3.40c). The right time for a conjunctival or full corneal cover had long been gone, and only a perforating keratoplasty procedure could help in this situation. The limbal position of the perforation and the size of the ulcer would have made the use of an oversized sclerocorneal graft necessary with the great danger of immunologic failure. In an attempt to at least save the still clear upper half of the patients cornea, only the lower half was resected "free hand" and the defect filled with a full thickness corneal graft (Fig. 3.40d). The further course was unexpectedly positive. Half a year later, the donor as well as the host cornea were both clear and the eye was clinically quiet (Fig. 3.40e). The mature cataract, which had developed in the course of perforation and keratoplasty, was secondarily successfully operated, and the patient gained reasonable vision with this previously almost lost eye without further surgical interventions.

Retrospectively, it was waited too long for the ulcer to heal with conservative measures only. A quicker emergency surgery with amnion, conjunctiva, or cornea to cover the large ulcer would have been less risky and would probably have spared some emotional stress of the patient and the surgeon. The unexpectedly good outcome in this case should not lead to the erroneous assumption that keratoplasty á chaud has a mostly good prognosis in ophthalmic zoster.

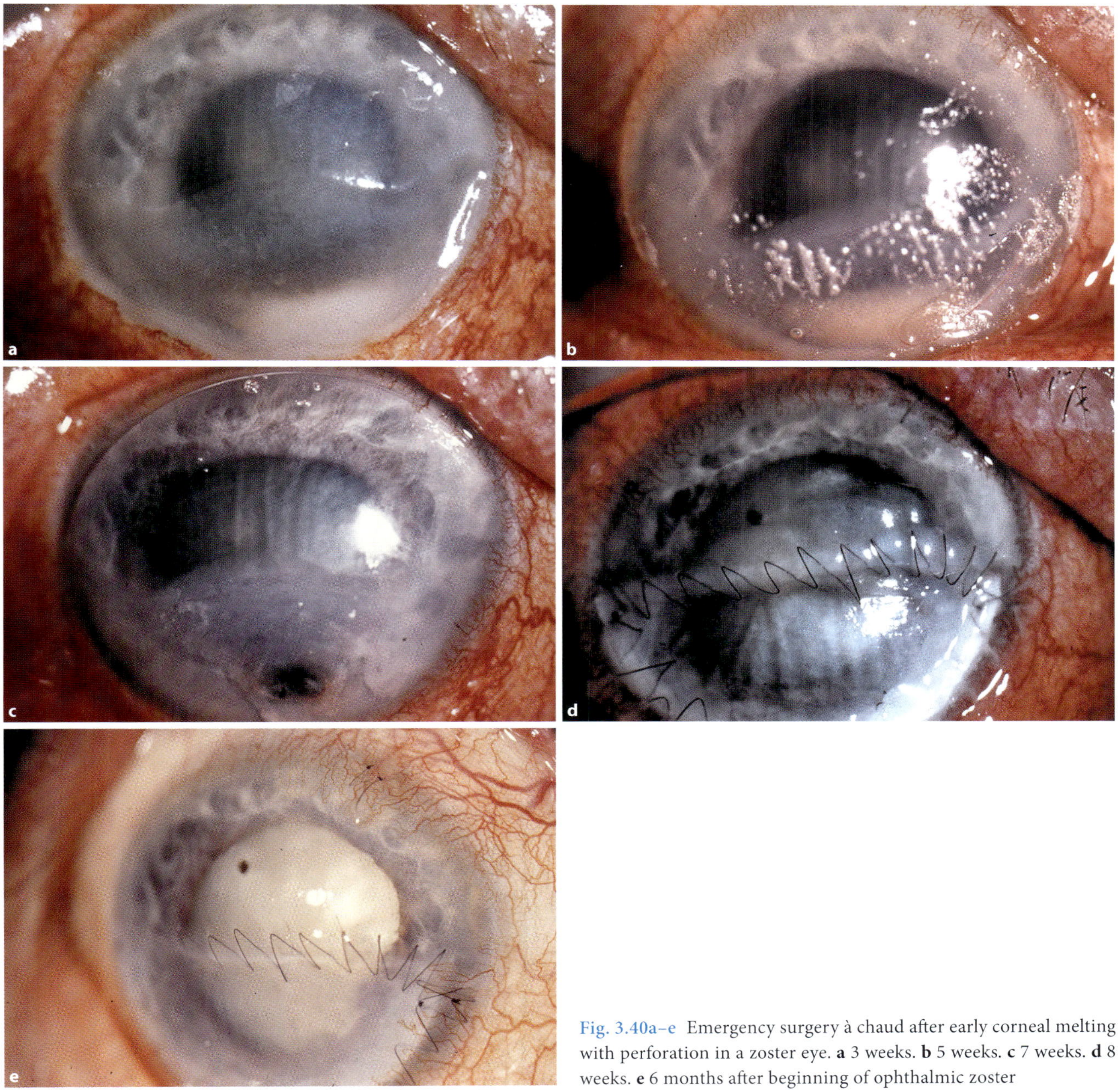

Fig. 3.40a–e Emergency surgery à chaud after early corneal melting with perforation in a zoster eye. **a** 3 weeks. **b** 5 weeks. **c** 7 weeks. **d** 8 weeks. **e** 6 months after beginning of ophthalmic zoster

## Analysis of Fig 3.41

Figure 3.41 shows how the case in Fig. 3.40 could have developed if the large basal ulcer would have been covered in time by a conjunctival flap. After an adequate consolidation time of 6–12 months, such an eye can safely be operated, especially if potent non-steroidal systemic immune-suppressive agents are available. The massive vascularization is no longer a major problem with substances like cyclosporine A or mycophenolate mofetil. The risk of immune reaction can be further reduced, and the chances for a clear long-term survival of the corneal graft can be increased by use of a well HLA-matched corneal transplant.

## Analysis of Fig 3.42

The case in Fig. 3.42 is rather special, but worthwhile demonstrating for principal reasons. It is common knowledge that keratoplasty wounds never reach the tensile strength of normal corneal tissue and that the life-long danger of wound rupture after blunt ocular trauma exists for every keratoplasty eye. However, this danger may be especially great in zoster eyes.

In the 1960s, a surgical treatment of zoster keratitis was occasionally tried and it was called "circumcision". The idea was to circumferentially cut all sensory nerves and thus block VZV from invading the cornea centrally to the circumcision line. Basically, simple

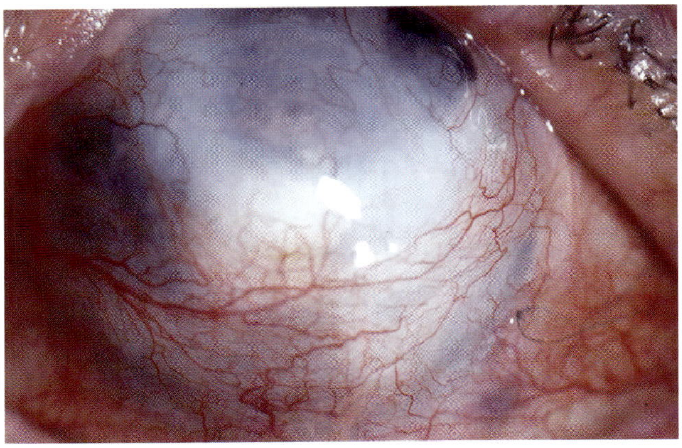

Fig. 3.41 Zoster eye, which received a conjunctival flap because of trophic corneal melting in the lower half of the cornea, now ready for *selective* keratoplasty

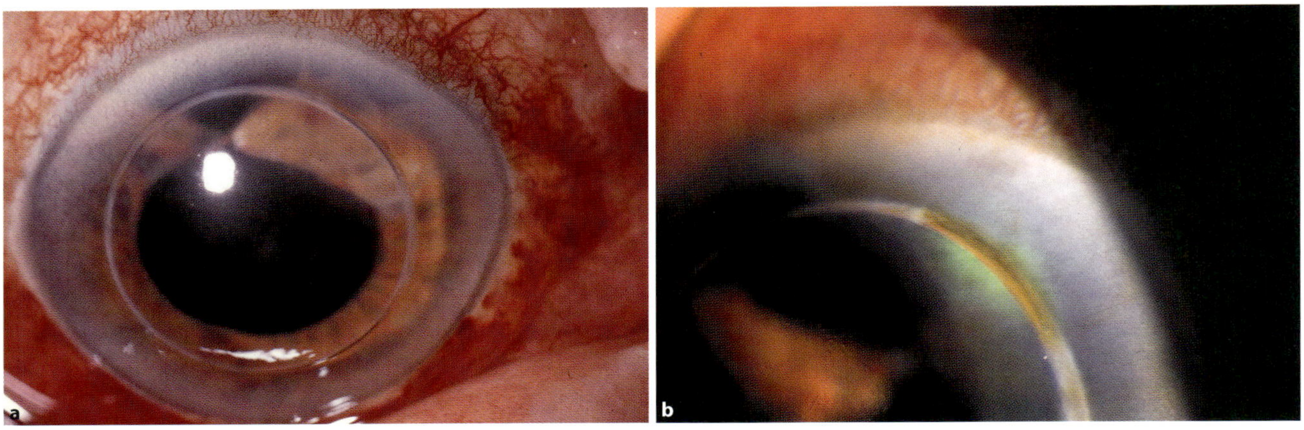

Fig. 3.42a,b Lysis of a corneal circumcision in a zoster eye following cataract surgery (see text)

trephination of the cornea down to the level of Descemets was performed, and sometimes Descemet´s was certainly perforated on this occasion, so that the resultant state was similar to that after perforating keratoplasty. The 90-year-old lady presented *22 years* after this procedure with a widely lysed corneal wound. She denied any trauma. 2 weeks previously, a corneoscleral cataract extraction had been performed. It seems then, that the minor trauma of lifting the corneoscleral flap in the course of cataract surgery was sufficient to open a "keratoplasty" wound in a zoster eye after 22 years. Such experience may be worthwhile to note in order to teach especially zoster patients with a corneal transplant to avoid even minor ocular trauma.

## References


Alino AM, Perry HD, Kanellopoulos AJ, Donnenfeld ED, Rahn EK (1998) Conjunctival flaps. Ophthalmology 105: 1120–1123

Mackensen G, Sundmacher R, Witschel H (1985) Late wound complications after circular keratotomy for zoster keratitis. Cornea 3: 95–98

Marsh RJ, Cooper M (1989) Ocular surgery in ophthalmic zoster. Eye 3: 313–317

Reed JW, Joyner SJ, Knauer WJ (1989) Penetrating keratoplasty for herpes zoster keratopathy. Am J Ophthalmol 107: 257–261

Soong HK, Schwartz AE, Meyer RF, Sugar A (1989) Penetrating keratoplasty for corneal scarring due to herpes zoster ophthalmicus. Br J Ophthalmol 73: 19–21

Tanure MA, Cohen EJ, Grewal S, Rapuano CJ, Laibson PR (2000) Penetrating keratoplasty for varicella-zoster virus keratopathy. Cornea 19: 135–139

Van Gelderen BE, van der Lelij A, Treffers WF, van der Gaag R (2000) Detection of herpes simplex virus type 1, 2 and varicella zoster virus DNA in recipient corneal buttons. Br J Ophthalmol 84: 1238–1243

# Differences Between VZV and HSV Ocular Disease

Section

3.10

The basic similarities (see Sect. 3.1) and the many dissimilarities between VZV and HSV ocular disease have already been discussed or shortly been mentioned in the preceding sections on HSV and VZV diseases. Therefore, for this concluding section it may suffice to compile the various aspects in an abbreviated form in Table 3.2. Some statements in this table do not fulfil the requirements of unequivocal scientific evidence. Instead, they express the author's belief on how to fit together clinical observations with a currently still partially hypothetical pathophysiological background.

Table 3.2 Some differences between VZV and HSV ocular disease

| Aspects | VZV | HSV |
|---|---|---|
| *Virus* | | |
| – Herpes virus subfamily | Alpha | Alpha |
| – Physical stability | Labile | More stable |
| – Replication | Slow | Quicker |
| – Preferred corneal target cells | 1. Keratocytes<br>2. Endothelial cells<br>3. Epithelial cells | 1. Epithelial cells<br>2. Endothelial cells<br>3. Keratocytes |
| *Primary infection* | | |
| – Clinic | Varicella (Sect. 3.2) | Rarely clinical (Sect. 2.12) |
| – Site of infection | Not determinative for site of zoster | Determinative for recurrent HSV disease |
| – Viremia | Important | Unimportant |
| *Latency* | | |
| – Site | Sensory ganglia | Sensory ganglia |
| – Cells offering latency resorts | Ganglia and satellite cells | Ganglia cells |
| – Latency control | Primarily immunologic | Not really known |
| – Stability of latency | Mostly high | 2/3 high, 1/3 low |
| *Recurrences* | | |
| – Clinic | Sects. 2.3–2.11 | Sects. 3.3–3.8 |
| – Primary trigger | Drop in anti-VZV immunity | Stress |
| – Hypothetical co-trigger | Possibly stress | Not known |
| – Number of recurrences | Normally only one | Mostly more than one |
| – Virus main transport | Intraaxonal and by viremia | Intraaxonal |
| – Site of disease | Variable | Site of primary infection |
| *Persistence in peripheral cells* | Easier than HSV | Occasionally |
| *Antiviral therapy* | Basically systemic | Topical and/or systemic |
| – ACV systemic therapy | 800 mg 5 qd | 400 mg 5 qd |
| – ACV ointment | 5 qd | 5 qd |
| – TFT eye drops | Inactive | 5 qd for superficial disease |
| – BVDU systemic therapy | 125 mg 1 qd | (not licensed, for HSV-1only) |
| – BVDU eye drops (invest.) | (5 qd) | (5 qd, for HSV-1 only) |

Table 3.2 (*continued*) Some differences between VZV and HSV ocular disease

| Aspects | VZV | HSV |
|---|---|---|
| *Steroids* | | |
| – Generally | To be avoided | No problems in combination with efficient antiviral therapy |
| – With deep ocular disease | Often necessary to preserve function, but only at lowest doses possible and only with efficient antiviral cover indicated for *all deep* ocular disease | Regularly indicated even at higher doses together with efficient antiviral cover |
| *Prophylaxis of recurrences* | | |
| – Generally | Normal immune status | "No stress" |
| – Medically | Not needed (except for states of severe immune incompetence) | ACV 400 mg 3 qd |
| – Vaccination | Promising and indicated | Not available |
| *General eye surgery* | | |
| – Trigger for recurrences | No | Theoretically yes, practically rarely |
| – Systemic ACV cover | No | Recommended |
| *Keratoplasty* | | |
| – Recurrences of viral disease | No | Frequent |
| – Antiviral prophylaxis | No | ACV for 1 year |
| – Trophic complications | Frequently severe | Rarely severe |
| – Syst. immune prophylaxis | MMF or CSA preferred, steroids increase trophic problems | MMF preferred, steroids trigger HSV recurrences |
| – General prognosis | Good, except kp à chaud | Very good, also after kp à chaud |
| *Some differences between recurrent viral disease types* | | |
| – Blepharitis | Dermatome V/1 | Variable |
| – Intermarginal blepharitis | Not in zoster | Circumscribed erosion |
| – Epithelial keratitis | Rare and transient | Frequent, long duration |
| – Dendritic k. | Short, plump, no microdestruction pattern | Larger and more structured, pathognomonic microdestructions |
| – Geographic k. | No (not even with steroids) | Regularly with steroids |
| – Interstitial keratitis | Nummuli frequent | Nummuli rarer |
| – Ulcerating interstitial keratitis | Early in severe zoster | More frequent with increasing number of recurrences |
| – Endotheliitis | Frequently first sign of ophthalmic zoster | Unusual as a first manifestation |
| – Trabeculitis | Clinically not identified | All grades of severity possible |
| – Acute secondary glaucoma | Clinically not so important | Regularly associated with intraocular HSV replication |
| – Focal serous iritis | | |
| – Pigment epithelial loss | Limited with only one disease attack | Lesions enlarge with every subsequent recurrence |
| – Vascular infarction | Frequent with stromal loss | Very rare |
| – Scleritis and sclerokeratitis | Relatively rare | Extremely rare |

## References


Ahonen R, Vannas A (1985) Clinical comparison between herpes simplex and herpes zoster ocular infections. In: PC Maudgal, L Missotten (eds.) Herpetic Eye Diseases. Doc Ophthal Proc Ser 44, pp 389–394

Beards G, Graham C, Pillay D (1998) Investigation of vesicular rashes for HSV and VZV by PCR. J Med Virol 54: 155–157

Croen KD, Ostrove JM, Dragovic LJ, Straus SE (1988) Patterns of gene expression and site of latency in human trigeminal ganglia are different for varicella-zoster and herpes simplex virus. Proc. Natl Sci USA 85: 9773–9777

Forrest WM, Kaufman HE (1976) Zosteriform herpes simplex. Am J Ophthalmol 81: 86–88

Kalman CM, Laskin OL (1986) Herpes zoster and zosteriform herpes simplex virus infections in immunocompetent adults. Am J Med 81: 775–778

Rubben A, Baron JM, Grussendorf-Conen EL (1997) Routine detection of herpes simplex virus and varicella zoster virus by polymerase chain reaction reveals that initial herpes zoster is frequently misdiagnosed as herpes simplex. Br J Dermatol 137: 259–266

Straus SE, Meier JL (1992) Comparative biology of latent varicella-zoster virus and herpes simplex infections. J Infect Dis 166 (Suppl 1): S13–S23

Thygeson P, Ostler HB (1979) Zoster and herpes simplex virus uveitis: a comparison. In: AM Silverstein, GR O`Connor (eds) Immunology and Immunopathology of the Eye. Masson, USA, pp 230–240

# Cytomegalovirus (CMV) Diseases of the Anterior Segment

*Rainer Sundmacher and Johannes Stammen*

Chapter

4

## Core Messages

- A connatal and two adult cases of *monosymptomatic* endotheliitis plus trabeculitis could be correlated with culturable CMV or the presence of CMV DNA in the aqueous humor.
- Cases with *Posner–Schlossman syndrome* are prime suspects for CMV disease of the anterior segment of the eye and should be accordingly investigated.

Intrauterine transmitted connatal viral ocular disease has been omitted as a topic for this book. The presentation and discussion would have had to include too many special fields of virology, obstetrics, and pediatrics, which are outside the scope of this atlas. Several intrauterine acquired virus infections may cause malformations and a variety of diseases. Sometimes also the eye becomes affected, e. g., the lens and also the cornea in the course of systemic rubella or CMV infection. The viral etiology can then mostly be easily suspected from the signs of general viral disease. Laboratory confirmation is also mostly not a problem. These *polysymptomatic* eye affections in the course of systemic intrauterine viral disease will not be further discussed here.

However, a special *monosymptomatic* connatal CMV disease of the eye will be presented because it fits well with the finding of monosymptomatic endotheliitis of suspected CMV etiology in adults. It seems that we are now able to define much more precisely as ever which type of inflammation of unknown origin in the anterior segment of the eye may be caused by CMV.

## Analysis of Fig 4.1

The newborn in Fig. 4.1 presented with a bilateral connatal *inflammatory* glaucoma with both corneae enlarged, but without the typical signs of idiopathic buphthalmus. There were no Haab lines, and the corneas were too opaque to disclose details in the eye. Intraocular pressure was 27 mm Hg RE and 50 mm LE. The suspected diagnosis was infectious endotheliitis and trabeculitis, with herpes viruses ranging among the most suspect viruses. CMV was grown from aqueous taps from both eyes on three occasions, the last time at the age of 10 months (Fig. 4.1c). Up to this time, all therapeutic attempts including trabeculotomies, medical glaucoma treatment, and also an antiviral trial with ARA-A, which was the only available experimental systemic antiviral agent in those years, had failed. The intraocular pressure was still high with the corneas further enlarged and scarred. There was no other help. The child remained blind bilaterally.

The intensive search for associated general viral disease remained constantly negative. The child was perfectly healthy except for the bilateral eye affection, and the child also developed somatically and mentally normal except for the incurable connatal blindness. The anterior chamber was not the only site where CMV was isolated from after birth. Virus was also repeatedly grown from conjunctival swaps and from the urine, though not regularly. A general CMV disease, however, was not present.

Therefore, this case was classified as the presumably first description of a *monosymptomatic severe CMV endotheliitis and trabeculitis,* with the infection acquired intrauterine, presumably rather late in the course of gravidity. The mother had never shown signs of clinical viral disease. However, she had high IgM-titers against CMV after birth.

The publication of this case in the proceedings of the first international herpes symposium certainly did not promote its knowledge.

Recently, a small series of observations has been published of CMV DNA findings in the aqueous humor of adults with endotheliitis and uveitis of unknown origin. Elevated intraocular pressure was also involved. Therefore, it becomes probable that monosymptomatic corneal endotheliitis associated with elevated pressure is a common feature of CMV infection of the anterior segment of the eye.

The clinical picture of connatal and adult diseases are quite different as far as acuity and severeness are concerned. Pathophysiologically, however, they follow an identical infection scheme. As endotheliitis with elevated pressure is still a somewhat imprecise description, which covers several viral etiologies and possibly also non-viral etiologies, the question is, whether additional signs exist which allow to more precisely predict which type of endotheliitis is a candidate for CMV etiology in adults. Two of my own cases of CMV DNA finding in monosymptomatic endotheliitis both fulfil the diagnostic criteria of Posner–Schlossman syndrome.

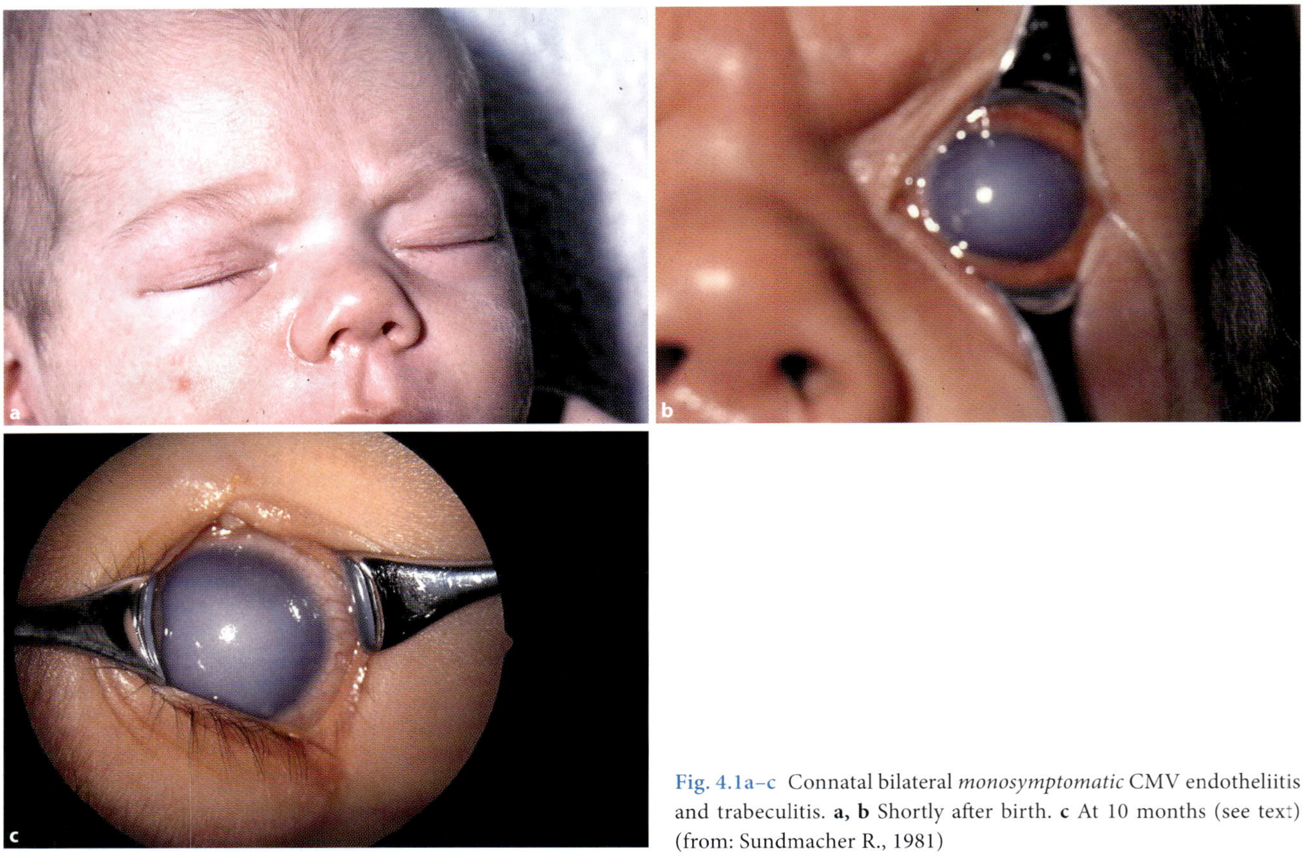

Fig. 4.1a–c Connatal bilateral *monosymptomatic* CMV endotheliitis and trabeculitis. **a, b** Shortly after birth. **c** At 10 months (see text) (from: Sundmacher R., 1981)

## Analysis of Fig 4.2

The 67-year-old male patient in Fig. 4.2 first presented with a 33-year long history of "recurrent iritis with increasingly severe secondary glaucoma, while the iritis was always stunningly mild with only very sparse precipitates".

This is a usual description of *Posner–Schlossman syndrome* with the typical course of glaucoma. In the first years or decades, glaucoma is only transient and quickly fades away with and without therapy. With symptomatic therapy (topical steroids), the attacks seem to have a shorter duration, which has led to the widespread conviction that some etiologically unclear acute "allergic" swelling of trabecular meshwork cells is the cause of disease, i.e., an immunologic trabeculitis of unknown origin.

We and others have favored the hypothesis of a viral etiology, especially of members of the herpes family. As HSV and VZV are typically causing endotheliitis and trabeculitis, they were prime candidates for etiology. HSV has been excluded. An etiologic role for VZV could never be unequivocally proven. It was some surprise when *CMV PCR was positive* in the aqueous humor of this patient on occasion of trabeculectomy, which became necessary, because the secondary glaucoma no longer responded to symptomatic therapy.

This is the second case after the newborn patient (Fig. 4.1) in which we could correlate trabeculitis and endotheliitis with a positive CMV finding in the aqueous humor.

## Analysis of Fig 4.3

The third case of endotheliitis and trabeculitis with a positive CMV PCR in the aqueous humor was found in a 30-year-old male who had suffered from yearly attacks of Posner–Schlossman syndrome for three years (Fig. 4.3). The disease had been classified as "some kind of atypical herpes disease with endotheliitis and glaucoma" and had already been treated as such with ACV plus steroids.

The complex history of these two adult patients is reserved for a separate publication after more follow-up time. For this atlas, it shall suffice to document the finding of intraocular CMV in two adults with endotheliitis and trabeculitis, and to elaborate a bit more on the clinical signs of this disease.

Posner–Schlossman syndrome is probably no clear-cut entity, i.e., it has more than one cause. This can be suspected from the observation that number, distribution, fine structure, and persistence of the endotheliitic precipitates are quite variable in Posner–Schlossman syndrome. The common link of *all* Posner–Schlossman syndromes, however, is the correlation of very subtle signs of endotheliitis – as evidenced by the typical endotheliitic precipitates – with a disproportionate acute rise in intraocular pressure by presumed trabeculitis.

If all cases from the potentially heterogenous Posner–Schlossman group are systematically punctured, and the aqueous humor investigated by PCR for the presence of herpes

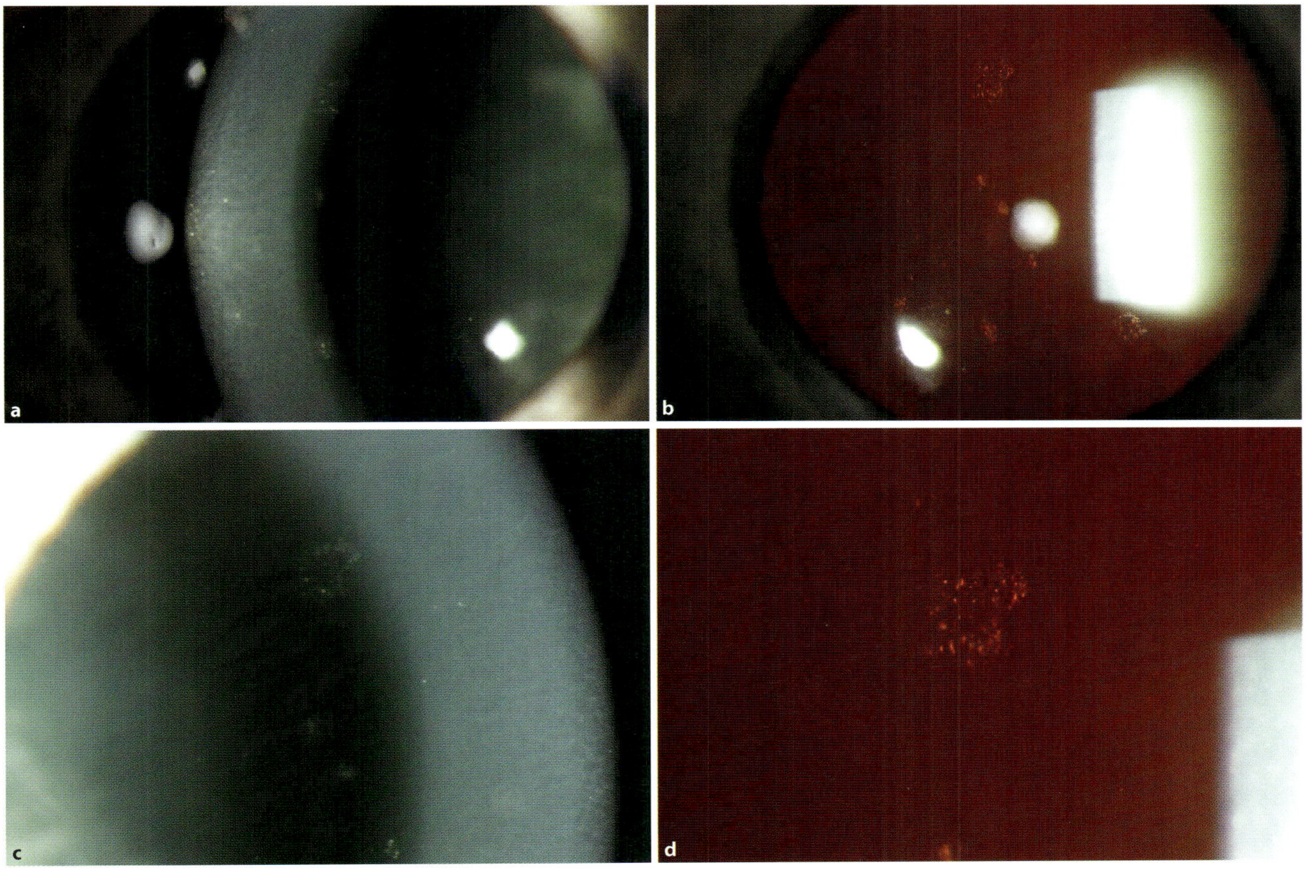


Fig. 4.2a–d Posner–Schlossmann syndrome of duration of 37 years: CMV PCR positive in the aqueous humor on occasion of trabeculectomy. Endotheliitic precipitates as seen with oblique beam (**a**,**c**) and with retro-illumination (**b**,**d**)

genetic material, we will quickly know what the actual correlation is between Posner–Schlossman syndrome and CMV. It may well be that only a percentage of cases are caused by CMV. It may also be that the biomicroscopic fine structure of the endotheliitic precipitates, as demonstrated above, has some additional diagnostic importance. Comparing the fine structure of the precipitates of the two adult CMV cases (Figs. 4.2 and 4.3), the similarity is stunning. The sparse fine endotheliitic precipitates are randomly distributed on the endothelium. They are composed of multiple fine granules, and these granules sometimes form a ring. This ring form suggests that a focally starting endothelial viral infection slowly spreads in all directions until it is halted by cellular immune reactions.

The second problem which has to be addressed after solving the diagnostic one is the therapy of CMV caused Posner–Schlossman syndromes. The question is whether or not the recurrences can permanently be inhibited by a systemic anti-CMV treatment. Our limited experiences with the two cases presented above have as yet not been encouraging but hope is reserved for the future.

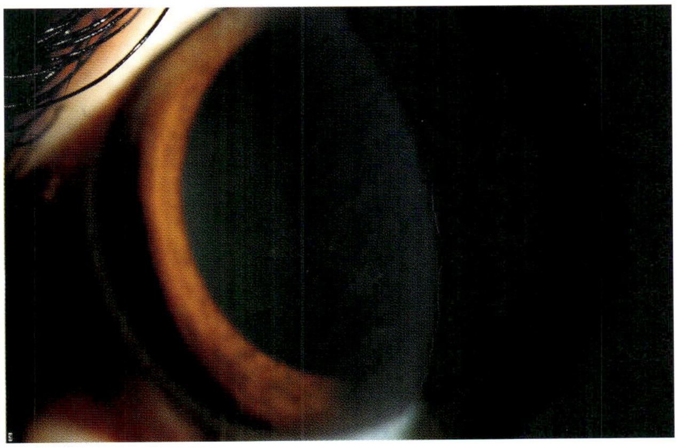

Fig. 4.3 Posner–Schlossman syndrome in a 30-year-old patient: CMV PCR positive in the aqueous humor

## References


Althaus C, Armsen B, Best J, Hintzmann A, Hudde T, Kersten A, Sundmacher R (1997) Endothelzelldichte bei AIDS-Patienten mit Cytomegalie-Virus-Retinitis im Langzeitverlauf. Sitzungsbericht 159. Versammlung Rhein.-Westf. Augenärzte, Düsseldorf. Zimmermann-Verlag, Balve, pp 167–170

Althaus C, Best J, Hintzmann A, Schimkat M, Hudde T, Cepin A, Sundmacher R (1997) Endothelial precipitates and laser flare photometry in patients with acquired immunodeficiency syndrome: a screening test for cytomegalovirus retinitis? German J Ophthalmol 5: 443–448

Chee SP, Bacsal K, Jap A, Se-Thoe SY, Cheng CL, Tan BH (2007) Corneal endotheliitis associated with evidence of cytomegalovirus infection. Ophthalmology 114: 798–803

Chee SP, Bacsal K, Jap A, Se-Thoe SY, Cheng CL, Tan BH (2008) Clinical features of cytomegalovirus anterior uveitis in immunocompetent patients. Am J Ophthalmol 145: 834–840

Grehn F, Sundmacher R (1982) Zur Pathogenese und Therapie des Posner–Schlossman-Syndroms. In: G Krieglstein, W Leydhecker (eds): Medikamentöse Glaukomtherapie. Bergmann, München, pp 95–99

Koizumi N, Suzuki T, Uno T, Chihara H, Shiraishi A, Hara Y, Inatomi T, Sotozono C, Kawasaki S, Yamasaki K, Mochida C, Ohashi Y, Kinoshita S: Cytomegalovirus as an etiologic factor in corneal endotheliitis. Ophthalmology, Print Electronic, 2007730

Koizumi N, Yamasaki K, Kawasaki S, Sotozono C, Inatomi T, Mochida C, Kinoshita S (2006) Cytomegalovirus in aqueous humor from an eye with corneal endotheliitis. Am J Ophthalmol 141: 564–565

Shiraishi A, Hara Y, Takahashi M, Oka N, Yamaguchi M, Suzuki T, Uno T, Ohashi Y (2007) Demonstration of "owl´s eye" morphology by confocal microscopy in a patient with presumed cytomegalovirus corneal endotheliitis. Am J Ophthalmol 143: 715–717

Sundmacher R, Neumann-Haefelin D, Mattes A, Cantell K (1981) Connatal monosymptomatic corneal endotheliitis by cytomegalovirus. In: R Sundmacher (ed): Herpetic Eye Diseases. Bergmann, Munich, pp 501–502

Suzuki T, Hara Y, Uno T, Ohashi Y (2007) DNA of cytomegalovirus detected by PCR in aqueous of patient with corneal endotheliitis after penetrating keratoplasty. Cornea 26: 370–372

Yamamoto S, Pavan-Langston D, Tada R, Yamamoto R, Kinoshita S, Nishida K, Shimomura Y, Tano Y (1995) Possible role of herpes simplex virus in the origin of Posner–Schlossman syndrome. Am J Ophthalmol 119: 796–798

Yamauchi Y, Suzuki J, Sakai J, Sakamoto S, Iwasaki T, Usui M (2007) A case of hypertensive keratouveitis with endotheliitis associated with cytomegalovirus. Ocular Immunol Inflamm 15: 399–401

# Suspected Epstein–Barr Virus (EBV) Disease of the Anterior Segment

Chapter 5

*Thomas Reinhard*

## Core Messages

- EBV specific antibodies (IgG) are found in the majority of healthy subjects and are therefore no direct evidence for presumed EBV etiology of eye disease.
- Since EBV DNA can also be found in healthy eyes, detection of its genome in eye fluids and tissues is not more than a hint at suspected EBV eye disease.
- Diagnosis of EBV caused eye disease is justified, if ocular symptoms and signs are observed in the acute phase of *primary* EBV disease together with EBV specific IgM antibodies.
- Diagnosis of *recurrent* EBV eye disease is far more equivocal. If in a case of "atypical herpes keratitis", e.g., only EBV specific antibodies are found and no antibodies against herpes simplex virus (HSV), varicella zoster virus (VZV), and cytomegaly virus (CMV), and if in addition a positive PCR proves the presence of EBV DNA in the disease area, then a causal role for EBV can be assumed with sufficient probability. Such a case is described.
- For therapy of deep recurrent EBV disease of the anterior segment of the eye, a combination of acyclovir (ACV) plus steroids is recommended.

## 5.1 General Pathophysiology and Epidemiology

Epstein–Barr virus primary infection leads to productive infection of cells especially in the oropharynx and nonproductive (latent) infection of circulating lymphocytes. Endogenous recurrences of disease seem to occur in various tissues. Productive as well as latently infected cells are detectable in healthy carriers. Like the other human herpes viruses, EBV causes a spectrum of inflammatory diseases following primary infection, presumably also via endogenous recurrences. As a specialty, EBV is involved in the pathogenesis of lymphoproliferative and other tumors, specifically endemic Burkitt's lymphoma and nasopharyngeal carcinoma. An association with Sjörgen's syndrome has also been suggested.

The primary infection with EBV leads to a virus carrier state (latency) that persists for a lifetime. Up to 85% of children have antibodies already by age four, and 82% of college students and military cadets in the United States were found positive for anti-EBV IgG.

In the acute primary phase, the hematologic picture consists of leukocytosis with more than 50% mononuclear cells and at least 10% atypical lymphocytes with a peak during the second week of illness. Then, fever, sore throat, and lymphadenopathy with frequent enlargement of spleen and liver are seen. Prodromal symptoms are chills, sweats, anorexia, malaise, headache, arthralgia, and myalgia. Presumed recurrent EBV disease in later life lacks all these acute phase signs and symptoms and is difficult to suspect and diagnose.

## 5.2 Laboratory Diagnosis

According to the widespread infection throughout the population, EBV specific IgG antibodies are frequently found. Primary infection with EBV leads to antibody formation against viral capsid antigen, early antigen and membrane antigen, followed weeks to months later by a serologic response to EBV nuclear antigen. Diagnosis of EBV disease of the eye can be easily made in the course of *primary infection* by demonstrating acute phase specific antiviral antibodies (IgM). Enormous diagnostic difficulties arise when *recurrent* EBV disease is suspected. Although PCR of EBV DNA has been well-established, detection of the EBV genome in ocular tissues unfortunately does not sufficiently prove the diagnosis of EBV eye disease. EBV genome was found in seven out of ten healthy eyes from deceased donors, and in five out of ten healthy eyes, it was present in the anterior chamber. This reduces the diagnostic value of positive PCR findings in the eye considerably and calls for additional diagnostic support, if a suspicion of EBV disease is to be substantiated. The most convincing additional finding would be a positive anti-EBV IgG titer in the absence of titers against HSV, VZV, and CMV, excluding the latter viruses from a causal relationship.

## 5.3 Ocular Manifestations

Nearly all reports of ocular and neurological EBV disease refer to the acute phase EBV infection (mononucleosis), i.e., to primary infection. In this situation, the causal role of EBV for general disease and all associated complications is undisputed. Ocular and neurologic complications in this phase are multiple, and their incidence is rare:

- Conjunctivitis with hyperemia and follicular reaction
- Nodular upper tarsal conjunctival mass formation with preauricular and cervical lymphadenopathy
- Dacryoadenitis
- Dendritic keratitis with microdendrites
- Nummular keratitis
- Episcleritis and scleritis
- Anterior uveitis
- Acute chorioidal lesions with yellow infiltrates, ranging in size from 50 to 500 micrometer
- Macular lesions of mostly 50-75 micrometer in diameter accompanied by mild vitritis
- Papilledema, papillitis, optic neuritis
- Ophthalmoplegia
- Facial nerve palsy
- Secondary cataract

All these complications can be easily associated with EBV etiology and they are treated together with general disease anyway. Therefore, they are not further addressed in this atlas.

The main focus of this chapter is: what do the suspected endogenous recurrences of EBV eye disease look like and how can they be treated?

EBV etiology may be suspected in any case of herpes-like eye disease, which is so *atypical* that it cannot be attributed to neither HSV nor VZV etiology.

What is meant by "atypical" is compiled in the following list:

- Insidious onset of disease, start of complaints cannot be defined
- No keratitis nor other eye disease in history, especially no herpes history
- Fairly white eye(s), i.e., rather chronic type of keratitis
- Nummular or similarly looking stromal infiltrates without any history of (adenoviral) conjunctivitis
- No reduction of corneal sensitivity
- Often associated endotheliitic precipitates with endothelial cell edema or frank corneal edema as signs of chronic endotheliitis
- Steroids reduce stromal infiltrates and endotheliitic signs, which may recur after withdrawal of the drug

In a case which fits exactly in the above description of *atypical chronic herpes keratitis* (Fig. 5.1), PCR investigation proved EBV DNA to be present in the aqueous humor, and in addition, antibody screening showed, that HSV, VZV, and CMV could **not** be the causal herpes viruses, but only EBV.

Although even this evidence may be called circumstantial evidence and no scientific proof, it is the best evidence available up to now. This case correctly describes at least one clinical manifestation of recurrent EBV disease in the anterior segment of the eye. Similar observations have already been previously reported. The objective now must be to alert the ophthalmological community to this diagnosis in order to detect and describe the possibly even broader complete spectrum of recurrent EBV eye disease.

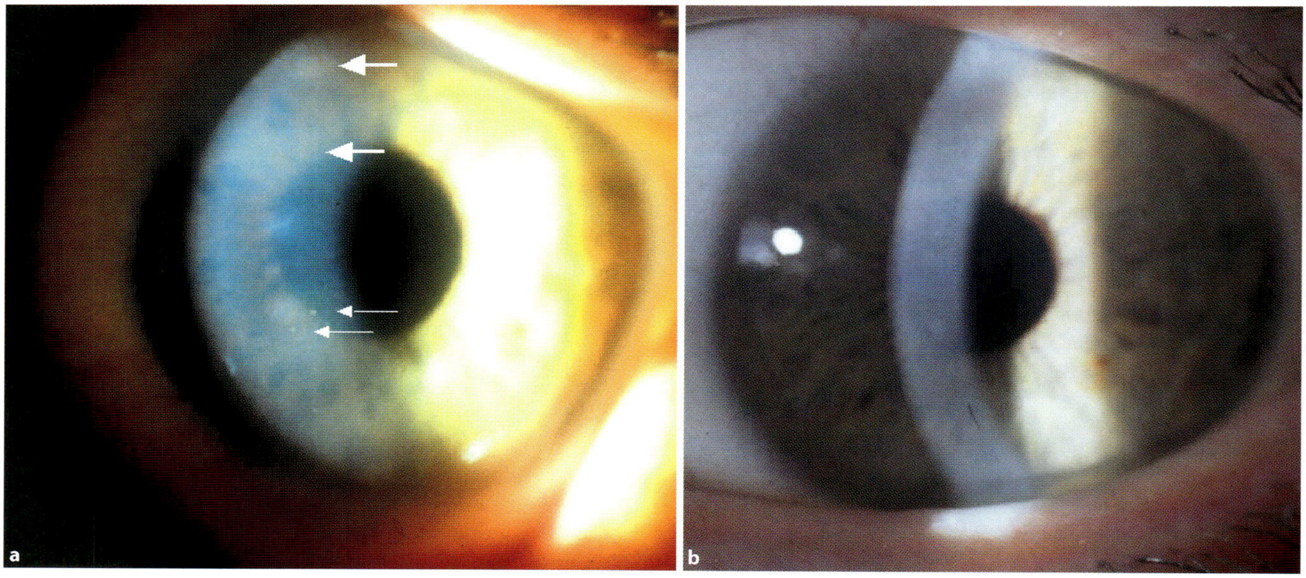


Fig. 5.1 **a** Right cornea of a patient with interstitial infiltrates (*large arrows*) and endotheliitic precipitates (*small arrows*) due to recurrent EBV infection (positive EBV-, but negative HSV-, CMV-, VZV-genome in the anterior chamber; IgG in the blood EBV- positive, and HSV-, CMV-, VZV-negative). **b** Resolution of most inflammatory signs within 4 weeks after topical acyclovir in combination with steroids (from: Reinhard et al., 2003)

## 5.4 Therapy of Recurrent EBV Disease of the Eye

Epstein–Barr virus is susceptible to systemic ACV. Resolution of microdendritic keratitis in the course of *primary infection* has been reported after 2 days of treatment with acyclovir. For stromal keratitis as a clinical manifestation of *endogenously recurring EBV disease*, the same therapeutic principles should hold true as for recurrent deep HSV and VZV disease, namely the principle of a combination therapy with an antiviral agent (ACV) plus steroids. Whether a topical combination therapy suffices in adequate cases, or whether a systemic combination therapy is to be preferred for terminating chronic recurrent EBV disease, remains to be seen. For theoretical pathogenetic reasons, a monotherapy with steroids should not be optimal.

## References


Alspaugh MA, Jensen FC, Rabin H, Tan EM (1987) Lymphocytes transformed by Epstein–Barr virus. Induction of nuclear antigen reactive with antibody in rheumatoid arthritis. J Exp Med 147: 1018–1027

Bernstein TC, Wolfe HG (1950) Involvement of the nervous system in enfectious mononucleosis. Ann Int Med 33: 1120–1138

Codosh J, Gan YJ, Sixbey JW (1996) Detection of Epstein–Barr virus genome in ocular tissue. Ophthalology 103: 687–690

Davie JC, Ceballos R, Little SC (1963) Infectious mononucleosis with fatal neuronitis. Arch Neurol 9: 265–272

Evans AS, Niederman JC, Genabre LC, West B, Richards VA (1975) A prospective evaluation of heterophile and Epstein–Barr virus-specific lgM antibody tests in clinical and subclinical infectious mononucleosis: specificity and sensitivity of the tests and persistence of antibody. J Infect Dis 132: 546–554

Grose C, Henle W, Henle G, Feorino PM (1975) Primary Epstein–Barr virus infections in acute neurologic diseases. New Eng J Med 292: 392–395

Henle W, Henle G (1970) Observation in childhood infections with the Epstein–Barr virus. J Infect. Dis 121: 303–310

Henle W, Henle G (1981) Serodiagnosis of infectious mononucleosis. Resident Staff Physician 27: 37–43

Horwitz CA, Henle W, Henle G, Rudnick H, Latts E (1985) Long-term serologic follow-up of patients for Epstein–Barr virus after recovery from infectious mononucleosis. J Infect Dis 151: 1150–1153

Jones BR, Howie JB, Wilson RP (1952) Ocular aspects of an epidemic of infectious moninucleosis. Proc. Univ Otago Med Sch 30: 1–4

Karpe G, Wising P (1948) Retinal changes with acute reduction of vision as initial symptoms of infectious mononucleosis. Acta Ophthalmol 26: 19–24

Librach IM (1956) Ocular symptoms in glandular fever. Br J Ophthalmol 40: 619–621

Matoba AY, Jones DB (1987) Corneal subepithelial infiltrates associated with systemic Epstein–Barr viral infection. Ophthalmology 94: 1669–1671

Matoba AY (1990) Review in Medicine: Ocular Disease Associatad with Epstein–Barr virus infection. Survey Ophtal 35: 145–150

Matoba AY, Wilhelmus KR, Jones DB (1986) Epstein–Barr viral stromal keratitis. Ophthalmology 93: 746–751

Meisler DM, Bosworth DE, Krachmer JH (1981) Ocular infectious mononucleosis manifested as Parinaud´s oculoglandular syndrome. Am J Ophthalmol 92: 722–726

Nelhaus G (1966) Isolated oculomotor nerve palsy in infectious mononucleosis: Neurology 16: 221–224

Oertel SH, Riess H (2002) Antiviral treatment of Epstein–Barr virus-associated lymphoproliferations. Rec Results Cancer Res 159: 89–95

Payrau P, Höel J (1958) Mononucleose infectieuse et kératite. Bull Soc Ophthalmol Fr 5-6: 381–384

Pflugfelder SC, Crouse CA, Atherton SS (1993) Ophthalmic manifestations of Epstein–Barr virus infection. Int Ophthalmol Vis Sci 33: 95–101

Pflugfelder SC, Crouse CA, Pereira I, Atherton SS (1990) Amplification of Epstein–Barr virus genomic sequences in blood cells, lacrimal glands, and tears from primary Sjögren´s syndrome patients. Ophthalmology 97: 976–984

Pflugfelder SC, Roessel TJ, Culbertson WW (1987) Primary Sjogjen´s syndrome after infectious mononucleosis. JAMA 257: 1049–1050

Pinnolis M, McCulley JP (1980) Nummular keratitis associated with infectious mononucleosis. Am J Ophthalmol 89: 791–794

Raymond LA, Wilson CA, Linnemann Jr CC, Ward MA, Bernstein DI, Love DC (1987) Punctate outer retinitis in acute Epstein–Barr virus infection. Am J Ophthalmol 104: 424–426

Reinhard T, Adams O, Sundmacher R (2003) Detection of the Epstein–Barr virus genome in the anterior chamber of a patient with chronic keratouveitis. Acta Ophthalmol Scand 81: 671–673

Rohrbach JM, Körber SM, Teufel T, Kortmann RD, Zierhut M (2004) EBV-induced polymorphic lymphoproliferative disorder of the iris after heart transplantation. Albrecht von Graefes Arch Clin Exp Ophthalmol 242: 44–50

Shaw EB (1950) Infectious mononucleosis of the central nervous system with bilateral papilledema. J Pediatr 37: 661–665

Tanner OR (1952) Ocular manifestations of infectious mononucleosis. Arch Opthalmol 51: 229–241

Usui MJ, Sakai J (1990) Three cases of Epstein–Barr virus-associated uveitis. Int Ophthalmol 4: 371–376

Wilhelmus KR (1981) Ocular involvement in infectious mononucleosis. Am J Ophthalmol 89: 117–118

Wong KW, D´Amico DJ, Hedges III TR, Soong HK, Schooley RT, Kenyon KR (1987) Ocular involvement associated with chronic Epstein–Barr virus disease. Arch Ophthalmol 105: 788–792

Wong KW, D´Amico DJ, Hedges III TR, et al. (1989) Ocular involvement associated with chronic Epstein–Barr virus infections. Br J Ophthalmol 73: 1002–1003

Yao QY, Rickinson AB, Epstein MA (1985) A re-examination of the Epstein–Barr virus carrier state in healthy seropositive individuals. Int J Cancer 35: 35–40

# Diseases of the Posterior Segment by HSV, VZV, and CMV

*Lutz L. Hansen*

Chapter

6

## 6.1 Epidemiology and Pathogenesis

Posterior herpes disease is rare in immunocompetent patients, yet it occurs in up to 40% of individuals with late stages of human immune deficiency virus (HIV) infection with severe immune suppression, and is then almost exclusively caused by the cytomegalovirus (CMV). It then follows, that the posterior part of the eye is much more often infected by the β subgroup of herpes viruses (CMV) than by α-herpes viruses (HSV, VZV). CMV retinitis is currently one of the most frequent single causes of posterior infection, at least in regions with high incidence of HIV, and with no access to modern antiretroviral treatment.

Posterior herpetic uveitis usually evolves by the endogenous reactivation of latent infection, but primary infection has also been described. Primary *manifestation* (i.e., first observed clinical disease, although the virus had already been present before latently) seldom occurs with HSV and VZV, but is often observed in conjunction with CMV. With HSV and VZV, clinical disease in the posterior segment develops when the virus, which is harbored within the central nervous system, spreads along the optic nerve fibers via retrograde axonal transport. The less neurotropic CMV, which can be acquired by blood and mucosal contact seems to be propagated by leukocyte associated viremia (monocytes, neutrophils). The lifelong persistent CMV is only reactivated in severely immuno-compromised individuals.

Patients with HSV or VZV infection often have a history of cutaneous or systemic infection, such as dermatomal zoster or herpetic encephalitis. The disease can also be triggered by various stimuli, such as neurosurgery, periocular trauma, epidural steroids, and immune suppression.

Virus-specific and host factors both define the course of the disease. Healthy (HSV, VZV) as well as immuno-compromised hosts (CMV, HSV, VZV) may be affected, but *typically* patients with HSV infection are immunocompetent. In patients with VZV infection, immune defects are suspected, but not always identifiable. CMV-infection definitely occurs only in severe immunodeficiency. Most forms of herpetic posterior uveitis are acute and fulminant, often resulting in serious complications. Milder chronic and less destructive forms of posterior uveitis are less common. Tissue destruction depends on a direct cytopathic effect, the secondary immune response, and occlusive vasculitis.

## 6.2 Phenotypic Clinical Features

Posterior herpetic disease is primarily classified by its *phenotypic* clinical appearance. One differentiates between *herpetic retinitis* (mild or moderate) and two severe, rapidly progressing forms, *acute retinal necrosis (ARN)* and *progressive outer retinal necrosis (PORN)*. Each of these three clinical forms can be caused with a certain probability by one or several herpes viruses (see Sect. 6.3: Virus Specific Features).

### 6.2.1 Herpetic Retinitis

Per definition, this clinical entity encompasses all diseases that are *not* characterized as acute retinal necrosis (ARN) *and not* as progressive outer retinal necrosis (PORN). Such a definition "per exclusionem" is a rarity in medicine and shows how difficult is the classification of herpetic posterior eye disease. Herpetic retinitis is very rarely seen with HSV or VZV infection. It is mostly CMV disease with a broad spectrum of courses ranging from mild retinochoroidopathy without much impact on visual ability (*i. e., non-necrotizing herpetic posterior uveitis*) to severe and devastating forms that may result in blindness *(necrotizing herpetic retinitis)*. Starting in one eye, it usually becomes bilateral within weeks or months if not adequately treated.

*Necrotizing herpetic retinitis* (Figs. 6.1 to 6.12) is characterized by white patches or areas of opacification, sometimes confluent, and more or less demarcated from the healthy retinal tissue (Figs. 6.1, 6.2c, 6.3a, 6.6a). These patches can start everywhere in the fundus without preference. Retinal hemorrhages are typically interposed between these patches, but can also occur as separate deep dot-and-blot bleedings, or as flame-shaped bleedings in the nerve fiber layer (Fig. 6.7). Vascular sheathing may be prominent but is not mandatory.

The optic nerve head may be involved in form of an isolated papillitis or in conjunction with retinal foci around the papilla. The concomitant inflammation of the vitreous and of the anterior part of the eye may vary widely leaving the view on the fundus ranging between unhampered and impeded, depending on the grade of cellular reaction which reflects the immunologic status of the host.

*Non-necrotizing herpetic posterior uveitis* is an uncommon form occurring in conjunction with herpetic infections of the α-subgroup (HSV, VZV). Few cases of acute chorioretinitis, multifocal chorioditis, and even choroidal granulomas have been described, and herpetic DNA has been found in idiopathic posterior uveitis cases like birdshot-like retinopathy and bilateral retinal vasculitis.

### 6.2.2 Acute Retinal Necrosis (ARN)

ARN (Figs. 6.13 to 6.17) is a relatively young entity in ophthalmology, first described in 1971 by Uruyama. It was initially seen only in immunocompetent patients, but we now know that it can also occur in immunocompromised patients. This phenotype of severe necrotizing retinitis can mostly be assigned to VZV, much less frequently to HSV, and seldom to CMV. It may occur without prodromi of cutaneous or systemic herpetic disease. Starting in one eye, the second eye may be affected in up to 70% of cases even years later. Adequate treatment of the first eye seems to be important for preventing outbreak of the ARN in the second eye.

Histopathological features of active ARN include diffuse necrotizing retinitis, occlusive vasculitis, optic neuritis, and papillitis associated with chronic panuveitis and characterized by dense plasmalymphocytic infiltration.

*Symptoms* in the acute phase consist of ocular discomfort (especially on eye movement) progressing to pain. Photophobia may ensue, floaters annoy the patient, and vision becomes blurred.

*Clinical findings* comprise a concomitant granulomatous iridocyclitis with large, granulomatous keratitic precipitates (Fig. 6.14a), cells, and flare in the anterior chamber, and cells in the vitreous (Fig. 6.14b). Intraocular pressure may be raised. Additional scleritis may enhance the redness of the eye.

Early affection of the retina is characterized by round or oval deep, yellow-white lesions with scalloped edges (Fig. 6.13a). These lesions usually start in the periphery and may be easily overlooked, misleading the clinician to diagnose anterior uveitis only. The patches spread peripherally and circumferentially over several days leading to large areas of retinal necrosis (Figs. 6.15–17). The necrotic lesions spare the posterior pole for the most part. Hemorrhages are less prominent than in herpetic retinitis. Arteriolitis and phlebitis complete the funduscopical aspect. Sometimes the feature of "cracked mud" appears (Fig. 6.17), caused by readily visible larger vessels within the white retinal necrosis. Mild optic edema is usually present and a relative afferent pupillary defect may indicate optic nerve involvement.

Later in the course, severe vitritis may obscure the retina. The retinitis starts to regress (usually within 4–5 days after beginning of antiviral treatment) from the leading edge, from around the venules, and from within the lesion, giving a "swiss cheese" appearance. The sloughing of retinal debris into the vitreous body worsens the vitritis, leaving holes in the peripheral retina which lead to retinal detachment after four to eight weeks in 75% of cases, even in patients with antiviral treatment. Fine salt-and-pepper pigmentation develops in areas of atrophic retina. Good vision may be maintained after prompt and vigorous therapy. However, most patients lose sight by smoldering progression of the retinopathy or optic neuropathy and vascular occlusion.

### 6.2.3 Progressive Outer Retinal Necrosis (PORN)

PORN was first described by Forster as a very severe variant of necrotizing retinitis in patients with AIDS. This devastating form apparently starts in the outer retinal layers and very quickly spreads out to whole thickness retinal disease. The degree of chorioretinal inflammation is less than one would expect from such profound necrosis. The causing agents seem to be HSV and VZV in severely immunocompromised patients.

*Clinical findings*. The painless loss of vision within days and without precursors is typical, and allows a differentiation to ARN.

The anterior chamber shows a minimal, non-granulomatous anterior chamber inflammatory reaction and no vitritis. A clear view on the fundus reveals one or more areas of retinitis in the posterior pole and mid-retina (Fig. 6.18a) without hemorrhages. The retinitis progressively spreads outwardly, often becoming confluent and involving the entire retina within a couple of days (Fig. 6.18b), even faster than in ARN. Retinal vasculopathy may be visible adjacent to the lesions. Bilaterality is observed in more than 70% of cases and it usually occurs within weeks or even simultaneously.

The devastating course to blindness can only seldom be impeded because of limited responsiveness to antiviral agents.

## 6.3 Virus Specific Features

### 6.3.1 Herpes Simplex Virus (HSV)

***HSV retinitis.*** is a rare disease and may vary from strain to strain. It comprises necrotizing and non-necrotizing herpes retinitis. History often reveals encephalitis weeks or years before the onset of retinal disease.

Retinal whitening, vascular occlusion, and papilledema have been described. The white necrotic lesions are less dense and fluffy than in CMV-retinitis, and inner retinal bleedings seem to be less frequent (Fig. 6.1), sometimes even absent.

***ARN syndrome***. While most ARN syndromes are associated with VZV, few culture-proven cases of HSV-associated ARN have also been published, and PCR of vitreous tap in ARN also revealed HSV-DNA. Early start of ocular pain with concomitant anterior inflammation may indicate HSV-associated ARN. Exsudative detachment appears more often than in VZV-induced ARN.

To the best of my knowledge, ***PORN syndrome*** has not been reported in conjunction with HSV infection.

### 6.3.2 Varicella Zoster Virus (VZV)

***VZV retinitis.*** has only been described as a mild, self-limiting form that develops rarely during chickenpox, mostly in adults and extremely seldom in children.

*ARN syndrome.* The cause of ARN is overwhelmingly VZV, and becomes even more probable if a history of chicken pox or cutaneous zoster is known. VZV-induced ARN may occasionally develop also before the outbreak of cutaneous zoster. In *immuno-compromised* patients, almost all cases are preceded by one or more episodes of shingles. Although, profound immunosuppression is not a pre-condition for VZV-induced ARN, the disease may be associated with a decline in cell-mediated immunity in general. General unspecific immunity tests usually give normal results pretending immunocompetence. An inverse relation between declining VZV-specific cellular immunity and an increase of VZV-associated diseases raises the possibility, however, of diminished or impaired cell-mediated immunity.

Symptoms and findings are described above, and no specific findings enable us to reliably discern between HSV and VZV as the causative agent. Both eyes are ultimately affected in 24–80% of cases.

*PORN syndrome* is apparently nearly always caused by VZV in patients with AIDS. It may be difficult to distinguish it from CMV retinitis, especially in the beginning. Multifocality, a lack of granular appearance, absence of extensive retinal hemorrhages, and an extremely rapid spread indicate VZV-induced PORN.

### 6.3.3 Cytomegalovirus (CMV)

***Pathogenesis and epidemiology.*** CMV differs from VZV and HSV in several aspects. It has less affinity to neural cells, and is disseminated by the bloodstream via monocytes and neutrophils. When CMV disease develops, viremia is always present. As with all herpes viruses, once infected with CMV, one carries the virus for life. It becomes dormant in a latent stage in leucocytes, from where it is reactivated if the cellular immunity becomes severely affected in immunocompromised patients. Humoral immunity is not involved in latency control. The retina is the main target organ, accounting for 75–85% of CMV-related disease, followed by the gastrointestinal tract, lung, and central nervous system.

Virions enter the target cells via endocytosis, probably facilitated by dendritic antigen-presenting cells. Replication of the virus in endothelial cells of the retinal vasculature compromises the retina-blood barrier. This facilitates the access of virions to glial and neural cells and thus the speed of the disease spread. Histopathologically, the lesions shows necrosis and bleedings in all retinal layers. Staining for CMV-specific antigens suggests that the infection progresses from the retinal vasculature horizontally through glial cells and vertically through Mueller cells, leading to full thickness necrosis.

*CMV retinitis* is by far the most frequent form of herpetic posterior disease. It occurs only in severely immunocompromised patients. The retinitis usually starts in one eye, but when it is finally detected, it is often already bilateral. About 50% of patients show no symptoms when retinitis first becomes apparent, since many lesions start from the periphery or mid-retina. As the eye is white and quiescent without view-impeding anterior or vitreous cells, the patient is unaware of his serious disease until the macula or the optic nerve become involved. Once a CMV-lesion has appeared, it usually doubles in area within one month.

The CMV lesion has several characteristic features that facilitate a correct clinical diagnosis in conjunction with the obligatory compromised immunocompetence. Four patterns are discernable: (1) a predominantly hemorraghic lesion (Figs. 6.6c, 6.7, 6.9), (2) a granular lesion (mostly peripheral retina) with few bleedings (Figs. 6.4, 6.5), a central atrophic area, and surrounding punctate satellite lesions, (3) a brushfire lesion, presenting a yellowish-white margin progressing to a sound retina and leaving a necrotic center (Figs. 6.10, 6.11). Less frequent is (4) the exudative form of "frosted branch angiitis" (Fig. 6.8). This classification is somewhat arbitrary, as several forms may appear concurrently. The progressive cause can only be stopped by improvement of the immunological situation (increase of CD4 cells above 200/μl), or by adequate antiviral CMV-treatment.

*ARN syndrome* is very atypical for CMV. It does not differ clinically from the VZV- and HSV-induced forms.

*PORN syndrome*, which only occurs in AIDS patients, is mostly induced by VZV in combination with CMV.

### 6.3.4 Epstein–Barr Virus (EBV)

There have been reports of chronic EBV infection in conjunction with posterior segment disease. Panuveitis with vitritis and macular edema, as well as multifocal choroiditis have been described. However, the etiology of EBV for these diseases is difficult to prove unequivocally, and posterior segment EBV diseases have thus remained controversially debated (see Chap. 5).

## 6.4 Diagnosis and Differential Diagnosis

Diagnosis and differentiation of herpetic posterior disease depends largely on the history and the lesions clinical appearance. In the presence of obvious immunoincompetence, CMV is by far the most probable causing agent. Thus, every effort should be made to detect HIV infection or any other type of immune suppression, so as not to bypass timely and appropriate treatment. Table 6.1 gives an overview on the differential diagnosis of herpetic posterior disease.

Since we are dealing with ubiquitous viruses, which persist in their host, antibody screening is of limited value. If we find a positive titer, it only tells us that this virus is present in the host. It gives us no information as to its potential etiologic role. If we have "negative" findings and do *not* find antibody titers against a certain herpes virus, then this virus can be excluded from

Table 6.1 Differential diagnosis of herpetic posterior disease

| Sign, disease | Immuno-competence | Findings | Additional examinations |
|---|---|---|---|
| Herpetic retinitis (CMV) | AIDS, CD4 ≤ 100/ml | – Grey-white flecks, slight or no vitritis<br>– Laminar bleedings<br>– "Cottage cheese and ketchup" | PCR from vitreous tap |
| Herpetic retinitis (HSV) | Normal | – Like CMV-retinitis (very seldom)<br>– Vitritis more pronounced than in CMV retinitis | PCR from vitreous tap |
| Acute retinal necrosis (VZV) | Normal, AIDS CD4 ≤ 60/ml | – Yellow white, confluent, starting peripherally<br>– Strong vitritis<br>– Rapid course<br>– Deep pain | PCR from vitreous tap |
| Progressive outer retinal necrosis (HSV, VZV) | AIDS CD4 ≤ 10/ml | – Yellow white, multifocal, starting centrally<br>– Only slight vitritis<br>– Very rapid course, early retinal detachment<br>– No pain | PCR from vitreous tap |
| Single cotton-wool-spots | Ischemic retinopathy, HIV-infection | – Fluffy, white, slightly prominent<br>– Late: granulated, silvery | FA: capillary occlusion |
| Branch vein occlusion | Normal | – Flecks are less extended<br>– Retinal vein engorgement<br>– Flame-shaped retinal bleedings | FA: black vein sign |
| Toxoplasmic retinochorioiditis | Normal<br>AIDS, CD4 ≤ 400/ml | – Grey-white, slightly prominent lesions<br>– Often solitary, seldom bleedings<br>– Strong vitritis | MRT (CNS-foci) |
| Candida-albicans vitreoretinitis | Normal<br>AIDS CD4 ≤ 400/ml | – White, prominent lesion, slightly anterior to retina<br>– Balls of vitritis | Serology, blood culture |
| Cryptococcosis | Final AIDS, GVHD | – Yellow, subretinal lesions<br>– Papilledema | CT, neurologist |
| Lues | Normal<br>HIV-infection | – Small white lesions<br>– Neuroretinitis | Serology, anterior uveitis |
| Ocular Non-Hodgkin Lymphoma | Normal | – Grey-white lesions, sometimes extended<br>– Moderate to strong vitritis with typical cell conglomerates | CT, neurologist |

Abreviations: CD4 = number of CD4-lymphocytes per mikroliter blood, CT = Computertomography, FA = fluoresceine angiographie, HIV = human immunedeficency virus, MRT = magnetic resonance tomography, PCR = polymerase chain reaction

the suspect list, and such knowledge may indeed help in the diagnosis and thus have a relative value. In ambiguous cases, mostly of ARN and PORN, a vitreous or anterior chamber tap will help to find DNA of the responsible virus and thus facilitate selection of the optimal antiviral drugs.

## 6.5 Therapy

### 6.5.1 General Guidelines

The goals of treatment in acute viral retinitis are: (1) arresting active viral infection in the retina, (2) preventing contralateral spread to the second eye, (3) minimizing secondary inflammatory intraocular damage, and (4) preventing and/or treating retinal detachment.

More or less specific drugs are available for all the herpes viruses that cause posterior disease. These drugs have been developed from acyclovir and ganciclovir, which were originally only applicable via intravenous administration. Two additional antiviral substances are used to treat CMV: foscarnet and cidofovir.

Nowadays, there are several other treatment modalities for derivatives of acyclovir and ganciclovir, including oral and intraocular delivery. Nevertheless, the low bioavailabilty of the oral drugs (acyclovir: valacyclovir, famciclovir; ganciclovir: valganciclovir) makes them still inferior to the intravenous route. Hence, the seriousness of the disease must be taken into account when considering oral therapy.

The retinis should begin to regress within three to 5 days

after initiation of the treatment. However, complete regression can often take over a month and highlight the need for long maintenance therapy.

Steroids should be applied with reservation and restricted to patients with strong vitritis, but should never be used in patients with immunodeficiency.

### 6.5.2 Herpetic Retinitis

If not occurring in immunocompromised patients, retinitis is best treated with aciclovir and its derivatives according to severity of the disease. Vigorous intravenous treatment with aciclovir (10 mg/kg 3 times daily for 5–10 days) is required when the macula is threatened. This is followed by oral aciclovir (5 × 800 mg/d) or the equivalent dosage of the derivatives famciclovir or valaciclovir. This treatment should be at least maintained for one year to prevent recurrences and bilateral disease. Whether lesions not threatening the macula can be treated using oral therapy alone is not known.

### 6.5.3 Cytomegalovirus Retinitis

The treatment of CMV retinitis depends on the state of the host. The following parameters must be taken into account: CD4 count, state of antiretroviral treatment, nonretinal CMV disease, an endangered macula, and the state of the second eye. The treatment effect is usually apparent within one week, leading to the disappearance of the fluffy white lesions which are replaced by an atrophic retina with a salt-and-pepper aspect. (Fig. 6.12a–c)

*Induction and Maintenance Therapy.* Treatment is best started with 5–7.5 mg ganciclovir/kg/d for 2–3 weeks followed by 5 mg/kg/d maintenance 5 d/wk. The last dose must be reduced in patients with renal failure, neutropenia, or thrombocytopenia. If CMV retinitis is reactivated during the maintenance phase, induction therapy must be repeated.

The second choice for induction is foscarnet, which is equally effective and reduces mortality in AIDS patients, but is nephrotoxic and requires more frequent infusions (induction 90 mg/kg/d twice a day for 2–3 weeks, followed by once a day as maintenance). Since its antiretroviral effect is beside the point ever since the introduction of highly active antiretroviral treatment (HAART), it is only used in patients with ganciclovir resistance.

Cidofovir is the third choice. Its efficacy is equal to that of ganciclovir and the patients need fewer infusions, which in turn makes this drug less discomforting (maintenance biweekly iv administration of 3–5 mg/kg). However, adverse reactions limit its use. In addition to the main side effects of nephrotoxicity and uveitis, cidofovir may lead to irreversible ocular hypotony.

*Alternative Therapy.* Intravitreal application of ganciclovir by injection (2 × 400 mg/week) or with an intravitreal implant is useful in patients with monocular diease and without CMV disease elsewhere when HAART has started but is still not fully effective. In such cases, it may be combined with oral valganciclovir to reduce the CMV viremia. The bioavailability of this derivative is too low for induction therapy.

Formivirsen is a new alternative in patients with multiresistant CMV strains. This antisense oligonucleotide can only be applied via intravitreal injection and may have considerable side effects in the eye (anterior and posterior uveitis, macular toxicity).

### 6.5.4 Acute Retinal Necrosis

*Immunocompetent patients* or those with only minor immunologic abnormalities should undergo intravenous aciclovir therapy (10–15 mg/kg/d for 5–10 days). After a response to antiviral treatment, a switch to oral aciclovir (800 mg five times daily) is suggested. This should be continued for at least three months, but some specialists recommend even longer periods lasting years. Newer drugs with a better bioavailabilty (valaciclovir, famciclovir) may replace aciclovir as oral treatment. It is important to emphasize that the risk of involvement of the fellow eye decreases with aciclovir, although a third of the patients remain at risk for a second eye infection.

In refractory cases, intravitreal antiviral therapy should be considered in conjunction with intravenous ganclovir and a vitreous tap for PCR studies.

Anti-inflammatory therapy suppresses intraocular inflammation and improves vitreous opacity. However, corticosteroids should be administered concomitantly (prednisone 1–2 mg/kg/d), and only after initiation of antiviral therapy. Tapering is recommended over 2–6 weeks.

Prophylactic laser coagulation has been recommended to prevent retinal detachment and may reduce its rate, but repeat treatments may be necessary because retinitis may still progress.

*Immunodeficient patients* seldom develop ARN. The cases reported so far were all AIDS patients, hence, a CMV infection should be suspected, prompting primary therapy with intravenous ganciclovir, as described above.

### 6.5.5 Progressive Outer Retinal Necrosis

PORN has only been described in patients with AIDS so far. Thus, it always includes the possibility of zoster virus and cytomegalovirus involvement. The suspicion of PORN ("indolent ARN" in severely immunodepressed patients) requires immediate systemic treatment with aciclovir and ganciclovir in doses as described above. A vitreous tap to detect the virus DNA should also be performed. Ganciclovir can be intravitreally injected at the same time (400 mg). If the patient has already undergone one course of ganciclovir treatment and a resistance is suspected, formivirsen should be attempted intravitreally. However, the prognosis remains very poor even after a prompt treatment.

### 6.5.6 Retinal Detachment

Antiviral therapy does not affect the frequency of retinal detachment. These detachments are characterized by large, relatively posterior breaks, as well as a high prevalence of vitreous traction and proliferative vitreoretinopathy. Some specialists recommend to apply a retinal barrier photocoagulation so long as the hazy vitreous does not prevent an adequate view of the fundus. Retrospective, non-controlled studies suggest a lower incidence of detachment among treated patients.

However, owing to the presence of multiple, posterior, ill-defined breaks associated with vitritis, the standard approach for patients with ARN, PORN, and necrotizing herpetic retinitis is *pars plana* vitrectomy with silicone oil tamponade. Only in quiescent CMV retinitis with retinal detachment may gas tamponade and laser coagulation suffice. Despite rates of anatomic success of 88–100%, final vision may be limited by optical atrophy or macular involvement.

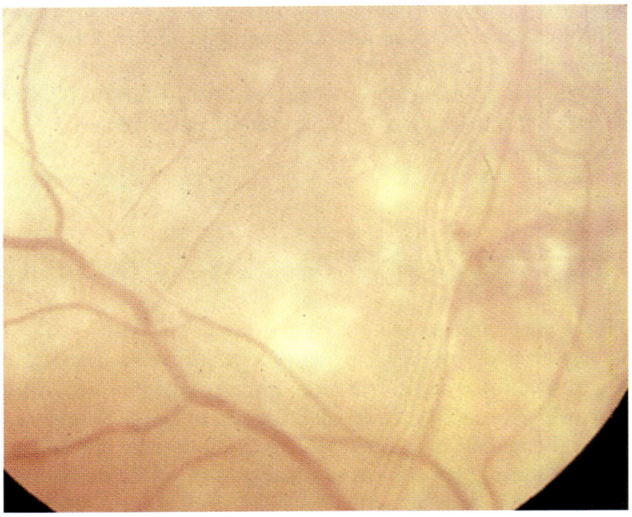

Fig. 6.1 Herpetic retinitis in a 35-year-old patient with AIDS and generalized HSV-infection. Subtle and poorly defined white patches with small satellite lesions and blood in the inner retina

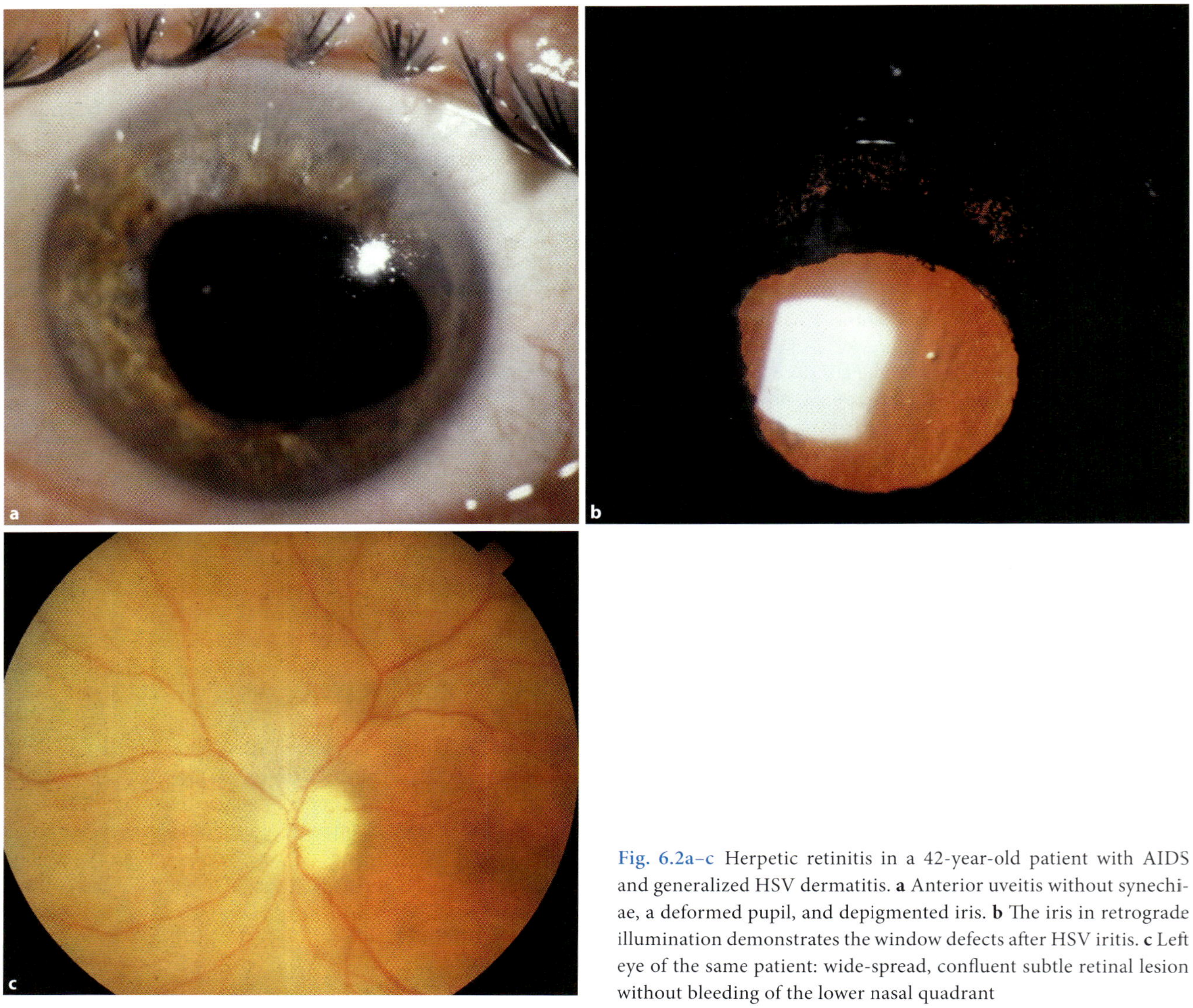


Fig. 6.2a–c Herpetic retinitis in a 42-year-old patient with AIDS and generalized HSV dermatitis. **a** Anterior uveitis without synechiae, a deformed pupil, and depigmented iris. **b** The iris in retrograde illumination demonstrates the window defects after HSV iritis. **c** Left eye of the same patient: wide-spread, confluent subtle retinal lesion without bleeding of the lower nasal quadrant

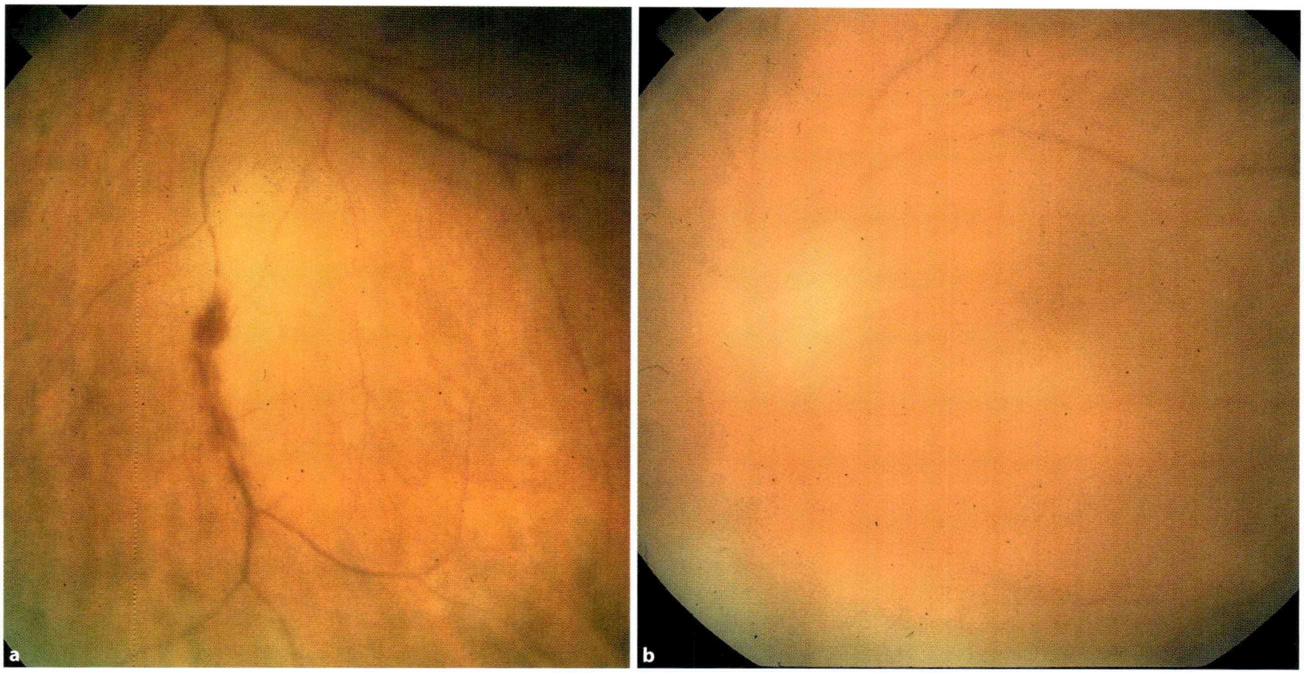

Fig. 6.3 **a** Suspected herpetic retinitis in a 54-year-old patient without signs of immunoincompetence. Poorly defined white lesion with overlying inflamed blood vessel and superficial bleeding. **b** Same patient 11 days later: signs of acute retinal necrosis have developed with considerable vitritis and confluent white lesions. The necrotic retinitis responded well to treatment with aciclovir. VZV was suspected as the inducing agent

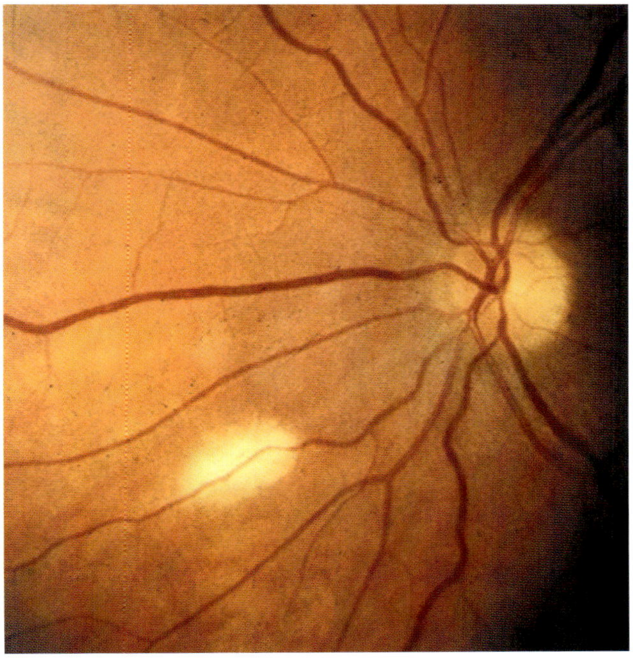

Fig. 6.4 CMV retinitis in a 38-year-old patient with AIDS. Clear view of the fundus reveals a small granular lesion without bleeding

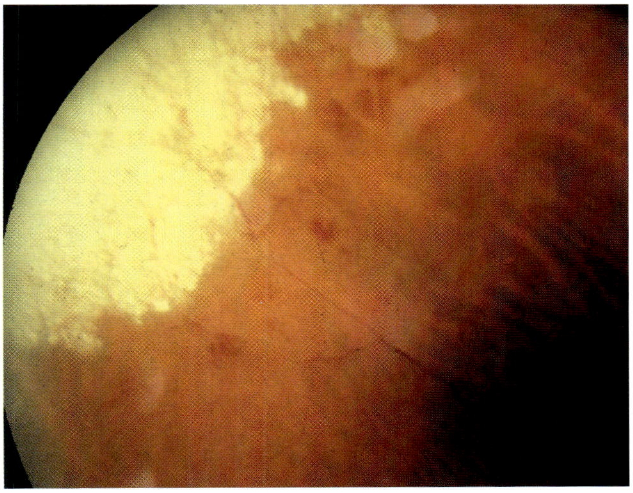

Fig. 6.5 CMV retinitis in a 43-year-old patient with AIDS without visual symptoms. Typical peripheral granular lesion and retinal bleedings at the central border. Clear view of the fundus

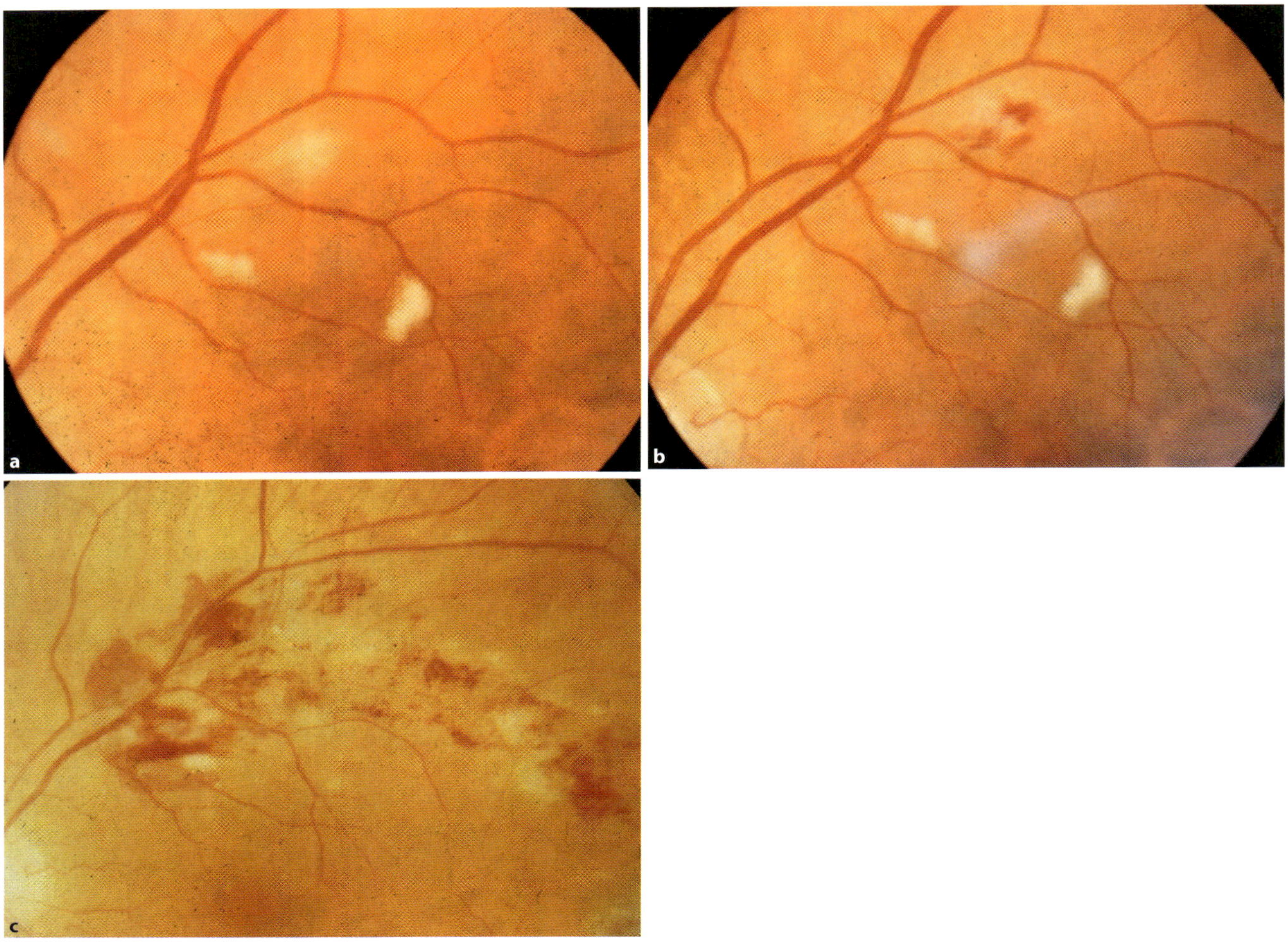

Fig. 6.6a–c CMV retinitis in a 32-year-old man. Development within 70 days without treatment. **a** Fresh CMV-lesion less than 7 days old. The subtle feathery lesion can easily be distinguished from two centrally located cotton wool spots. **b** Same lesion one week later: first bleedings have appeared, cotton wool spots are unchanged. **c** Same lesion after ten weeks: enlargement, still active lesion without scarring, cotton wool spots have disappeared

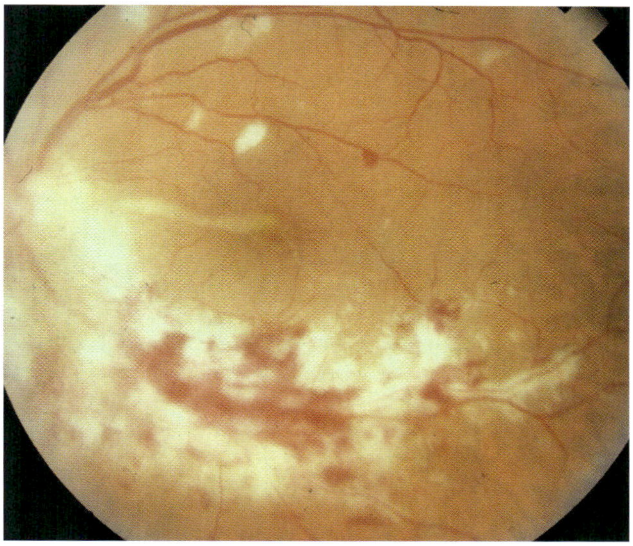

Fig. 6.7 CMV retinitis in a 40-year-old patient with AIDS. Typical central lesion ("cottage cheese with ketchup") with necrotic patches, vasculitis, superficial bleedings, and edema endangering the fovea

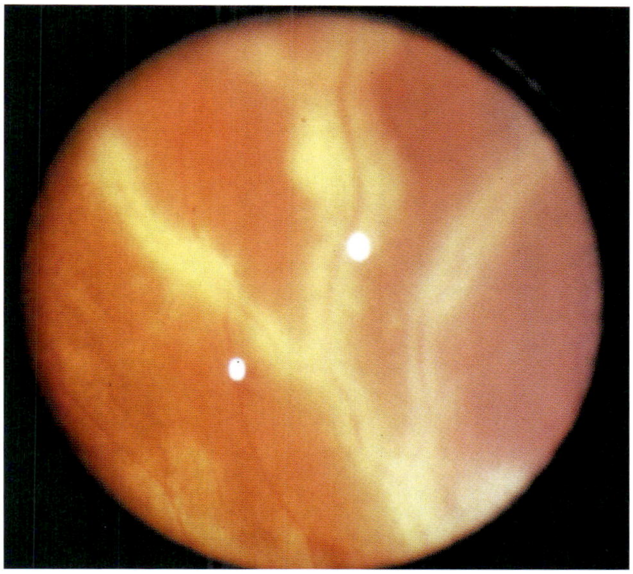

Fig. 6.8 CMV retinitis in a 27-year-old female, drug-addicted AIDS patient. Exsudative lesion with frosted branch angiitis

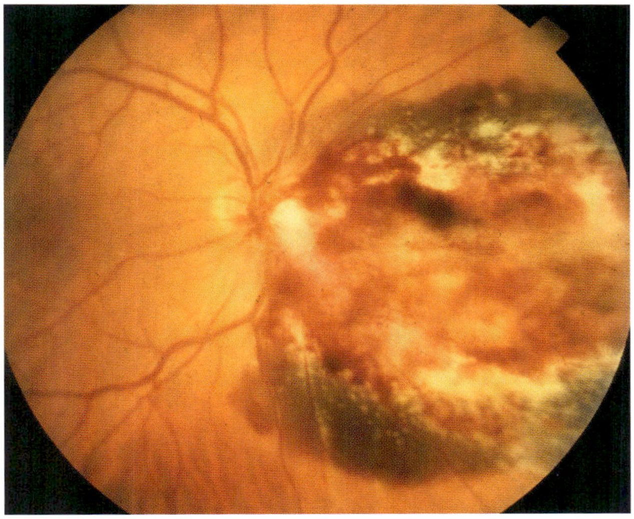

Fig. 6.9 CMV retinitis in a 34-year-old AIDS patient. Large central CMV-lesion with dominating bleedings, comprising dark deep subretinal and central superficial bleedings with interspersed fresh necrotic patches

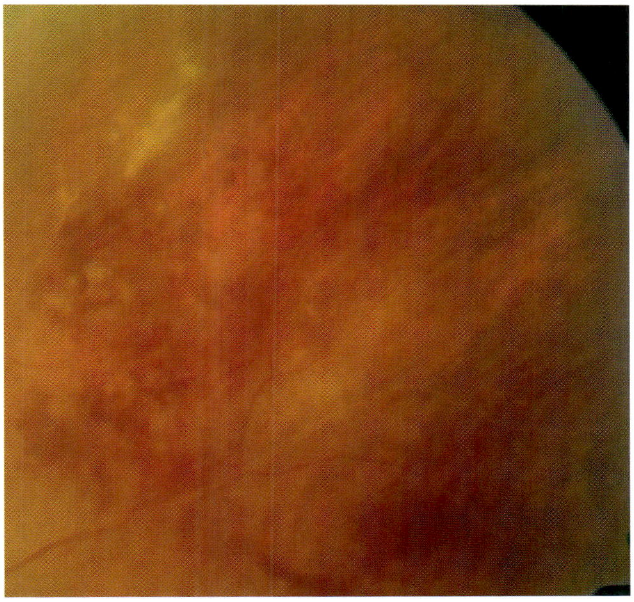

Fig. 6.10 CMV retinitis in an immunosuppressed patient after bone marrow transplantation. Regressing peripheral lesion with large superficial bleedings, an active border and vasculitis

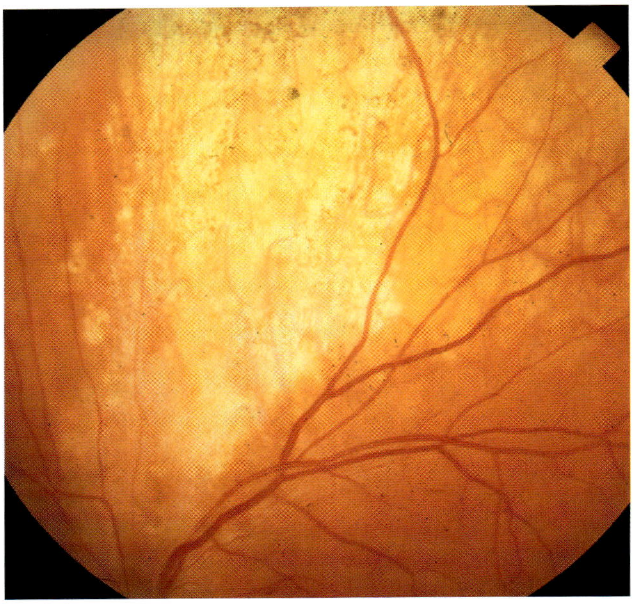

Fig. 6.11 CMV retinitis in a 39-year-old patient with AIDS. The smoldering retinits shows only a slightly active border leaving behind a “pepper-and-salt” scar

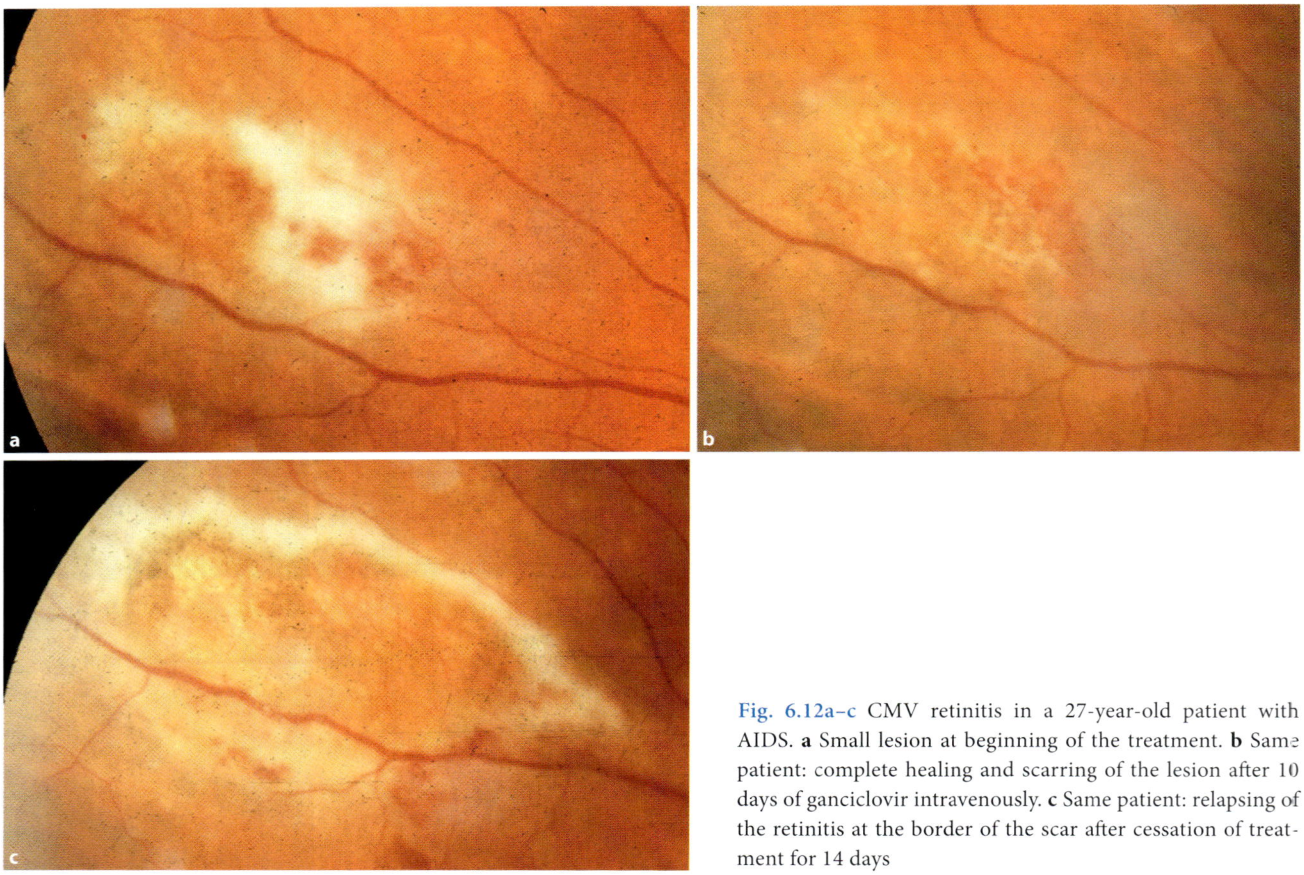

Fig. 6.12a–c CMV retinitis in a 27-year-old patient with AIDS. **a** Small lesion at beginning of the treatment. **b** Same patient: complete healing and scarring of the lesion after 10 days of ganciclovir intravenously. **c** Same patient: relapsing of the retinitis at the border of the scar after cessation of treatment for 14 days

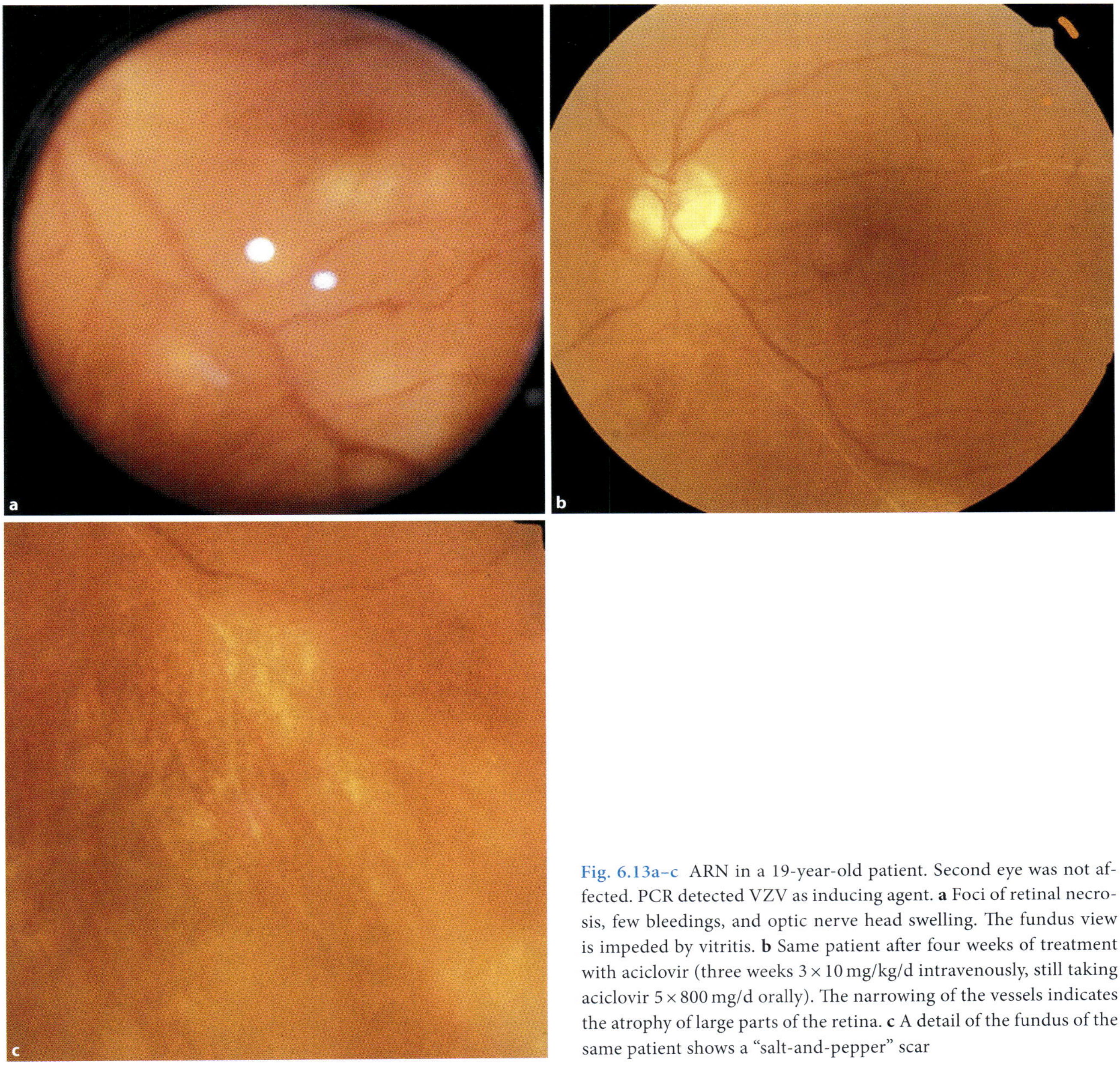

Fig. 6.13a–c ARN in a 19-year-old patient. Second eye was not affected. PCR detected VZV as inducing agent. **a** Foci of retinal necrosis, few bleedings, and optic nerve head swelling. The fundus view is impeded by vitritis. **b** Same patient after four weeks of treatment with aciclovir (three weeks $3 \times 10$ mg/kg/d intravenously, still taking aciclovir $5 \times 800$ mg/d orally). The narrowing of the vessels indicates the atrophy of large parts of the retina. **c** A detail of the fundus of the same patient shows a "salt-and-pepper" scar

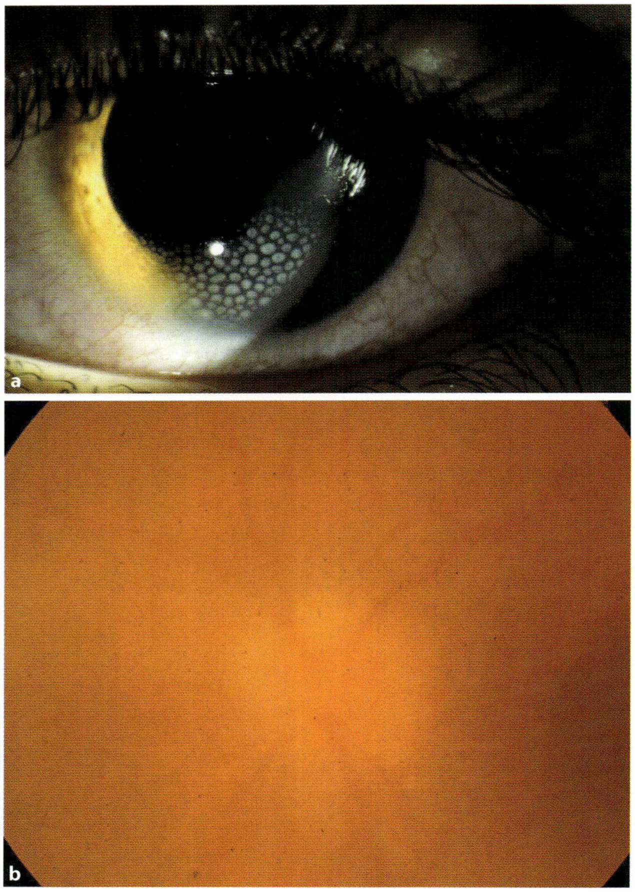

Fig. 6.14a,b ARN in a 16-year-old otherwise healthy girl with pain, drop of VA to 0.2. Second eye not affected. PCR reveals HSV as causing agent. **a** Keratic precipitates. **b** Posterior pole of the same patient is free of retinal lesions, but the periphery shows a confluent retinal necrosis (not to be seen). A heavy vitritis obscures the view on the papilledema

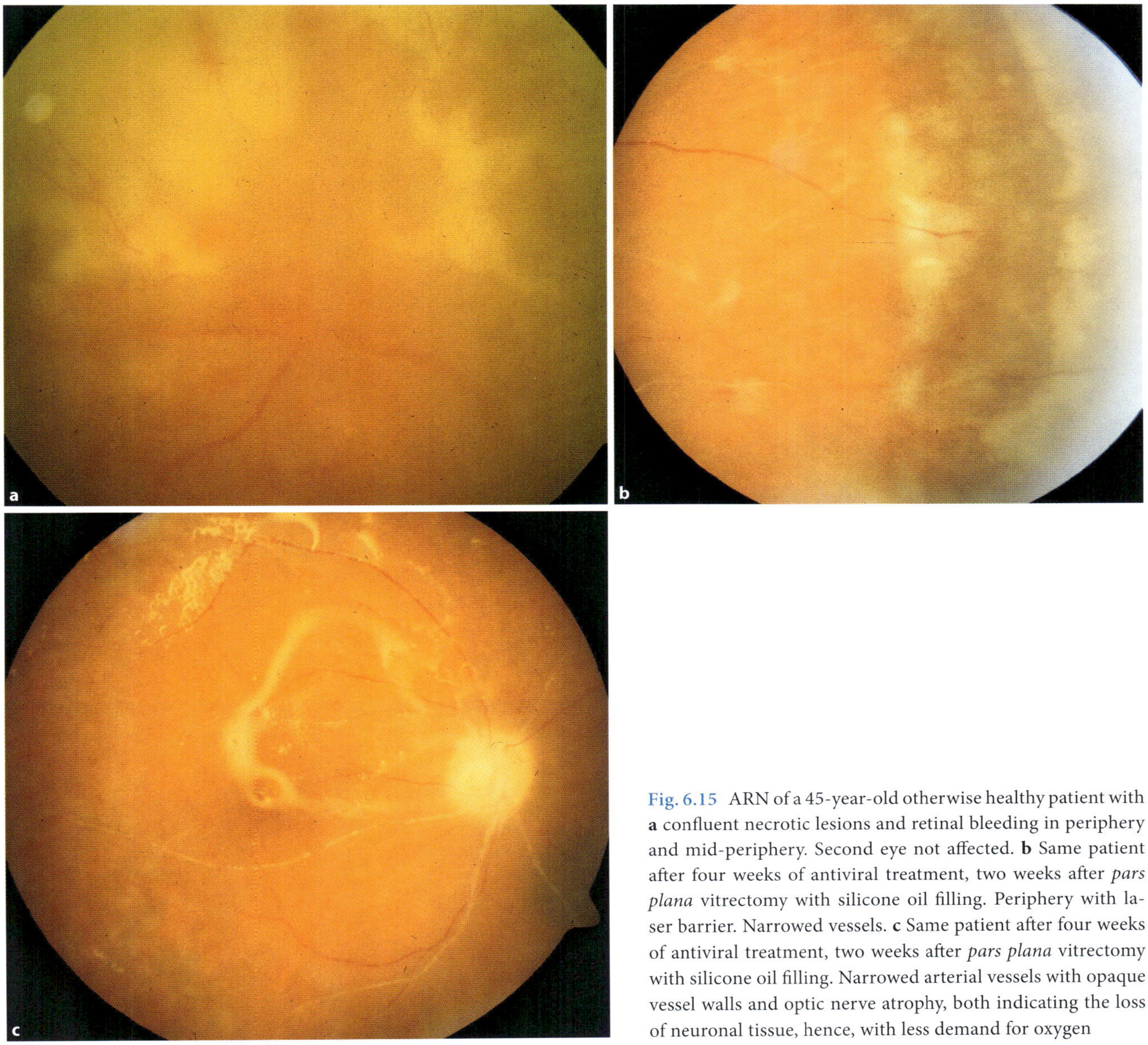

Fig. 6.15 ARN of a 45-year-old otherwise healthy patient with **a** confluent necrotic lesions and retinal bleeding in periphery and mid-periphery. Second eye not affected. **b** Same patient after four weeks of antiviral treatment, two weeks after *pars plana* vitrectomy with silicone oil filling. Periphery with laser barrier. Narrowed vessels. **c** Same patient after four weeks of antiviral treatment, two weeks after *pars plana* vitrectomy with silicone oil filling. Narrowed arterial vessels with opaque vessel walls and optic nerve atrophy, both indicating the loss of neuronal tissue, hence, with less demand for oxygen

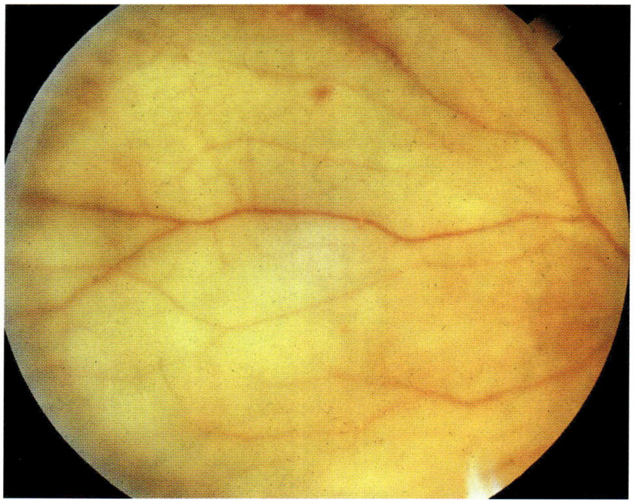

Fig. 6.16 ARN in a 42-year-old patient with AIDS and generalized herpes simplex infection. Mild vitritis, confluent patches of retinal necrosis with few bleedings, and cracked mud appearance

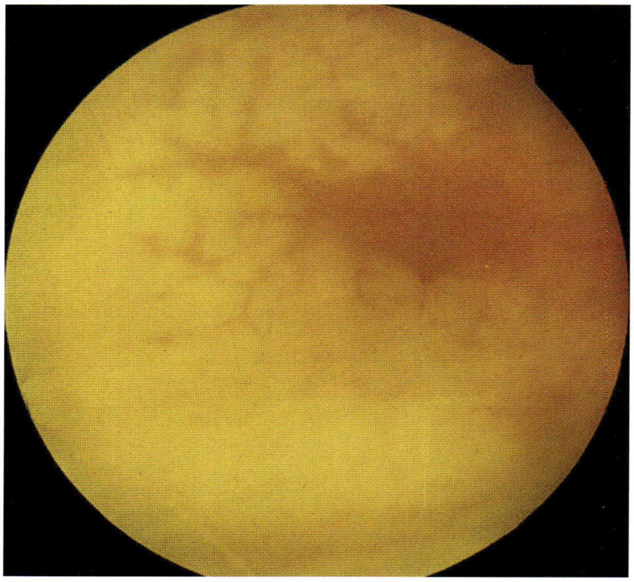

Fig. 6.17 ARN of a 74-year-old otherwise healthy patient. Widespread retinal necrosis with cracked mud appearance, only few bleedings. Second eye not affected. VZV proven as inducing agent

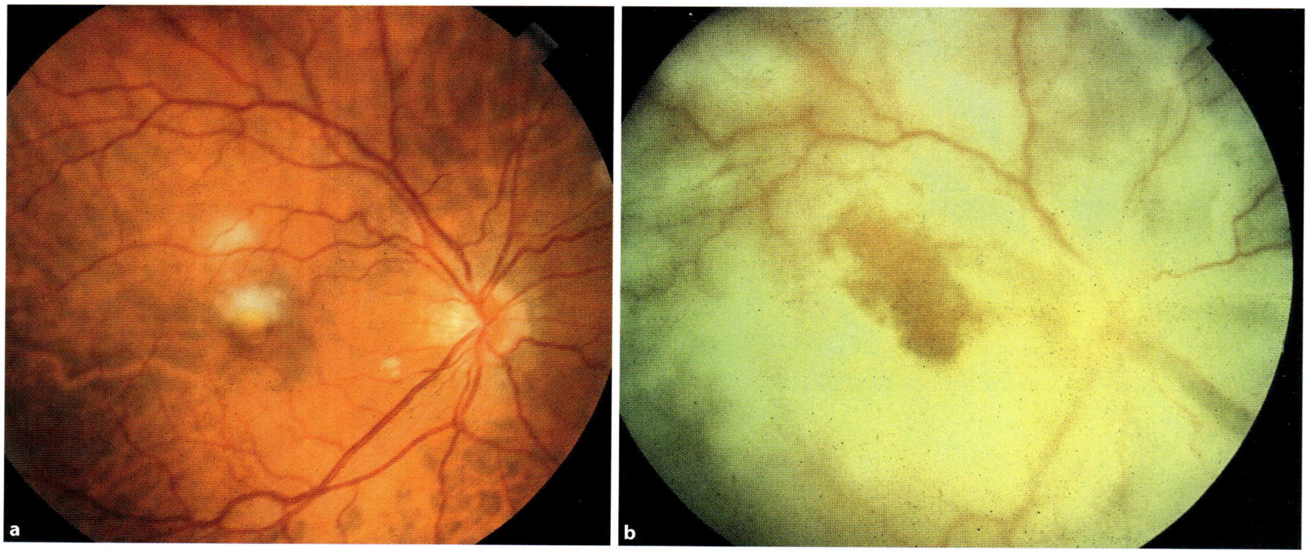


Fig. 6.18a,b PORN in a 42-year-old male with AIDS without any pain. **a** Initial central outer CMV retinitis without bleeding. **b** Same patient after 10 days without treatment: full thickness extension of the retinitis and affection of the complete retina. Clear fundus view indicates CMV infection

## References


Browning DJ (2003) Acute retinal necrosis following epidural steroid injections. Am J Ophthalmol 136: 192–194

Chang S, Young LH (2007) Acute retinal necrosis: an overview. Int Ophthalmol Clin. 447: 145–154

Culbertson WW, Dix RD (1996) Varicella-Zoster Virus Diseases: Posterior Segment of the Eye. In: Pepose JS, Holland GN, Wilhelmus KR. Mosby (eds) Ocular Infection and Immunity, pp 1131–1154

Gerling J, Neumann-Haefelin D, Seuffert HM, Schrader W, Hansen LL (1992) Diagnosis and management of the acute retinal necrosis (ARN) syndrome. Germ J Ophthalmol 1: 388–393

Hansen LL (1993) Retinale Erkrankungen bei AIDS. Ophthalmologe 90: 239–249

Hansen LL (2000) HIV-Infektion und Auge. Ophthalmologe 97: 718–736

Holland GN, Tufail A, Jordan MC (1996) Cytomegalovirus Diseases. In: Pepose JS, Holland GN, Wilhelmus KR. Mosby (eds) Ocular Infection and Immunity, pp 1088–1129

Margolis TP, Atherton SS (1996) Herpes Simplex Virus Diseases: Posterior Segment of the Eye. In: Pepose JS, Holland GN, Wilhelmus KR. Mosby (eds) Ocular Infection and Immunity, pp 1155–1167

Matoba AY (1996) Epstein–Barr Virus Diseases. In: Pepose JS, Holland GN, Wilhelmus KR. Mosby (eds) Ocular Infection and Immunity, pp 958–969

Rochat C, Polla BS, Herbort CP (1996) Immunological profiles in patients with acute retinal necrosis. Graefes Arch Clin. Exp Ophthalmol. 234: 547–552

Tran TH, Stanescu D, Caspers-Velu L, Rozenberg F, Liesnard C, Gaudric A, Lehoang P, Bodaghi B (2004) Clinical characteristics of acute HSV-2 retinal necrosis. Am J Ophthalmol 137: 872–879

Wiegand TW, Young LH (2006) Cytomegalovirus Retinitis. Int Ophthalmol Clin 46: 91–110

Zamir E (2005) Herpetic Posterior Uveitis. Int Ophthalmol Clin 45: 91–110

# Subject Index

Printing and Binding: Stürtz GmbH, Würzburg